Virus Hunters

COVID's Diagnostics Dividend:
Better Health Testing in a Post-Pandemic World

by David Kerrigan

Preface

A nasal swab.
The wait for the result: Positive or Negative.
The relief or the worry.

This is the scene that played out millions of times per day across the world in 2020/2021 as the COVID-19 pandemic gripped the world.

But few, if any, of the people anxiously waiting for their test result paused to consider the mammoth effort that enabled this testing to take place. The fact that we could accurately detect a new pathogen, at global scale, just months after its initial discovery, is a scientific and logistical triumph. And it's a triumph we mustn't waste.

Most people taking a test probably didn't dwell on the technology involved, being more concerned with when this would all end than whether the diagnostic advances inspired by COVID-19 could make the pandemic a turning point in the relationship between humans and viruses. Almost everyone I talk to is very fed up with COVID-19. But now is precisely the right time to look for positives, to leverage what we've learned, and apply those lessons to other diseases as well as to avoiding, or at least better managing, future pandemics.

In 2020, viral testing technologies changed the world, enabling mass, rapid, accurate diagnosis. This contributed to the saving of hundreds of thousands of lives. So now we need to ask, how can further such developments be encouraged and accelerated, so that similar approaches can be used to anticipate and limit the health damage from mutating or new pathogens with pandemic-causing potential?

As an early sign of positive dividends, late in 2021, just as the Omicron wave receded in Europe, I was able to acquire 3 different laboratory-grade portable PCR-type tests, for use *at home,* that perhaps offer a glimpse of what improved testing could be like in the future – testing that can save lives the world over.

About The Author

David is an analyst and speaker specialising in the impacts of technology on society. He is a regular speaker on topics ranging from AI and Innovation in Business to Autonomous Vehicles, Technology in Healthcare and the Future of Retail.

As well as being a frequent guest lecturer at Stanford Continuing Studies, The Irish Management Institute and Technological University Dublin, David also works with select commercial clients including Mastercard and Enovation Solutions.

© September 2022

Also by the Author

The following books are available in Paperback and Kindle formats from Amazon:
- Your Phone Can Save Your Life (2015)
- Life As A Passenger (2017)
- The New Acceleration (2018)
- When Humans Stop Shopping (2020)
- Better Online Presenting (2020)
- Unlock Your Learning (2021)

Colour Images and References

Higher Resolution colour images of all figures are included at the accompanying website: https://david-kerrigan.com/virushunters

Disclaimers

Nothing in this book constitutes medical advice. Always discuss any health concerns you have with a qualified healthcare professional.

I have no commercial relationship with any diagnostic or device vendor mentioned. All devices and tests were purchased with my own funds and not supplied for review or inclusion by any vendor. All images are copyright their respective owners.

Contents

Preface ii
   About The Author iii
      Also by the Author iii
   Colour Images and References iii
      Disclaimers iii
Chapter 1: Introduction 1
   Testing Goals 1
   What's Ahead 2
      Part 1 - Viruses and Testing Fundamentals 2
      Part 2 - Core Testing Technologies 3
      Part 3 - The Future of Testing 3
      Part 4 - Future Directions and Conclusions 3
      Terminology 4
   What We Won't Cover 4
   A Matter of Size 5
   Learning to Talk about Testing 5
   The Disease Burden 6
      Improving Testing 7
      Learning for the Future 7
Chapter 2: Viruses and Epidemiology 9
   Finding Viruses 9
   Humans vs Viruses 11
   Viruses: An Overview 11
      Small but Mighty 11
      Size and Structure 12
   Classifications/What's in a Name? 14

    Relationships Matter 15
    Virus Taxonomy 15
Coronaviruses..**16**
    SARS-CoV-1 and MERS vs SARS-CoV-2 18
    SARS-CoV-2 Composition and Structure 19
Other Virus Families...**19**
    Influenza 20
    HIV 21
The Virome **22**
Epidemiology **23**
Pathogenesis and Virus Response................................**24**
    Individuality..24
Viruses: One of Our Biggest Challenges **25**
    The Need for Diagnostics 25
Chapter 3: The Ascent of Diagnostics **27**
A Brief History of Diagnostics/Into the Limelight.......**27**
    A Century of Foundational Progress............................27
The Need for Speed **29**
Laboratory Diagnosis...**29**
    Expanding Horizons 30
The Pandemic Imperative **31**
    The Commerce of Disease 31
    COVID Diagnostics Investments 31
    Testing Capacity 34
Scale of Testing **35**
    Inequalities 36
    Testing Commerce..37
Chapter 4: Testing Fundamentals **39**
Testing Basics **39**

Why Test? 40
Diagnostic vs Screening testing 40
Screening & Testing Harms 41
Testing Trade-offs (Test*CASE*) 44
Cost 44
Accuracy 45
Speed 45
Ease 45
Understanding Testing 46
Sensitivity and Specificity 46
Testing for SARS-CoV-2 47
Types of Testing - Overview 48
Testing the Tests 48
Labs and Kits 49

Chapter 5: Sample Collection 53
Sampling Trade-offs 54
Sampling Decisions 55
The Target Pathogen 55
Self-Collection 56
Specimens & Sites 56
Lower Respiratory Specimens 57
Upper Respiratory Samples 57
Evolving Thinking 58
Oral Options 58
Combined Sites 60
Development Focus 61
Self Collection vs Professional Collection 63
Instructions 64
Tears 67

Location and Time to Result (TTR) 67
Swabs 69
   Swab Composition 69
Breath Tests 70
Scent Dogs for Covid 71
Chapter 6: Nucleic Acid Amplification Tests (NAAT) 73
The Emergence of PCR 73
PCR Targets (Primers & Probes) 75
The "RT" Part 76
The PCR Process 76
   The Real Time "Q" part 78
   PCR CT value 79
   RT-PCR Assays for SARS-CoV-2 79
Extending PCR Testing 80
PCR Accuracy 82
   PCR Costs 82
NAAT Beyond PCR 83
   Isothermal Amplification Technologies 83
   LAMP 84
Next Steps for NAAT 85
Chapter 7: Antigen Tests (Ag-RDT) 87
   Antigens and Antibodies 88
Lateral Flow Tests (LFTs) 88
   Samples 89
   LFT Design 89
   Sizes and shapes 90
   Reading Devices: Quantitative Results 91
Suitability Debate 92
   Environmental Impacts 96

Chapter 8: Antibody Testing (Ig-RDT) 97
Antibody Basics 97
Types of Antibodies (IgM, IgG and IgA) 98
Detection Antigens 100
Vaccines and Antibodies 101
More on Timing & Seroconversion 102
Waning/Longevity 103
Antibody Tests 104
Specimens and Collection 105
Types of Serological Testing 105
Beyond Blood 107
Assessing Antibody Tests 108
Test Accuracy 109
Beyond Antibodies: Cell-Mediated Immunity 110
T-Cells and Immunity Memory 111
Testing for T-Cells 112
Ongoing Research 112
Chapter 9: Honey, I Shrunk the Lab 115
From Lab to POC and Domestic Testing 115
From Lab to POC 116
From POC to Home - Diagnostic Devices 121
Design for Consumers 121
Is that a Lab in your Living Room? 123
Cue 123
Detect 126
Circle 127
Lucira 128
More Molecular 131
Chapter 10: Wearables: Sensors as Diagnostics? 133

Diagnostics to Wellness **133**
How It Works **135**
    PPG 136
    Respiratory Rate 139
    Temperature 140
Early Warnings: Trackers **142**
Diagnosing the Sensors **144**
    Influenza Studies 144
    COVID-19 Studies 145
    Accuracy and Regulation 149
Other Sensors **150**
    Passive Exposure Sensor 150
    Acoustic Epidemiology and Diagnostics 151
    Patient Friendly 153
    Glucometers and Antibody Testing 153
Chemistry vs Devices **154**

Chapter 11: Emerging Diagnostic Innovations **155**
Flow Cytometry **155**
Future Diagnostics **156**
CRISPR **157**
    CRISPR Multiplex and Microfluidics 158
    Low Cost CRISPR for RLS 159
    CRISPR Therapeutics 160
Next Generation Sequencing (NGS) **161**
    Sharing Sequences 162
    NGS Devices 162
    Nanopore Sequencing 163
    NGS Applications 164
    Combinatorial Barcoding 165

- **Microfluidics** 166
  - The Broad Promise of Microfluidics 166
- **Other Tech: Biosensors, Aptamers and More** 168
  - Biosensors & EIS 168
  - Aptamers 170
  - Other Biosensors 171
- **Blood: Beyond Theranos** 172
- **From Diagnostics to Prognostics** 173
  - cfDNA 174
  - Proteomics 174
  - Genome Wide Association Studies 176
- **Other Diagnostic Technologies** 176

Chapter 12: Variants, Surveillance & Timing 179

- **Moving Targets** 179
  - Mutations, Variants and Strains 180
  - Mutation Mechanisms 180
  - SARS-CoV-2 Mutations 182
- **Diagnostics & Variants** 184
  - PCR Tests and Variants 185
  - Antigen Tests and Variants 186
  - Variants and Sample Collection 186
- **Monitoring Variants** 187
- **Wastewater Surveillance** 188
  - Surveillance 190
  - Self-reporting 191
- **Organisational Testing** 191
- **Early Warning Systems** 192
  - CDC and Forecasting 193
  - Machine Learning and Predicting Viruses 193

Influenza and Global Cooperation **194**
Timing **194**
    Incubation, Infectiousness and the Asymptomatic
        Challenge 195
    Timing and Types of Test..196
Other Testing & Surveillance Examples.....................**198**
    Langya..199

Chapter 13: Reducing the Disease Burden 201

Healthcare Inequality..**201**
The Disease Burden **202**
    Malaria 202
    Tuberculosis (TB)..204
    HIV 204
    Enteric Viruses 205
Polio **206**
Healthcare Equity **207**
Diagnostics in Resource Limited Settings..................**208**
    WHO POC Guidelines for SARS-CoV-2 209
    Affordable LFTs 212
When Neglected Diseases Aren't.................................**213**
    MonkeyPox Testing..213
Drug Resistance **216**
What Happens Next?...**217**

Chapter 14: Conclusion..219

A Pandemic of Questions **219**
Our Relationship with Viruses.....................................**220**
    Multiple Sclerosis 221
    Alzheimers...221
Current Testing Choices **221**

Testing Futures 222
Awareness and Preparedness 222
Personal Health vs Public Health 223
   Public Health Policy 223
The Diagnostic Dividend 224
Harnessing the Pandemic 225

Appendices 226

Appendix 1: Common DNA & RNA Viruses 227

Appendix 2: Sampling Options in More Detail 229
Nasal Options: Depth Matters 229
Nasal & Oral Options 229
   3 Noses 230
   Comparisons 232
Swab Composition & Transport 233
   Swabs and Transport 234

Appendix 3: COVID-19 Tests 235

Appendix 4: The SARS/MERS Immunology Dividend 237

Abbreviations/Glossary 238

Further Reading & References 241

Acknowledgements 242

References 243

'Our key message is: test, test, test'

Dr Tedros Adhanom Ghebreyesus

WHO, Director General

March 2020

Chapter 1: Introduction

"Whatever sets forth the union of chemistry and medicine tends to promote not only the good of science but also the welfare of mankind"

Henry Bence Jones (1813–1873)[1]

Finding the invisible invaders that make hundreds of millions of people sick, and cause millions to die each year, deserves more of our attention than it has had to date.

Testing is humanity's first line of defence against the countless pathogens that threaten our existence. Diagnostic test results determine the vast majority of medical treatment decisions (60-80%[2]) and, in 2020, test results were the basis of unprecedented worldwide restrictions on freedom of movement, saving perhaps millions of lives albeit with catastrophic impacts on livelihoods. So how do we ensure that tests are fit for purpose?

Outside of medical circles, few people are familiar with diagnostic testing and its true importance, its inherent challenges and the cutting-edge scientific struggle to make it ever faster, cheaper and more accurate. The COVID-19 pandemic has thrust testing into the spotlight as never before, made technical diagnostic terms part of daily vocabulary and perhaps also given us one of the best opportunities in history to transform global health.

Improving accuracy and speed in identifying infectious agents has the potential to reduce the global disease burden, save countless lives and protect economic growth. Thanks in part to the extra investment and focus arising from the pandemic, there's never been more interest in diagnostics, but we must not let our progress slip as the COVID-19 threat loses its urgency for many - we must instead redouble our efforts to ensure we build on the progress of recent years truly to secure the diagnostics dividend.

Testing Goals

Finding viruses isn't easy. As we'll see in Chapter 2, these tiny microbes, some as small as 20nm (that's 20 nanometres – for scale, a human hair is about 60,000nm wide), can make us severely ill or even kill us. To further complicate the task of finding them, there are hundreds of different types of virus that can infect humans, as well as millions that aren't known to cause disease in humans but may be present in other animals.

In order to combat viruses, we need to be able to find them and identify them and do so quickly enough to enable medical interventions (if they exist) in serious cases. An ideal diagnostic test is accurate, fast, affordable and readily available, leading to an effective intervention.

Achieving that ideal is not necessarily easy or cheap - it requires a complex chain of research, logistics, technology and education. The closer to the patient we can complete a test, the faster the result can be known - but testing outside laboratories can reduce the accuracy. Luckily, the breakthrough technologies we'll discuss in this book promise to bring us closer to testing ideals that will save millions of lives.

What's Ahead

This volume is an attempt to summarise the current state of testing and, more importantly, what we can learn for the future, after two of the most eventful years in the history of diagnostic virology. The focus is on presenting a detailed yet accessible overview of the tests that have defined the COVID-19 pandemic, the emerging technologies and techniques that give us hope for the future of testing and identifying the key diagnostic dividends from what has been a tumultuous few years. My earnest hope is that the advances and learnings spurred by the urgent imperative of the COVID-19 pandemic can lead to lasting benefits to global health; some consolation for the lives and livelihoods lost since 2020.

The book is arranged in 4 parts:

Part 1 - Viruses and Testing Fundamentals

- Chapter 1 begins with a brief overview of the importance of testing.

- In Chapter 2, we'll look at the common types and structures of viruses, setting the scene for the rest of the discussion as we go on, in later chapters, to review how best to detect pathogens of concern.

- Chapter 3 provides some background on the development of viral diagnostics to date and on the extraordinary scale of testing seen in 2020-22.

- Chapter 4 will outline the fundamentals of testing practices - the pre-analytical considerations that play a crucial role in the choice and accuracy of tests.

- Chapter 5 focuses on the critical sample collection phase that precedes most actual tests.

Part 2 - Core Testing Technologies

- Chapter 6 describes the category of molecular tests known as Nucleic Acid Amplification Tests (NAAT).

- Chapter 7 discusses Rapid Antigen Tests (primarily Lateral Flow tests).

- Chapter 8 moves the discussion on to Antibody tests to detect prior infections and immunity.

Part 3 - The Future of Testing

- Chapter 9 looks at Point of Care (POC) and Self-Testing developments

- Chapter 10 looks at digital diagnostics, including wearable technologies

- Chapter 11 explores some emerging test techniques and technologies

Part 4 - Future Directions and Conclusions

- Chapter 12 highlights the challenge of variants and how it impacts monitoring and test timings

- Chapter 13 reminds us of the global disease burden and the urgency beyond COVID-19

- The Conclusion sums up what I see as the key learnings and resulting opportunities

Terminology

Viral diagnostics is a very complex field and is replete with acronyms, medical and technical terminology. The topic can be intimidatingly jargon-filled as you dig deeper, but I believe it's so important that it's worth making the effort to understand a little more about the viral challenges to humanity, without becoming fully immersed in molecular biology. Taking the time to better understand some of the techniques involved may help you make more informed personal well-being decisions and advocate for fairer public health policies. I've attempted to keep the jargon to a minimum whilst keeping the discussion accurate and informative, with a full glossary provided in an Appendix for easy reference.

COVID-19 vs SARS-CoV-2

Although often commonly referred to as "Covid tests", I'll refer to such tests more precisely as being for SARS-CoV-2, the virus that causes the disease known as COVID-19. As we'll see, someone can be infected with, and transmit, the SARS-CoV-2 virus without displaying any of the symptoms of COVID-19. Where I refer to SARS-CoV-1, this refers to the causative virus of the disease *Severe Acute Respiratory Syndrome* (SARS), the last outbreak of which was in 2003.

What We Won't Cover

The vast range of target substances (analytes) of interest in a diagnostic procedure means clinicians and virologists need a wide range of test types, and we'll discuss the main ones that are used in hunting viral targets. However, we won't look at adjacent but equally important diagnostic branches such as imaging (X-Ray, CT, MRI, Mammograms, Ultrasounds etc.), nor will we look in any detail at bacterial pathogens.

There are already numerous books examining the impacts of the COVID-19 pandemic and I'm sure there are many more to come. In this book, we won't talk directly about the development of COVID-19 related vaccines or therapeutics (treatments), nor the merits of the various public health policies (such as mask wearing) pursued around the globe. Nor will I attempt to cover the economic, social or practical challenges of advising or requiring someone to isolate on the basis of a test result. The focus is on what we can learn from the COVID-19 era to improve the performance and accessibility of diagnostic testing for viral threats in the decades ahead - with the prize of millions of lives to be saved.

A Matter of Size

The story of viral testing is one of extremes - diagnostic tools have never before been deployed at this scale to find such a small target. At the staggeringly large end of the scale, there have been more than 3 *billion* lab tests for SARS-CoV-2 carried out worldwide in the last two years; at the hard-to-comprehend opposite end of the scale, the culprit, SARS-CoV-2, averages around 60 nanometres in diameter - you could fit about 1,000 virions (entire virus particles) side-by-side on the width of a human hair.

The human effort put into finding this virus is also unprecedented in size: according to Finddx[3], just two years since the start of the pandemic, more than 1,000 types of molecular and antigen-based immunoassay tests to detect SARS-CoV-2, including at least 400 Rapid Diagnostic Tests, are now commercially available worldwide. Production capacity for these tests has been ramped up to over 1 billion units per month in the US alone.

Yet many of the biggest benefits we need to derive from these efforts also focus on size reductions - we need to make the testing machines smaller and reduce the costs of testing, which involves using less reagents (chemicals) in each test. Making testing devices smaller, so that they can be used for testing outside laboratories, has outsized potential for good. Making the cost of testing smaller is also a crucial consideration to improve equality of access to testing - tests that are not affordable at mass scale exclude access for billions of people in low- and middle-income countries (LMIC) and the Resource Limited Settings (RLS) that persist in richer countries.

Learning to Talk about Testing

Prior to 2020, I think many people were more concerned about a computer virus than a biological one. The arrival of the disease we now know as COVID-19 changed that. The normally unsung but critical disciplines of clinical pathology and public health have been thrust into the limelight as never before. Previously obscure technical virology terminology has become part of the daily lexicon, though there have been challenges around the reliability of information on topics such as test accuracy.

In this book, I want to take some time to talk about common viruses, some differences between them, how variations affect testing for them and about society's response to the threat they pose. Viral testing has suddenly come to have an important role in our lives and in our society. In fact, it's hard to think of anything in history that has moved so suddenly from the scientific margins to being part of millions of peoples' daily activities and concerns.

Daily case numbers from tests, both reported by the millions of people using testing kits at home and from national testing schemes which determined the need to impose restrictions on normal activities, suddenly became the most discussed indicator on the planet.

The Disease Burden

Notwithstanding the focus on COVID-19, and amid concern about other similar potential future pandemics, respiratory pathogens are not our only adversary - we must reconsider the other health challenges that kill millions each year across the world - Influenza, HIV, TB, and Malaria, as well as challenges such as sexually transmitted diseases (STDs) - and look to apply COVID-19-related diagnostic advances to these domains as well. And that's without considering the neglected diseases we'll discuss later that can also benefit from novel diagnostics advances.

I'll use SARS-CoV-2 as the primary example of a viral target, but we'll refer to other viruses as we go, emphasizing the need to expand the COVID-19 - spurred pandemic progress in diagnostics to other viral threats; existing, neglected and future. So, although most of the examples given will draw on current developments relating to SARS-CoV-2, the bigger prize is the application of what we've learned in the last two years to improvement of diagnostics across the spectrum of pathogens that inflict *largely preventable* misery and death around the world. The COVID-19 pandemic showed the positives of progress that can be made with the right level of focus and investment, but again brought into sharp relief the inequalities of global healthcare access. The decisions made now, and in the coming few years, at national and global health policy levels, coupled with the funding choices for new technologies, will largely determine how much equitable progress humanity can make in reducing the global disease burden.

Importance of Testing

Many different diseases present initially with similar non-specific symptoms, such as fever, with testing often the only way to determine the cause. Similarly, with many infections lingering in asymptomatic or presymptomatic states, tests are the only medical tools available to screen for the presence of non-obvious pathogens.

Fast and accurate diagnosis of viral infections enhances the ability of Health Care Professionals (HCPs) to make decisions on appropriate treatment of patients, evaluate disease progression and prevent inappropriate treatments, such as the misuse of antibiotics. Knowing the identity of the pathogen present also allows implementation of suitable infection control and assessment of antiviral treatments that may affect the prognosis of patients.

As we'll discuss more in Chapter 3, there has been massive progress in the field of diagnostic technologies in the last century. However, many challenges remain to improve access across the globe to accurate tests. New technologies that make testing more accurate, smaller, lighter, cheaper and even electronic instead of chemical, will shift the balance more in favour of humans as we battle increasing zoonotic viral outbreaks - where a virus jumps from an animal reservoir to the human population and causes serious illness.

Improving Testing

Prior to 2020, significant efforts were already underway to improve diagnostic testing for a variety of diseases, building on decades of work that has seen laboratory testing advance, and the emergence of Point of Care (POC) and even some domestic self-testing. Many of these nascent projects were vastly accelerated and their potential to benefit society has been brought forward many years thanks to COVID-19.

COVID-19 lockdowns, and pressures on health services, have impeded the diagnosis of other diseases, ironically just as the world undergoes more testing than at any time in history. With all the focus on COVID-19, there has been an underlying concern among medical professionals about other diseases going undetected and about the consequences of such late diagnosis and resulting delayed treatment.

There's also a concern that we may move towards too much testing - might our new abilities to test in novel ways trigger a new wave of "worried well", constantly using new testing tools to seek out real and imagined threats, and adding to the burden on health services? As with any tool, the correct use of whatever new testing capabilities we develop is key to maximising the upside.

Learning for the Future

I'm particularly interested in discussing what we can learn from the diagnostic advances of the COVID-19 pandemic to improve global health and to better prepare for future outbreaks. There are myriad other areas of adjacent study outside this scope - vaccines and therapeutics to name two. But diagnostics can benefit from lessons in those disciplines too.

With the benefit of hindsight, we can now regret that efforts to create a vaccine for SARS were halted just as early trials in animals got underway, due to the lack of an urgent need as the 2002-2004 outbreak ended. However, had we continued to invest in coronavirus vaccine research, we might have been better equipped for SARS-CoV-2. Similarly, if work on better testing for SARS-CoV-1 had continued at that time, more types of testing would have been available faster for SARS-CoV-2.

Let's begin our discussion with some basic detail on our viral adversaries, and the mind-boggling variety of tiny viruses that surround us.

Chapter 2: Viruses and Epidemiology

To design effective tests and treatments for viruses, we need to understand them as best we can. We need to learn more about their composition, their characteristics and their evolution. As we do that, we see already that they may be involved in many conditions not previously thought to be viral - a topic we'll return to later. But before we look at the techniques and technologies we have to detect viruses, let's examine some basic information about viruses, and our relationship with them.

Finding Viruses

Although they've been present on Earth for far longer than humans, viruses have really only come to our attention in the last 100 years or so. As medical science evolved, we've come to understand more about these tiny entities, thanks to breakthroughs in microscopy and, laterally, genetics.

Prior to 1900, scientists had speculated on the potential existence of pathogens too small to be seen using even the most advanced microscopes of that era. In the early 1890s, researchers found that infected tobacco leaves remained infectious after passing through a filter designed to remove bacteria and, in 1898, Dutch microbiologist and botanist Martinus Beijerinck named the pathogens "*Contagium vivum fluidum*" or virus[4]. Just 10 years after the first discovery of a plant-infecting virus (tobacco mosaic virus), the first identification of a virus infecting humans (yellow fever) occurred in 1901.

In the 120 years since then, many thousands of viruses have been identified, infecting not just humans, but most other species too. Only about 200 or so viruses are known to directly infect humans and to cause noticeable disease. Viruses that can jump between species and move from animals to humans (zoonotic viruses) have come to be of particular concern as a source of serious infection in recent decades, with animal sources implicated in all recent epidemics of SARS (2003) and MERS (2012).

As we'll discuss more in the next Chapter, the second half of the 20th century has seen the rapid acceleration of virus detection, and most of the documented species of animal, plant, and bacterial viruses were discovered during these years. But while new viruses are currently being identified at an increasing rate, researchers believe we've, as yet, discovered less than 1% of them. A review in 2008 documented that 335 new infectious diseases had emerged in the period between 1940 and 2004 and their threat to global health was actually increasing[5]. Over the past ten years in particular, the number of known and named viruses has exploded, owing to advances in the technology for finding them[6]:

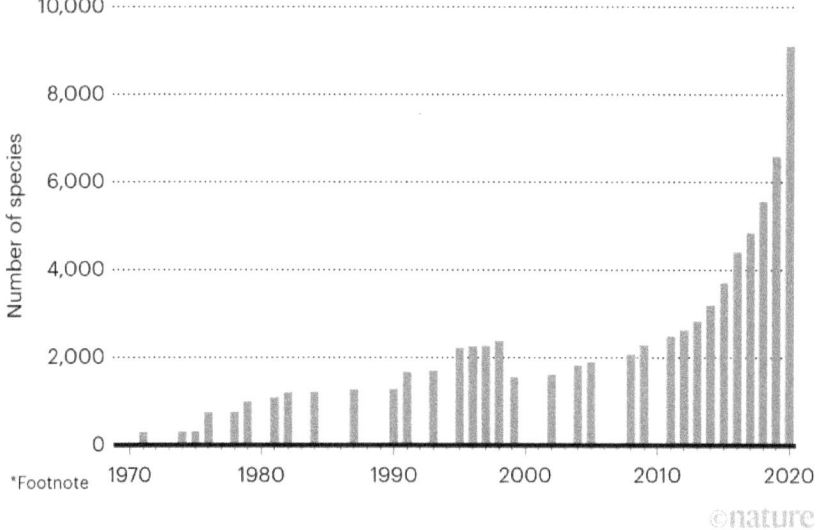

Figure 1: Number of Virus Species discovered [7]

Although the illustration above shows increasing numbers of viruses being discovered, especially in the past decade or so, the pace of discovery is still accelerating: as an example of the speed at which new viruses are now being discovered thanks to increases in computational power, a two-week intensive investigation project in 2021 identified over 130,000 novel RNA viruses, including 11 new species of coronavirus, by searching over 5 million publicly available biological samples, using 22,250 virtual processors[8]. For more detail on the history, discovery and emergence of viruses, see this 2012 Royal Society article[9].

Humans vs Viruses

The human relationship with viruses is a complex one that in many ways remains poorly understood. Although some viruses affect the health of their hosts, most have very little or no known impact - but the 2020's COVID-19 outbreak has proven these tiny things pose a giant challenge to humanity.

Despite the saturation coverage and personal impacts on lives over the course of the COVID-19 pandemic, most people outside the biological sciences understand little regarding viruses. We've heard daily about the spread of SARS-CoV-2 and words like *variants*, but in terms of understanding our enemy, we depend on the molecular biologists who are dissecting and documenting our invisible nemeses, nucleotide by nucleotide (nucleotides are the basic building blocks of RNA and DNA), working to develop tests, treatments and vaccines. In the next sections, we'll introduce some of the key concepts and terms that will form the basis of our discussion of how we go about identifying viruses with diagnostic tests.

Viruses: An Overview

Viruses are the most numerous biological entities on the planet and there is evidence that probably all organisms in the biological world may be infected by at least one virus[10]. Every litre of seawater contains more viruses than there are people on the planet - each litre is populated with up to 10 billion viruses - and viruses infect not just humans and animals but even other microbes such as bacteria. Our understanding of how human interactions with viruses impact us is evolving, but examples of very prevalent human diseases caused by viruses include the common cold, influenza, chickenpox, and cold sores. Many serious diseases such as rabies, Ebola, AIDS, avian influenza, SARS and COVID-19 are also caused by viruses. There is also emerging evidence that a virus, EBV, plays a significant role in Multiple Sclerosis[11] - more on that topic in Chapter 14.

Small but Mighty

Viruses are sometimes compared to, or confused, with *bacteria*, especially as both are too small to see and can make humans sick with similar symptoms. Technically though, bacteria are quite different. Bacteria are living organisms that, although small, are relatively much larger than viruses: the smallest bacteria are about 0.4 microns (μm)[12] in diameter while viruses range in size from 0.02 to 0.25μm. More importantly though, unlike viruses, bacteria do not depend on host cells and can reproduce on their own. From a treatment point of view, antibiotics can be effective against bacterial infection but not viral infections. It's also worth noting that viruses can actually infect bacteria (viruses that infect bacteria are called *bacteriophages or phages*), just as they can infect humans, animals and plants.

Viruses rely on external forces for transmission - fluid or air being the most common, or sometimes insect *vectors* (carriers). At a basic level, a virus is an infectious particle that reproduces by invading and commandeering a host cell so the virus can use the cell's machinery to make copies of itself. A complete virus particle, known as a *virion*, consists of nucleic acid surrounded by a protective coat/shell of protein called a *capsid*. Some viruses (including Influenza, HIV and SARS-CoV2) are further encased in an outer envelope that aids their access to host cells. In simple and innocuous-sounding terms, even the most harmful virus is just some protein enveloping a molecule of nucleic acid genetic instructions. As we'll see in later Chapters, these proteins and nucleic acid are central to almost all viral diagnostic endeavours.

Size and Structure

Viruses are so small that it's hard to comprehend just how small they are. So, while early microscopes gave scientists the ability to see bacteria, it wasn't until the invention of the electron microscope that it was possible to see anything except the largest viruses - most viruses are smaller than the limit of resolution of a traditional light microscope, which is about $0.3\mu m$ (300nm). Without a microscope the limit of what's visible to the naked eye is about $100\mu m$. Compared to everyday tiny particles such as a grain of sand ($40\mu m$), viruses are a fraction of that size.

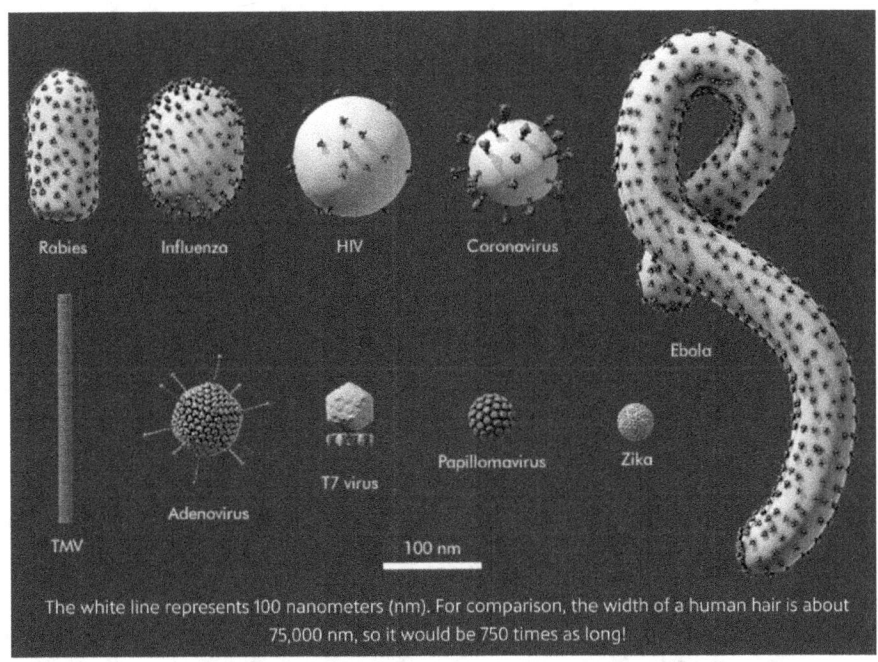

Figure 2: Comparative Viral sizes. Source: PBS[13]

As mentioned, there are vast numbers of viruses on our planet so it's important to remember the sheer variety of viruses - even within viruses, depending on the type of virus, the typical size can range from ("large") poxviruses at 0.3μm, to 0.1μm (*"medium"*) Influenza viruses and retroviruses, to 0.01 μm (*"small"*) Picornaviruses, (including polioviruses) and circoviruses. A SARS-CoV-2 virion typically ranges from 0.07μm to 0.09μm. Despite their tiny size though, each virus is packed with genetic code: the size of viral DNA genomes ranges from 1.7 kilobases (kb) for some circoviruses to over 200 kilobase pairs (kbp) for 'larger' herpesviruses and poxviruses.

And they're not only small in terms of size, but also in terms of weight. Research on COVID-19 infections show that "although each infected person carries an estimated 1 billion to 100 billion virions during peak infection, their total mass is no more than 0.1 mg"[14].

Despite the tendency to think of viruses as a somewhat homogenous group, there is a very diverse range of not only sizes but shapes and structures, known as morphologies. These are important to the identification and classification of viruses. The differences in structure also influence the most reliable target for tests – some virus structures present more potential targets for tests. The 4 most common morphological types are: Helical, Polyhedral, Spherical and Complex.

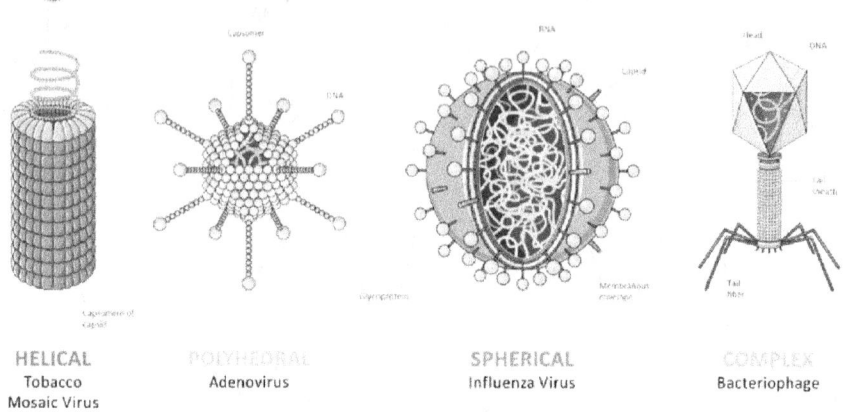

Figure 3: Common virus morphologies. Source: Artasensi et al, 2021[15]

As we look to understand these tiny entities better, we need to move on from size and structure to composition. Viruses contain one type of nucleic acid - either RNA or DNA; never both. Diseases caused by RNA viruses include the common cold, influenza, SARS, COVID-19, hepatitis C, Ebola, rabies, polio, and measles, while examples of DNA viruses include Herpes simplex virus, varicella-zoster virus, Monkeypox, cytomegalovirus and Epstein–Barr virus. See Appendix for more examples of RNA and DNA viruses.

As we discover the existence of more viruses and understand more about their structures and composition, we can better classify them, uncover their similarities and differences, and begin to predict their evolution.

Classifications/What's in a Name?

Taxonomy – the discipline of classifying and naming things – is the bedrock of nearly all sciences, and, perhaps particularly so in fields as complex as virology. A virus taxonomy is a framework for analysing viruses, cataloguing them and deciphering the relationships between them, which helps in tracking their evolution.

As a topic, virology quickly becomes far too detailed for anyone not wishing to pursue a career in the field, but I do think there's some merit in appreciating at a high level the diversity of what we're dealing with, if only to understand a little of the scale of challenge faced by those seeking to diagnose and treat us. It's important to discuss here the sheer breadth of viruses that exist, while remembering it doesn't include the ones we haven't yet identified. As we talk about approaches to diagnosing viral pathogens and the wider benefits I believe will emerge from the intense hunt for SARS-CoV-2 that began in 2020, we need to be mindful too of the less notorious viruses that may pose a risk in the future through mutation, as well as those that may be discovered to be a causative agent we don't yet fully appreciate.

Relationships Matter

Understanding the relationship or otherwise between different viruses is also crucial in directing our efforts to better know or treat them. There Is immense practical value, for example, in knowing that the novel coronavirus, now known as SARS-CoV-2, that emerged in late 2019 is closely related to the SARS-CoV coronavirus identified in 2002/3. With that knowledge, it has been possible to repurpose existing antiviral drugs for the treatment of COVID-19 and to follow the lead that monoclonal antibodies, generated from the cells of a patient infected with the 2003 coronavirus, may be useful in the treatment of COVID-19 patients in 2020:

In 2003, researchers at the company developed an antiviral, known as PF-00835231, that could block the main protease of a coronavirus that emerged in 2002 and causes severe acute respiratory syndrome (SARS). But by the time they were ready to test it in patients, the SARS outbreak had been contained. PF-00835231 is structurally similar to a peptide that binds within SARS's main protease. That binding site in SARS is identical to the one in SARS-CoV-2, so Pfizer researchers thought the molecule could work against the new virus. Tests showed they were right[16].

Virus Taxonomy

The International Committee on Taxonomy of Viruses (ICTV) is the agency responsible for maintaining a universal system for classifying viruses[17]. As of 2021, 6 realms, 10 kingdoms, 17 phyla, 2 subphyla, 39 classes, 65 orders, 8 suborders, 233 families, 168 subfamilies, 2606 genera, 84 subgenera, 10434 species have been defined by the ICTV. This situation is constantly changing, and the interested reader should consult the ICTV website (http://www.ictvonline.org) for the latest updates and a fully interactive/searchable resource.

The following table shows the number of species classified, as of 2021, into the 6 realms:

Viria Realm:	Ribo	Duplodna	Monodna	Varidna	Adna	Ribozya
Number of Species:	4317	3731	1463	272	31	15

Figure 4: The 6 Virus Realms sorted by number of species. Source: ICTV

Of this vast number of virus groups, most interest in recent years has been directed towards coronaviruses due to outbreaks SARS, MERS and COVID-19 which are all caused by this family of viruses, members of the Riboviria realm:

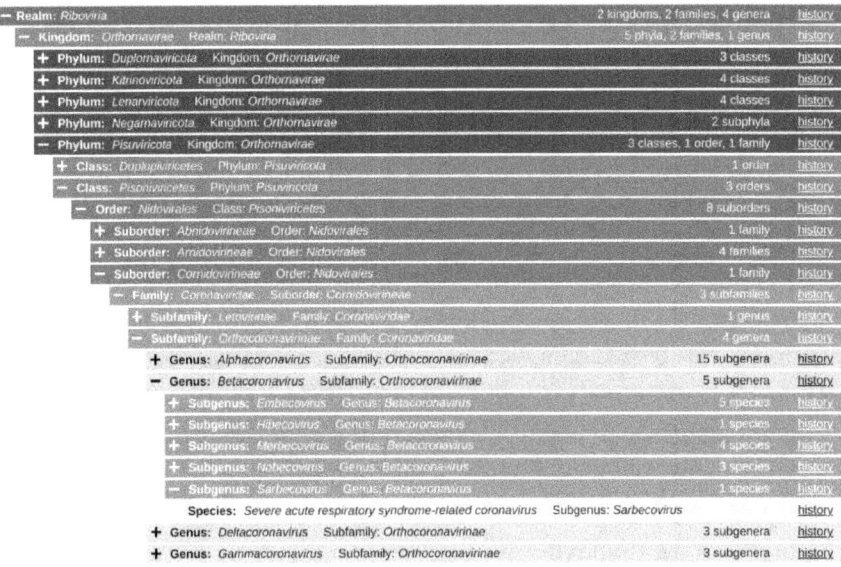

Figure 5: The expanded Taxonomy view showing the classification of species: SARS-CoV

Coronaviruses

In the early days of what became known as the COVID-19 pandemic, the virus was referred to by its family name, Coronavirus. However, there are many different coronaviruses - for most people outside the world of microbiology/virology, any awareness of Coronaviruses likely comes from SARS-CoV-1 which, in 2003, caused the Severe Acute Respiratory Syndrome (SARS) outbreak, or MERS-CoV which caused Middle Eastern Respiratory

Syndrome (MERS) in 2015, or, of course, SARS-CoV-2, which causes COVID-19. However, SARS-CoV-2 is not the third coronavirus to infect humans - it is in fact the 7th. The other four, HKU1, OC43 (originally from rodents), NL63, 229E (from bats) are associated with mild symptoms and usually dismissed as a "common cold", although they only cause about one third of common colds. (Other viruses associated with common cold symptoms included rhinoviruses, respiratory syncytial viruses and adenoviruses).

Discovered in the 1960s, coronaviruses possess a distinctive morphological feature, consisting of a ring of spike proteins on the outer surface of the virus, giving the appearance of a halo or corona when viewed via an electron microscope (see below). In addition to inspiring the name of the coronavirus genus, the spike proteins are also essential for infection of host cells. In the case of SARS-CoV-2, the spike protein binds to a receptor (angiotensin-converting enzyme 2 or ACE2) on epithelial cells found in human lungs. From a diagnostic point of view, these spike proteins are a vital element of many tests as we'll see later, as well as forming a key part of many vaccine designs.

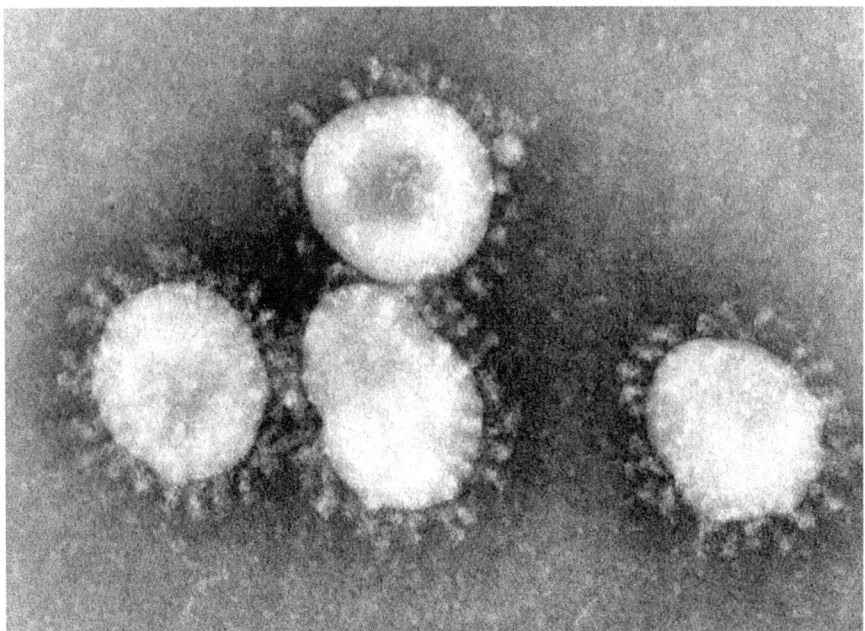

Figure 6: Electron Microscope view of a Coronavirus (229E) - Source: CDC Public Domain Image

Technically, Coronaviruses (CoV) are enveloped, positive-stranded RNA viruses. As seen in the taxonomy above, the subfamily Coronavirinae contains the four genera Alpha-, Beta-, Gamma-, and Delta-coronavirus. Delta and gamma groups affect mostly avian species, while alpha and beta (shown below) primarily affect mammals, particularly bats, and including humans. A coronavirus found in bats, RaTG13, is the most closely related (phylogenetically or from an evolutionary point of view) coronavirus genome to SARS-CoV-2 with approximately 96.2% genetic similarity.

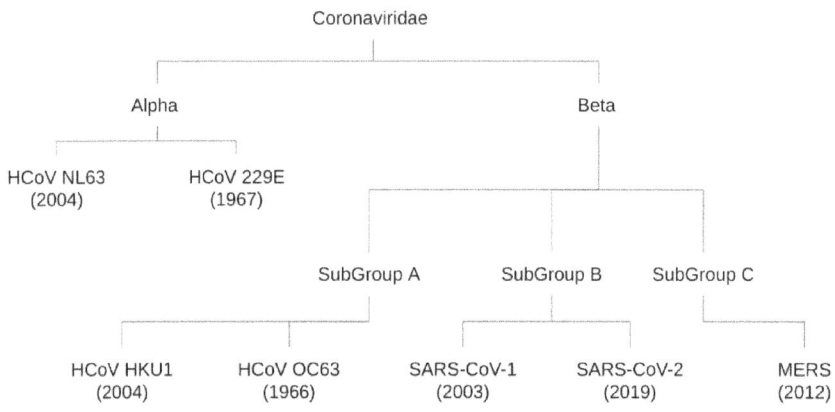

Figure 7: Alpha and Beta Coronaviruses that affect humans and their discovery date

SARS-CoV-1 and MERS vs SARS-CoV-2

Although they didn't become global pandemics, the 2003/2012 outbreaks of SARS/MERS highlighted the very real dangers of zoonotic coronaviruses and also boosted research into coronaviruses. Both SARS-Cov-1 and MERS-CoV have a similar genetic size to SARS-CoV-2 (c.30,000 nucleotides from the four building blocks of RNA - adenine (A), cytosine (C), guanine (G), and uracil (U)). SARS-CoV-2 shares about 80% nucleotide sequence identity with SARS-CoV and about 50% with MERS-CoV.

Highlighting the benefits of understanding viral relationships, this high level of similarity of the sequence revealed a common pathogenesis (the manner of development of a disease) which assisted scientists with therapeutic targeting for SARS-CoV-2[18]. Both SARS-CoV (c 15%) and MERS-CoV (c 34%) had substantially higher case fatality rates (CFR) than SARS-CoV-2 (<3%, still TBC).

Learnings from successful attempts to control the earlier outbreaks were the basis of most initial public health interventions when SARS-CoV-2 emerged, and the discontinued work on treatments and vaccines from 2003/2012, no longer needed then, in 2020 kick-started efforts to tackle the novel coronavirus. Thus, the study and classification of virus and viral evolution is a critical weapon in preparedness for future threats and that must be a key learning from the COVID-19 pandemic.

SARS-CoV-2 Composition and Structure

Focusing in on the composition of the cause of the recent pandemic, SARS-CoV-2 is a spherical virus, about 60–100nm in diameter, and it contains single-stranded, positive-sense RNA.

Structurally, SARS-CoV-2 contains four structural proteins, that include spike (S), envelope (E), membrane (M), and nucleocapsid (N) proteins. These proteins are key targets for diagnostics, and we'll refer to them again in later Chapters.

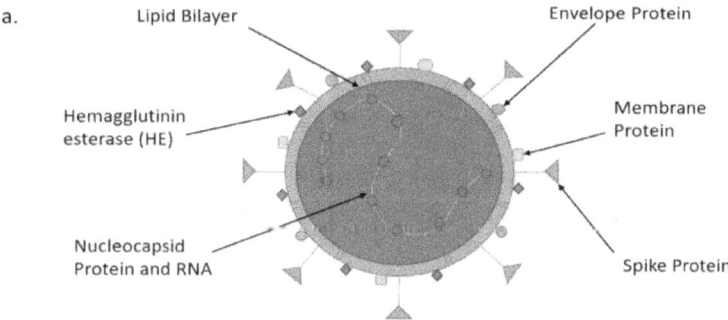

Figure 8: Structure of SARS-CoV-2 Source: Bioengineering 2021[19]

Other Virus Families

Away from the recent pandemic limelight there are, of course, many viruses that have long been causing varying degrees of human distress. Although they are from distinctly different virus categories than coronaviruses, there are transferable learnings from recent diagnostic breakthroughs that apply regardless of the virus categorisation. To help put SARS-CoV-2 in context and highlight how it differs from other familiar viruses, let's briefly consider Influenza and HIV. An appreciation of the differing structures of what we refer to homogeneously as "viruses" is useful to better understand firstly, the diagnostic challenges, and then the therapeutic ones.

Influenza

For most people, Influenza as a disease needs little introduction. In the last 100 years or so, the flu group of viruses (A, B, C and D) has probably been the deadliest microscopic force on the planet, causing 4 pandemics with a combined death toll of over 50m, along with perhaps 500,000 seasonal deaths each year[20]. Though a mild disease for most people, Influenza infections can cause especially high morbidity and mortality rates in the elderly (65 or older). Because of its familiarity and widespread occurrence, it was the reference point for many people who described COVID-19 as similar to flu, due to the overlapping symptoms in many cases. However, at a more technical level, they are very different viruses and tests designed for one will not find the other.

Influenza Composition

Coronaviruses and Influenza viruses share the same top-level taxonomic designation but quickly diverge from there due to their very different structure:

> **Riboviria** > **Orthornavirae** > Negarnaviricota > Polyploviricotina > Insthoviricetes > Articulavirales > Orthomyxoviridae > Alphainfluenzavirus > Influenza A virus

> **Riboviria** > **Orthornavirae** > Pisuviricota > Pisoniviricetes > Nidovirales > Cornidovirineae > Coronaviridae > Orthocoronavirinae > Betacoronavirus > Sarbecovirus > SARS-CoV

At around 80μm, influenza virus is similar in physical size to SARS-CoV-2, though the influenza genome is less than half the size of SARS-CoV-2 at about 13.5kb. Unlike the key proteins N and S that we noted above for SARS-CoV-2, the key proteins when discussing influenza are usually the hemagglutinin (HA) and neuraminidase (NA), as it is variations in these that give rise to names such as H1N1 and H3N2, which are the *variants* most common in humans. In influenza, there are eighteen different kinds of hemagglutinin (H1 to H18) and eleven different kinds of neuraminidase (N1 to N11).

From the outside, the two viruses initially look a little similar. The key external visual difference is that the flu relies on the combination of the HA/NA proteins to enter a cell, while SARS-CoV-2 relies on its Spike (S) protein. Internally though, a crucial difference is that the Influenza virus RNA is in 8 strands versus a single strand in SARS-CoV-2. We'll return to this crucial difference later when we talk about variants and viral evolution in more detail.

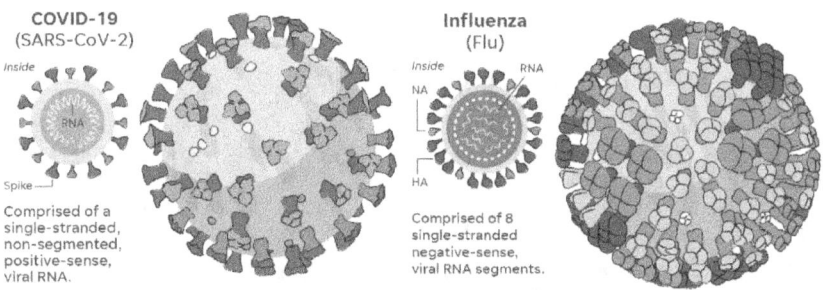

Figure 9: SARS-CoV-2 compared to Influenza. Images from USA Today[21]

HIV

The examples above are all respiratory viruses, so as a final example of common RNA-based viruses, let's look briefly at HIV. According to a UNAIDS (United Nations on HIV/AIDS) update in 2018, it is estimated that there are 37.9 million individuals living with HIV all over the world, with a cumulative 32 million people dead from AIDS-related illnesses[22].

Belonging to another, different taxonomic category, HIV is a spherical virus, physically about 20% larger than a SARS-CoV-2 virion but containing only 9749 nucleotides:

> **Riboviria** › Pararnavirae › Artverviricota › Revtraviricetes › Ortervirales › Retroviridae › Orthoretrovirinae › Lentivirus › Human immunodeficiency virus 1

From a transmission, diagnostic and symptomatic point of view, HIV has little in common with the respiratory diseases we've been talking about so far. Transmission is typically via sexual activity, parenteral (e.g., blood transfusion or needle-sharing) or perinatal (mother-baby) and initial symptoms (fever, headache, muscle pain, rashes, sore throat and mouth sores, and swollen lymph nodes) are so mild as to be missed or confused with other causes. Usually, if it is not diagnosed and treated (Antiretroviral therapies-ART-have transformed HIV infection into a chronic disease), HIV turns into AIDS in an average of 10 years.[23] Studies searching for vaccines have not been successful yet though a vaccine candidate has entered phase 1 trials in late January 2022[24], using the mRNA technology that came to prominence for some COVID-19 vaccines.

Beyond these examples, although we don't have space here to explore many more viral infections, it's important to remember the extent of different diseases they can cause across the entirety of the human body.

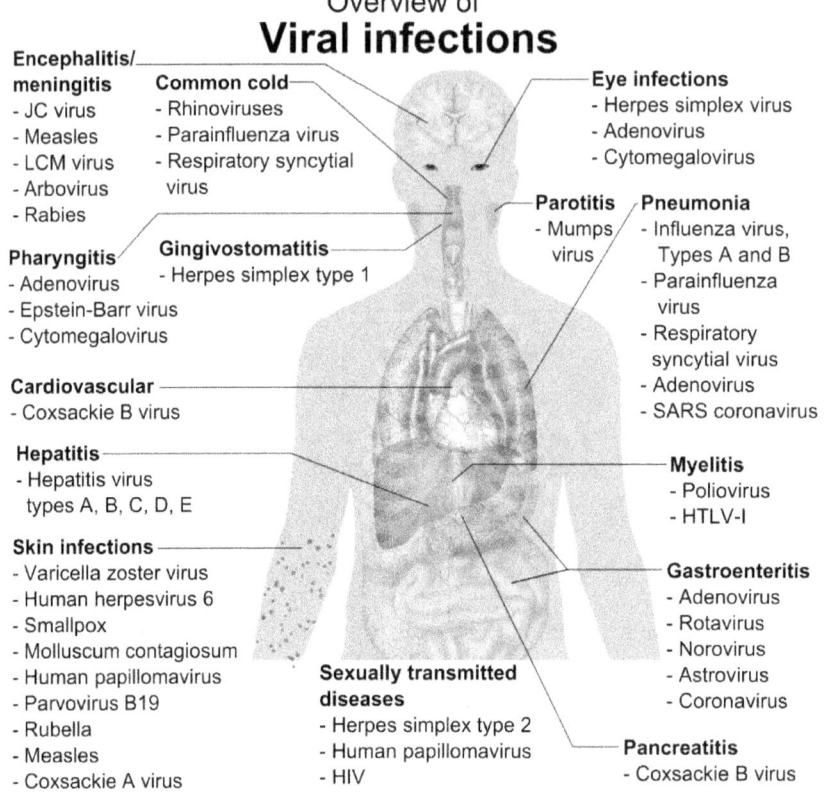

Figure 10: *A simplified overview of the main viral infections and the most notable involved species. Source: Häggström, Mikael (2014)*[25]

The Virome

"Biologists estimate that 380 trillion viruses are living on and inside your body right now— 10 times the number of bacteria"

Scientific American[26]

To set the stage for discussing human efforts to identify viruses, we've just briefly discussed 3 topical/common viruses (SARS-CoV-2, Influenza and

HIV). Much of the commentary, mid-COVID-19 pandemic, was about how and when we might "live with the virus". However, it's worth pointing out that we already live with many, many viruses. In the case of SARS-CoV-2, "living with the virus" will mean being able to quickly and accurately diagnose it compared to diseases with similar presentations, monitoring its mutations and adjusting treatments as necessary.

But as we refine the tools we have to diagnose viruses, we will undoubtedly uncover many more viral relationships, both positive and harmful. We've known for decades that humans have a complex relationship with vast quantities of microorganisms. Most early studies of this human *microbiome* were focused on bacteria. However, we now know that there is also a significant viral component, referred to as the human *virome* - the collection of all viruses found on or in humans. Scientists have found viruses in every part of the human body - from saliva and blood to breast milk to cerebrospinal fluid, as well as on our skin, in our gut, and urine/faeces. Studies[27] have shown that each individual has a highly personal virome.

While many viral pathogens have clearly defined negative interactions with humans, causing acute or chronic infections, many more have undefined impacts or latent/asymptomatic infections. In a further layer of complexity, there are viruses (known as prokaryotic viruses or bacteriophages) in the human virome that act to control their larger microbial neighbours; bacteria - without the presence of viruses, our relationship with bacteria would be drastically altered, with unpredictable consequences.

Recent advances in genetic sequencing (which we'll talk about more in Chapter 11) are key to understanding the virome. With so many viruses to comprehend, the ability to analyse them quickly at a genetic level will become increasingly important.

Epidemiology

Viral epidemiology is the branch of medical science that deals with the transmission and control of virus infections in humans. The diagnostic techniques we'll explore in the upcoming Chapters are an integral part of understanding the wider picture of viral behaviour.

With all the emphasis on virus transmission during the COVID-19 pandemic, it's interesting to consider the ways other viruses spread: People who cohabitate (whether intimately or not) share about 25 percent of the viruses in their viromes. As well as human-to-human transmission, and transmission via fomites (surfaces), another pathway is through disease-bearing organisms, known as vectors, such as aphids or mosquitoes.

Most of the familiar viruses, including influenza viruses, SARS-CoV-2, chickenpox, smallpox, and measles, spread in the air via coughing and sneezing. Enteric viruses such as norovirus and rotavirus (that cause gastroenteritis), are transmitted by hand-to-mouth contact or in food or water. Depending on the means of spreading, epidemiologists may advise public health measures and/or pharmaceutical interventions (e.g. vaccination) to break chains of transmission. For viral outbreaks in animal populations, large-scale slaughtering may be advised to stop transmission as has been seen in Foot and Mouth (caused by Aphthovirus of the family Picornaviridae) or Avian Flu outbreaks.

Pathogenesis and Virus Response

When discussing viruses, a key term is *pathogenesis*. A pathogen is any bacterium, virus, or other microorganism that can cause disease, and pathogenesis is the term to describe its progress - the sequence of events from entry of the virus into the body, *tropism* (i.e. what cells it infects), multiplication and spread, the development of tissue damage, and the production of an immune response. This progression may yield specific markers that are useful in diagnostics. The *virulence* of a pathogen refers to the proportion of infections that produce serious disease.

Individuality

Not everyone responds to a viral infection in the same way - there may be significant variation from individual to individual in the severity, timing and/or the duration of symptoms. According to the book, Viral Infections of Humans[28], the following host factors influence the occurrence, course or severity of disease:

- Age at onset of disease
- Sex
- Race
- Genetic Factors
- Pre-existing level of specific or nonspecific immunity
- Iatrogenic immunosuppression
- Behaviour and Lifestyle
- Coinfections
- Pre-existing chronic conditions or pregnancy
- Nutritional status
- Psychological Status

Viruses: One of Our Biggest Challenges

As many bacterial threats have succumbed to treatment with antibiotics (despite the growing concern around antibiotic resistance undermining and even reversing this progress), viral infections have come to pose a proportionately greater threat to global health than at any time in history. While there are some antiviral treatments, there are no broad-spectrum equivalents that work, as antibiotics do for bacteria. Although we focus here on viral infections of human medical significance, the reader should be aware that viruses are also a major threat to livestock and plant species, and therefore of great importance in human nutrition and food supply.

The Need for Diagnostics

Scientists know more than ever about viruses but, in many ways, are still only at the point of knowing more precisely how little is known. Finding and correctly identifying these tiny threats is a massive scientific challenge – as we'll see in the upcoming chapters, a few key breakthroughs have enabled accurate identification of more viruses, more quickly, giving much cause for optimism. In the next Chapter, we'll explore these and the extra challenge of diagnosing at population scale.

Chapter 3: The Ascent of Diagnostics

"Time to result was slow and it was often said that the patient was dead or better by the time the result was received. Over the intervening years, diagnostic advances have transformed the field by allowing accurate results in a clinically useful time frame."

Mary Louise Landry, MD, Yale School of Medicine[29]

A Brief History of Diagnostics/Into the Limelight

As we learn more about the structures, composition and pathogenesis of viruses, central to our improving understanding of them is the development of technologies to quickly find and analyse these tiny pathogens. Before the emergence of diagnostic capabilities, physicians had to make treatment decisions based only on visible evidence, which is often non-specific.

Although we can now see even the smallest viruses on electron microscopes and examine every element of their genome with sequencing technology, it hasn't always been that way. And while these kinds of technologies are critical in the analysis phase, solutions for finding and identifying viruses "in the field", in a timely manner to help patients, are likely to be one of the more significant legacies of the COVID-19 pandemic.

If we go back far enough (to the 18th century), the primary diagnostic techniques available included tasting patients' urine. Thankfully, the sophistication of diagnostic techniques has come a long way since then and continues to develop at breakneck, and even increasing, speed. The clinical laboratory did not become a standard fixture of medicine until the beginning of the 20th century; around 1900, dedicated laboratory facilities replaced doctors using optical microscopes in their own offices and myriad chemical tests were developed - quantitative analytical methods for several urine analytes also came into existence around then[30].

A Century of Foundational Progress

"In the final analysis, only an antibody response in the host constitutes definitive evidence of infection with a specific virus."

Principles of Internal Medicine, 1962[31]

Compared to recent times, prior generations of health care professionals had a very limited toolkit to identify pathogens, and even then, lacked the ability to do so in a useful timeframe. I want to look to the future, to identify the dividends we should be seeking based on the acceleration and developments of the last two years, but I think it's useful firstly to very briefly acknowledge the scientific advances of the last 120 years that have set the scene. For more detail, the meticulously researched book, *To Catch a Virus*[32], provides an exceptionally detailed summary of the key milestones, following the growth of diagnostic virology from its beginnings over a century ago to the present: the scientific discoveries, the blind alleys, the missteps, the epidemics that gave urgency to the quest, the technological advances we now take for granted.

For our purposes here in briefly exploring the background, the turn of the 20th century saw a defining breakthrough in the development of medical science - investigators demonstrated the causative agent of yellow fever passing through a filter designed to stop the passage of bacteria, thus proving the existence of a smaller pathogen that could infect humans - the virus.

Despite this advance however, it was another three decades before the influenza virus was finally identified in 1933, long after the pandemic of 1918. It would be another half century to the 1980s before diagnostic technologies, with the advent of the molecular techniques we'll discuss in Chapter 6, matured to the point of being able to provide a viral identification in a clinically useful timeframe to influence the management of an acute patient.

Cultures & Antibodies

Bereft of the technological ability to see sub-microscopic viruses, pathologists for much of the 20th century had to rely on culturing viruses in animal hosts or finding antibodies in blood samples to identify infectious agents. Indeed, for decades, lab-based serological (blood tests) identification of the presence of antibodies was preferred to culturing viruses, though both approaches were too slow to guide treatment, even if any was available. While modern diagnostics can guide a choice between antibiotics and antiviral treatments, the urgency in those days might have been to determine if an animal had been rabid or if a patient had chickenpox (varicella virus) or the more worrying smallpox (variola virus).

The middle years of the 20th century saw rapid advances. While only 20 human-specific viruses were known in 1948, an additional 70 were identified in the following 10 years[33]. In 1962, Yale Medical School created the first postgraduate course in "Diagnostic Virology"[34] and the increased availability of the electron microscope brought the ability to see many more viruses for the first time. Of particular relevance to our discussion, is the 1965[35] discovery of a new group of RNA viruses, coronaviruses, which were named for the corona-like or "crown" spikes seen electron microscopically.

The Need for Speed

The *time to result* (TTR) is a key concern for diagnostic tests, as we'll refer to frequently. And while the first two thirds of the 20th century saw the fundamental abilities to isolate and even see viruses, from then on there was an increasing interest in techniques to speed up the diagnostics for what were largely newly discovered viruses.

The World Health Organisation (WHO) published a manual for Rapid Viral Diagnostics in 1979, highlighting four techniques that were improving the speed of diagnostics[36]:

- Electron Microscopy
- Immunofluorescence
- Enzyme-linked immunoassay (ELISA)
- Radioimmunoassay

Just a few years later in 1985, arguably the biggest breakthrough in diagnostics would be discovered - Polymerase Chain Reaction (PCR), the beginning of the now widespread era of nucleic acid amplification tests (NAAT) that we'll review in Chapter 6.

Laboratory Diagnosis

"An accurate virus diagnosis invariably requires laboratory testing of clinical specimens for the presence of virus, viral antigens, or specific antibodies. The past few decades have seen a major revolution in the operation of virus diagnostic laboratories and in their role in clinical patient management. Virus isolation has been largely replaced by sensitive nucleic acid detection assays and the measurement of specific antibodies at a very high level of sensitivity and specificity".

Chapter 10 - Laboratory Diagnosis of Virus Diseases
Fenner and White's Medical Virology (Fifth Edition)[37]

Centralised commercial laboratories or facilities attached to larger hospitals have become the preferred approach to analysing clinical specimens for the presence of a virus or specific antibodies. Laboratory techniques have advanced greatly in recent times, mainly with the advent of molecular methods. Older methods such as Cell culture, Cytology and Histopathology are no longer used in most settings.

The 2000s saw the rise of molecular testing (primarily PCR, but more on that in Chapter 6) that provided accurate results with relatively high speed and acceptable cost. Lab automation allowed for high throughput, with a wide range of assays available to screen for all common pathogens. Improvements in technologies like ELISA for the detection of antigens and antibodies (see Chapters 7 and 8) mean that laboratories have an array of diagnostic tools necessary to identify a wide range of pathogens.

Expanding Horizons

As well as looking at the techniques and technologies of testing, another key topic for us is *where* the testing takes place. Already, before the COVID-19 pandemic, emphasis was shifting away from sole dependence on laboratory testing, driven by the benefits, that new technologies enabled, of moving testing closer to the patient, alongside trends around convenience and even "worried well" people seeking tests to "self-diagnose" without the need for a Healthcare Professional (HCP) to order or provide a test.

The miniaturisation of laboratory testing technologies is vital to address the inequitable distribution of diagnostic capacity and access to testing. As the ability to move testing closer to the point of care (POC) brings the potential to test in Resource Limited Settings (RLS) and Low/Middle Income Countries (LMIC), giving laboratory-grade results without access to a laboratory, it also promises to reduce the burden on laboratory-based testing, even in ostensibly well-served areas.

Moving beyond POC, we'll also explore in later Chapters the move towards at-home testing - the ability to conduct a test and get a result in a domestic setting, as opposed to at-home collection, where a patient may self-collect a sample that is then sent to a laboratory for analysis. At-home testing is already increasingly common for non-viral reasons such as blood glucose levels but can also be used for drug screening, food sensitivities and cholesterol.

There is some hesitancy among medical professionals and regulators about the use of at-home testing. In the US, the FDA offers consumer guidance and reminds users of the importance of seeking professional advice, as well as providing a list of approved at-home tests[38]. However, as the quality of at-home tests improves, they do seem poised to become a crucial on-going part of healthcare, at least on a triage basis, with confirmation via laboratory-based tests if necessary.

The Pandemic Imperative

If there were gradual shifts in the diagnostic world underway before 2020, nobody foresaw the utterly changed landscape we're now talking about in 2022, less than three years later. The emergence of SARS-CoV-2 saw an explosion of research interest in viral diagnostics. A search on PubMed.gov (the US National Institutes of Health's National Library of Medicine) for articles relating to "SARS-CoV-2 Test" during the period 2020-2021 returns over 18,000 results[39].

The research interest in diagnostics has been matched by the commercial interest. The critical need to develop tests to identify the novel coronavirus spurred Governments around the world to promote unprecedented investments into diagnostics. The growth in the availability of diagnostic tests by type and volume during the COVID-19 pandemic represents a scientific and logistical triumph.

The Commerce of Disease

The human cost of COVID-19 has been immense, with millions of excess deaths and many survivors suffering from long COVID - and that's without counting the impact of delayed diagnosis/ treatment of other diseases, the mental health implications and economic cost of lockdowns. The IMF estimates that COVID-19 cost over $13 trillion[40]. Economies will take years to recover but there is a need, nonetheless, to have a debate about healthcare costs; investing in public health measures may be more palatable now to policy makers previously hobbled by a prevention paradox[41] - spending money to stop something that *might* happen isn't popular when more visible priorities aren't funded, especially where the expenditure has little apparent benefit at an individual level. After the COVID-19 pandemic, however, it may be easier to see the merits of investing in preventative policies at a societal level as the costs of failing to prepare have been laid bare.

COVID Diagnostics Investments

In April 2020, the US National Institutes of Health used $1.5bn of Congressional funding to establish the Rapid Acceleration of Diagnostics

(RADx) initiative to support the development, production scale-up, and deployment of accurate, rapid tests. As well as increasing short term testing capacity, the programme also aims to support the development and production of innovative diagnostic technologies as well as strategies for making testing available to diverse, vulnerable, and underserved populations. Similar funding programmes were set up in other jurisdictions, such as the EU[42].

In a clear indication of the separate importance of diagnostics, RADx was a distinct programme from the public-private Accelerating COVID-19 Therapeutic Interventions and Vaccines (ACTIV) initiative announced earlier in April[43]. RADx essentially added focus, urgency and funding to build on long-existing efforts such as the Point-of-Care Technologies Research Network[44], which was established in 2007 by the National Institute of Biomedical Imaging and Bioengineering (NIBIB) and had focused on STDs, HIV and Cardiovascular testing, as well as the underlying diagnostic technologies.

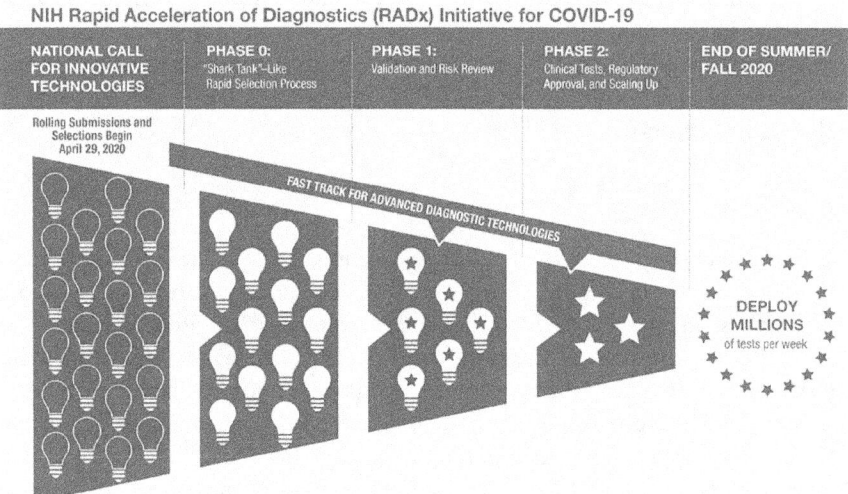

Figure 11: the RADx approach to speeding diagnostic developments. Source: NIH

The RADx initiative is split into 4 primary strands[45]:

Strand	Focus	Budget	Projects funded as at Feb 2022
RADx® Tech	To speed the development, validation, and commercialization of innovative point-of-care and home-based tests, as well as improve clinical laboratory tests, that can directly detect the virus.	$666 million	22
RADx® Advanced Technology Platforms (RADx-ATP)	To increase testing capacity and throughput by identifying existing and late-stage testing platforms for COVID-19 that are far enough advanced to achieve rapid scale-up or expanded geographical placement in a short amount of time. These efforts will focus on scaling up technologies, including improving existing high-throughput platforms, to increase performance.	$191 million	
RADx® Underserved Populations (RADx-UP)	To understand the factors associated with disparities in COVID-19 morbidity and mortality and to lay the foundation to reduce disparities for those underserved and vulnerable populations who are disproportionately affected by, have the highest infection rates of, and/or are most at risk for complications or poor outcomes from the COVID-19 pandemic.	$512 million	122
RADx® Radical (RADx-rad)	To support new, non-traditional approaches that address current gaps in COVID-19 testing. The program will also support new or non-traditional applications of existing approaches to make them more usable, accessible, or accurate. These may lead to new ways to identify the current SARS-CoV-2 virus as well as potential future viruses.	$187 million	50

Testing Capacity

Thanks to Government initiatives (such as the US RADx model) and the substantial investment in manufacturing and laboratory capacity, the amount of testing available globally is higher than at any time in history. Looking at the US, testing capacity and availability of rapid tests has hit 1 billion tests per month.

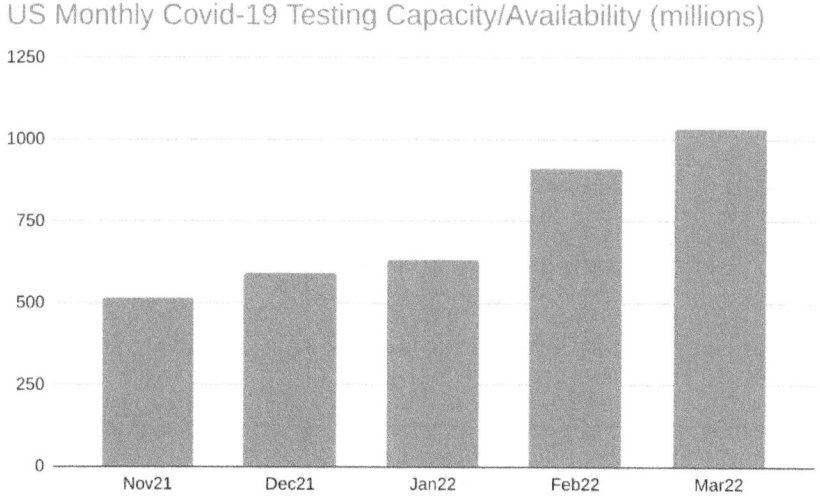

Figure 12: US Monthly testing capacity as at Q1, 2022[46].

Although consumers who struggled to get access to testing at various points during the pandemic may express frustration about availability, the scale at which tests are being produced is pretty impressive from a standing start. In Ireland, with a population of about 5 million, the health services moved from distributing about 20,000 at-home tests per week in October 2020 to sending out over 350,000 per week by January 2021[47].

Production of rapid tests now far exceeds the laboratory testing capacity available. In the US, combined PCR testing capacity across all labs stands at around 2.5 million tests per day. For comparison, just one of the dozen or so companies producing Antigen tests, iHealth[48], has increased output to 300 million per month[49]. Abbott produced almost 1 billion Binax Now antigen tests in 2021, while US Department of Defense funding has enabled Australian firm Ellume to create a US production extension for about 20m tests per month[50].

Scale of Testing

The dawn of 2020 saw the first murmurs of concern among epidemiologists and public health officials about a novel virus, but PCR was still an obscure scientific term confined to molecular biologists and lab technicians - few members of the public were aware of what 2021's most commonly used acronym actually meant (we'll explore PCR in Chapter 6). Most of the world's population had no intention of putting any diagnostic tests up their noses and virtually nobody in the world had antibodies for the soon to be named SARS-Cov-2, let alone any way to test for them.

The number of tests carried out during the COVID-19 pandemic is absolutely vast. People who have never in their lives been tested, are carrying out daily tests. Globally, clinical laboratories have performed approximately 3 billion molecular diagnostic tests for SARS-CoV-2[51]. By way of context, during the 2009 H1N1 pandemic, the CDC developed and shipped over one million tests throughout the United States just two weeks after the virus was discovered[52].

The website, Our World in Data[53], publishes graphs updated daily (as well as making the full data set available for free download to anyone who wants to run their own analysis[54]) comparing global reporting on testing. Visit their website to watch an animated version of graphs like this one showing the number of tests per thousand people carried out each day.

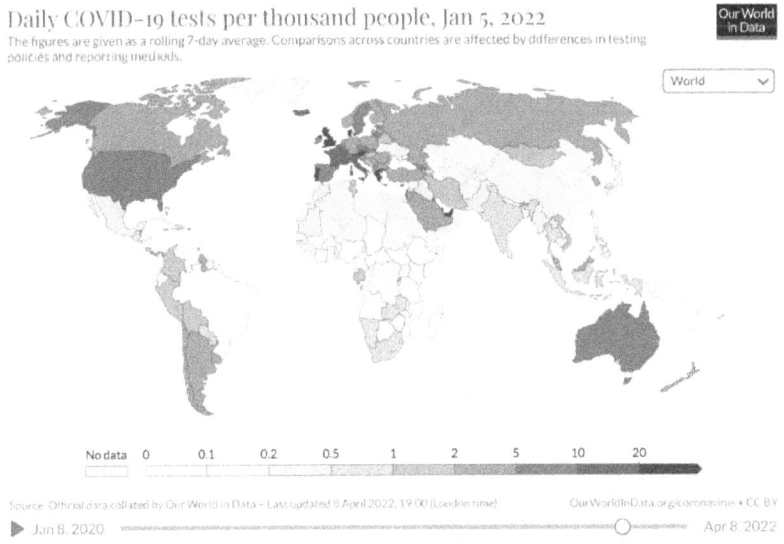

Figure 13: Daily Covid Testing in January 2022. Source: Our World In Data

Taking England as an example, with a population around 56m, people were carrying out over 1.1m rapid at home tests per day in late 2021.

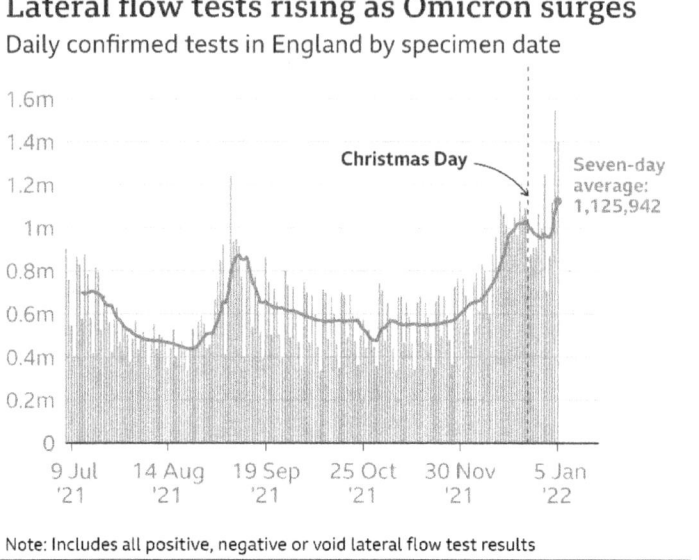

Figure 14: UK daily testing, as reported by BBC[55]

Inequalities

While the total number of tests carried out during the COVID-19 pandemic is enormous, the distribution of testing remains deeply uneven. So far, only 21.1% of tests administered worldwide have been used in low- and middle-income countries (LMICs), despite these countries comprising 50.8% of the global population.

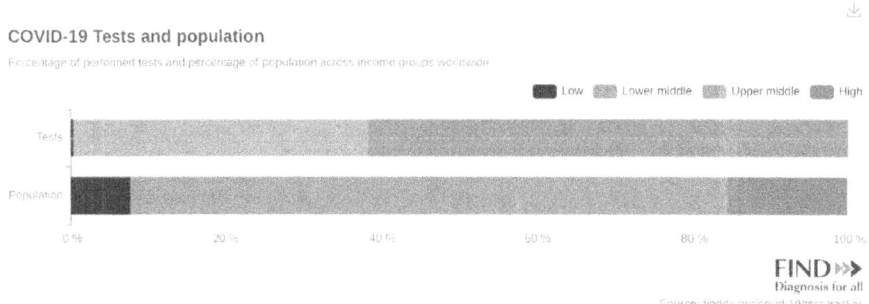

Figure 15: Disparities in testing by income[56]

Note: For those looking for more statistics on testing, Arizona State University has an excellent dashboard with numerous metrics freely available[57].

Testing Commerce

As pointed out in *To Catch a Virus*[58], commercial considerations have long been involved in driving disease diagnostics. The first agent identified as a virus, the tobacco mosaic virus, was of concern due to its threat to the tobacco crop. Investigations into Foot-and-Mouth disease were driven by the reduction of cattle breeding and milk production. Now, healthcare has grown to be big business and testing is a competitive commercial sector. Analysts predict that the global market for POC diagnostics (a subset of the larger invitro-diagnostics market) will grow from around $25bn to $43bn from 2021 to 2026[59].

To take some examples of third quarter financial results in 2021 for suppliers of COVID-19 testing, the figures reflected the massive demand for rapid tests in particular. Quidel made $406 million[60], while Abbott revenues amounted $1.9 billion globally from COVID-19 tests[61].

Although cheaper than developing new therapeutics, developing and commercialising tests is expensive. While some may feel that the big pharma companies are profiteering from COVID-19 testing, allowance should be made for the uncertainties of demand as waves come and go, as well as for the huge costs to scale up production capacity. I do believe it's important, though, that where public funding is provided to private companies to scale production capacity, there is an equitable use of any excess capacity in the future towards the provision of additional testing in RLS/LMIC.

During the COVID-19 pandemic, the cost of tests has varied widely. In the US, typical pricing for a twin-pack of rapid tests is around $20, while in France the cost of tests is capped at €5.20. In many other countries, tests were distributed freely to many citizens; the UK Government spent £2bn per month on mass testing.

Chapter 4: Testing Fundamentals

"Reliable viral diagnostics depend on preanalytical issues such as choice of the correct sample material, optimal sampling time with regard to the course of the disease and the duration/ conditions of sample transport to the laboratory".

Lennette's Laboratory Diagnosis of Viral Infections[62]

What we generally refer to as a "test" is in fact a complex chain of steps, including those that precede the actual test itself. Incorrect decisions or operations at any point in the process may render the test and any result unreliable. The final sensitivity of tests in a real-world setting depends on various factors, including the timing and type of specimen to be analysed, the collection technique, and the quality of test materials used to perform assays. Before we move on to look at the test technologies themselves, here we'll discuss the steps leading up to an actual test.

Testing Basics

The seemingly simple concept of testing someone to see if they have a disease is, in fact, a multifarious process requiring several decisions to be made based on the context, motivation, resources available and underlying assumptions. Just as a doctor may order an X-Ray in some circumstances and an MRI in others, different types of viral diagnostics may be chosen based on what's being sought, what tests are available, costs etc. The suitability of rapid at home tests compared to laboratory tests has been a contentious issue in many countries during the COVID-19 pandemic.

While testing during a pandemic may be an obvious requirement, in normal circumstances, a number of questions should be considered when deciding if a test is appropriate and, if so, which testing pathway should be chosen. Among the factors are:

- Why is the test being considered - what actions will come from the result?
- How will the person be tested - what sample needs to be collected and by whom?
- How will the sample be tested - what technology will be used for the test and where?

- When are they to be tested - will the timing impact the result and/or the resultant actions?
- How soon is the result required and how reliable is it - is speed or accuracy more important?
- Is the result binary or quantitative?
- Is some patient discomfort acceptable?
- How much will the test cost?

These fundamental questions will determine the testing strategy and will vary from case to case and situation to situation. Above all, an understanding of the trade-offs between each parameter is vital to achieve the best outcome in a given context.

Why Test?

The reason why a decision to perform a test is made is a crucial factor in deciding what type of test is most suitable. A test may be to identify the presence or absence of a pathogen with a view to determining a clinical intervention or, as we've seen since 2020, to determine if an asymptomatic person should be advised to isolate. More broadly though, testing decisions may be influenced by the availability or otherwise of treatments, or they may be part of screening or research efforts.

Different diseases follow a different course of infection (*pathogenesis*) - different viruses will be detectable at different times, in different specimens and pose varying levels of threat. Understanding the characteristics of different approaches to testing, different techniques and different tools is the focus of this and the next Chapter, and we'll go on to examine the question of test timing in Chapter 12, after we've covered more about the types of test technologies available.

Diagnostic vs Screening testing

Typically testing is motivated either by a suspicion of the presence of a pathogen that needs to be confirmed or identified (diagnostic testing), or by a desire to identify the presence of a disease in someone considered to be at risk but not showing any obvious signs of infection (screening).

While diagnostic testing is usually a determinant of treatment (or Non-Pharmaceutical Intervention - NPI - such as isolation), screening may be used for quantifying disease prevalence, public health policy or statistical purposes. Screening can also be intended to identify conditions that may at some point in the future give rise to disease but do not currently constitute a threat.

Although there has been much discussion about asymptomatic and pre-symptomatic testing in the case of COVID-19, we cannot assume that any future epidemics will follow the same pattern. As we look to build on our diagnostic capabilities based on recent advances, we must avoid the trap of narrowing our thinking due to recency bias. This also applies to the type of result that tests can return - in some infections, a quantitative result may be important, not just a binary outcome.

Beyond Binary

The focus on COVID-19 testing was almost entirely on the binary distinction between positive and negative (not detected). Although certain types of test (primarily RT-qPCR that is described in Chapter 6) can report quantitatively (i.e. how much SARS-CoV-2 was found), a simple yes/no was sufficient information for the majority of tests where the outcome was patient isolation or not. With a new pathogen like SARS-CoV-2, too little was known about the relative importance of viral load in determining likely outcomes and guidance of immature treatment protocols to emphasize a quantitative result.

In other testing scenarios, the *amount* of an analyte found may be significant rather than just the presence - for example the presence of a target above or below a threshold may not trigger an intervention, and in essence constitutes the same as a negative test, while a large deviation from the expected amount may be important. For example, too much Prostate Specific Antigen (PSA) may trigger concern, while a small amount is expected. Conversely, either an unusually high or low result from a Red Blood Cell (RBC) count would alert a healthcare professional.

As we consider potential applications of technologies that have come to the fore during the COVID-19 pandemic, it's vital to consider if it's possible, practical and desirable to elicit results on a more quantitative basis. For example, if we learn that there's a significant viral load threshold that would inform a particular treatment, should that be a desirable capability requirement for future at-home testing or would it suffice to have qualitative tests at home and leave more granular readings to laboratories?

Screening & Testing Harms

Testing to determine the presence of potentially dangerous entities may seem obviously beneficial, but it's worth pointing out that screening programmes in the past have resulted in disappointing and even negative outcomes.

Screening programmes are usually initiated by public health authorities looking to identify the prevalence of a potential pathogen or condition in populations where there are no obviously detectable symptoms. By identifying invisible threats, screening is intended to enable earlier treatments. But, while screening can be beneficial, it should only be undertaken with careful regard for the potential harms of testing. Non-invasive tests generally pose no risk to patients, but over-diagnosis or misdiagnosis, as well as the creation of psychological harms, may indicate against widespread testing in some situations. As we'll see in Chapter 9, increasingly sensitive test technologies will become available for domestic use in the coming years, which may lead to an increase in the detection of previously undetected pathogens and consequent concern, even where there is no imminent danger.

Screening can, for example, identify abnormalities that might never cause a problem in a person's lifetime. An example is prostate cancer screening; it has been said that "more men die with prostate cancer than of it."[63]

Value Framework for Diagnostics

Although much of the focus on assessing diagnostics is rightly on the objective accuracy of the assay, there are multiple other factors to consider when designing and deploying diagnostic tools. Ultimately, the ability of the test to inform and influence clinical decision making, to improve patient outcomes, is usually paramount. In the case of infectious diseases, public health priorities may dictate testing policies. However, in many other cases, where diseases are non-transmissible and/or slow moving, the decisions on use of diagnostics may not be as straight-forward.

Even when the sample collection or test itself poses no risk to a patient, the testing process can involve significant harms, which need consideration when assessing diagnostics for possible use. Asch et al. observed that clinical impact alone is an insufficient measure of value for diagnostics because diagnostics also have the potential to affect patients' sense of psychic value, whether or not test results affect treatment. For example, a diagnostic test for dementia may have relatively little impact on treatment or outcomes but may have a substantial effect on the patient's psychic value[64]. Conversely, taking a test can be a psychologically important tool for people struggling with a sense of powerlessness or fear - it's a tangible action. So, a decision to test is not always a simple choice.

In the 2010 paper, *Understanding the Medical and Nonmedical Value of Diagnostic Testing*[65], the authors proposed that, regardless of type, diagnostics have the potential to create value along three dimensions:

- **Medical value** - reflects a diagnostic's ability to inform clinical treatment recommendations

- **Planning value** - refers to a diagnostic test's ability to inform patients about choices on reproduction, work, retirement, long term health, financial plans, and so on.

- **Psychic value** - captures how diagnostics can directly change patients' sense of satisfaction and may yield either positive (good news) or negative (bad news) value.

Diagnostic results have consequences beyond determining a treatment plan, and can have significant impacts on the patient - e.g., the anxiety of knowing you may have a disease that can have severe outcomes. Even self-testing can deliver bad news. I recall clearly when I did a 23andMe DNA test how insistent the website was that I be prepared for potentially hard-to-take results. It repeatedly asked if I was sure I wanted to see the results and it counselled me to open them in a supportive environment and to seek professional advice in the event of worrisome findings.

In a seminal work on screening, the World Health Organisation in 1968 published the "Principles and practice of screening for disease", often known by its authors names as the Wilson and Jungner criteria[66]. Their principles were as follows:

- The condition sought should be an important health problem.
- The natural history of the condition, including development from latent to declared disease, should be adequately understood.
- There should be a recognizable latent or early symptomatic stage.
- There should be a suitable test or examination.
- The test should be acceptable to the population.
- There should be an agreed policy on whom to treat as patients.
- There should be an accepted treatment for patients with recognized disease.
- Facilities for diagnosis and treatment should be available.
- The cost of case-finding (including diagnosis and treatment of patients diagnosed) should be economically balanced in relation to possible expenditure on medical care as a whole.
- Case-finding should be a continuing process and not a "once and for all" project.

Despite being over 50 years old, a 2018 review[67] found that the principles were "remarkably enduring". There have, however, been numerous suggested revisions and so in 2008, with the emergence of new genomic technologies, the WHO published updated screening criteria[68]:

- The screening programme should respond to a recognized need.
- The objectives of screening should be defined at the outset.
- There should be a defined target population.
- There should be scientific evidence of screening programme effectiveness.
- The programme should integrate education, testing, clinical services and programme management.
- There should be quality assurance, with mechanisms to minimize potential risks of screening.
- The programme should ensure informed choice, confidentiality and respect for autonomy.
- The programme should promote equity and access to screening for the entire target population.
- Programme evaluation should be planned from the outset.
- The overall benefits of screening should outweigh the harm.

Testing Trade-offs (Test*CASE*)

Once a decision to test is made, the focus can turn to choosing the right type of test for a given situation, which is itself a multi-dimensional challenge. I refer to it as a Test*CASE* - as an easy mnemonic to remember 4 of the key parameters: Cost, Accuracy, Speed and Ease.

Cost

Cost is a very relative term when it comes to testing. While many rapid tests can be produced affordably, higher accuracy tests are often very expensive. However, even an "expensive" test can be dramatically cheaper than the costs incurred by treatment for a case that might have been easier to prevent from progressing if caught earlier. Although, on the one hand, the absolute figures for wide-spread subsidies for mass testing are eye-watering, on the other hand, with the daily cost of mechanical ventilation in ICU running to €1500[69] per patient, mitigations that reduce the numbers ending up in ICU are, aside from the obvious human cost, easy to justify.

Accuracy

Assuming such a thing existed, in a scientifically ideal world, you'd likely always opt for the most accurate test. But in reality, the importance of other factors may sometimes see a more pragmatic compromise to get an acceptable level of accuracy as quickly and cheaply as possible - waiting for the nearly-perfect (e.g. a lab-based PCR test) may be the enemy of the good-enough (a self-use rapid test).

Speed

All modern testing methods represent remarkable speed compared to earlier techniques such as growing cultures, but the need for speed varies. For a virus that is not readily transmissible and poses little immediate danger to its host, a relatively slow test result may be acceptable, while in an ED a rapid result may be crucial in defining a treatment.

Ease

Aside from availability, speed and accuracy considerations, even the relative ease of sample collection may influence the test type most appropriate for a situation. For example, a less invasive sample type that is tested using a 90% accurate assay is of more practical use than a very invasive test giving 93% accurate results, but which patients tend to object to.

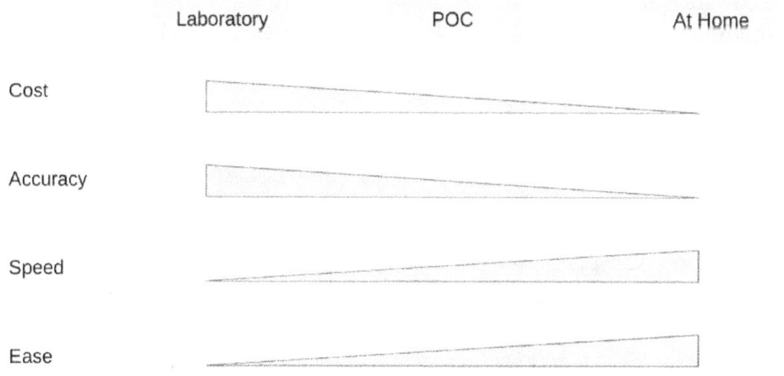

Figure 16: Testing Trade-offs by Location of Testing

Note: Cost are shown as highest at central lab due to infrastructure/ machine costs, though individual cost of test may be low when large pools of samples are processed efficiently in batches.

Understanding Testing

The COVID-19 pandemic led to an unusually public discussion of previously obscure technical terms related to testing. It has also highlighted policy/approach conflicts where people concerned with economic and collateral health impacts advocated faster, less accurate tests, compared to those who advocated more conservative policies relying on slower, more reliable tests but which might increase isolation requirements while awaiting results.

It's worth emphasizing again that future development of testing should not be considered solely in the context of the COVID-19 pandemic. That sort of recency bias might lead to unhelpful decisions when applied to a broader context. With COVID-19, a highly transmissible respiratory disease, it was important to break chains of transmission whilst still facilitating economic and special activities. In a different situation - say where there's no immediate risk of transmission and a fast but less reliable result could lead to serious harm - a more cautious approach may be advised.

Improving public understanding of testing is important. While regulators take special care to review the instructions for use of at-home tests, a challenge remains around educating people about the reliability level of tests. Human nature may lead people to put a misplaced level of trust in a technical-looking test if it gives them the result they want. So, if a user with mild COVID-19 symptoms takes a test and it gives a negative, they may continue socialising and end up infecting others, rather than questioning the validity of the test or how well it was carried out.

Sensitivity and Specificity

Digging a little deeper into the broad term "accuracy", the interpretation and performance of any diagnostic assay are judged by two essential criteria, *sensitivity* and *specificity*. Sensitivity refers to the correctly identified positive results, given as a percentage. If a test has 98% sensitivity, it will correctly identify as positive c.98 out of every 100 samples that are actually infected, and return c.2 false negatives. Specificity refers to correctly identified negative results. Likewise, if a test has 98% specificity, it will correctly identify as negative c.98 out of every 100 samples that aren't infected and return c.2 false positives.

A clear understanding of a test's sensitivity and specificity is an important factor in selecting the most appropriate one for a given situation. However, it is not a fixed value - the numbers quoted by test manufacturers will usually refer to the assay performance on high quality samples taken at the easiest time for a test to perform well. We'll come back to the timing of tests later in Chapter 12.

Testing for SARS-CoV-2

The COVID-19 pandemic provides many examples of the challenges of testing - a novel virus such as SARS-CoV-2, with, in a major departure from SARS-CoV-1, significant levels of pre-symptomatic and asymptomatic transmission, required new tests and new research into the vagaries of testing timing, sample collection and transmission attributes.

For most of the pandemic's duration, there were few proven treatments available, and so testing was primarily to identify and control infection/transmission rather than defining treatment paths. As antiviral treatments such as Paxlovid[70] are approved for use, testing will be used to inform treatment. In March 2022, the US President announced[71] a "test-to-treat" programme: *people can get tested at a pharmacy and if they're positive, receive antiviral pills on the spot at no cost.*

The European Centre for Disease Prevention and Control (ECDC) outlined its guidance to member states on testing strategies for SARS-CoV2 in September 2020[72], advocating objective-driven and sustainable testing strategies for COVID-19 that support the overall public health response to the pandemic and help mitigate its impact on vulnerable populations and healthcare systems, while ensuring that societies and economies continue to function.

The high-level objectives were:

Objective	Tactic
Control transmission	testing of symptomatic individuals and contacts of COVID-19 cases
Monitor incidence and trends and assess severity over time	(multiplex) testing for SARS-CoV-2 and co-infections, e.g. with Influenza
Mitigate the impact of COVID-19 in healthcare and social-care settings	screening for nosocomial (hospital-acquired) infection
Rapidly identify all clusters or outbreaks in specific settings	Screening in at risk workplace or educational settings
Prevent (re-)introduction into regions/countries with sustained control of the virus	Follow-up screening, border controls and antibody testing

Clearly, the different objectives may require different test characteristics, speed, administration and cost profiles. Almost all countries have ended up deploying a multitude of test types to address the different testing needs.

Types of Testing - Overview

We'll spend Part 2 of this book talking in detail about the major types of tests and how recent advances may see improvements in the capabilities, reach and use of testing. Here it's useful to briefly introduce some key elements that affect this chapter's discussion of testing trade-offs.

To understand testing methods, it is helpful to recall the structure of the coronavirus SARS-CoV-2, as we described in Chapter 2, which causes the disease COVID-19.

Three major categories of test have been deployed at various points in the COVID-19 pandemic, depending on their availability, cost and the then-current testing goals of public health officials. The tests commonly available for SARS-CoV-2 can detect either:

- the RNA of the virus – detected by a *molecular/NAAT* - widely referred to as PCR
- the viral proteins of the virus – detected by *antigen* tests - widely referred to as Rapid tests
- our immune system's response to the virus – detected by *antibody* tests

As we'll discuss later, there are pros and cons to each type of test; one may be more appropriate than another, depending on the test setting. Before tests get to be performed on the public, however, there is typically a rigorous regulatory process to test the tests.

Testing the Tests

When tests form the basis of important decisions, be they clinical or socio-political, it's vital to know how reliable the tests are. While this will primarily relate to the accuracy of the result, regulators will also be concerned about any potential harms that could be caused by the test (whether administered correctly or incorrectly), as well ensuring the integrity of any ingredients required for the test such as primers or reagents. It's likely that existing regulatory frameworks in place for testing will be reviewed based on the learnings from the COVID-19 pandemic, as existing approaches will fail to provide for new technologies, use cases and situations.

As I write this towards the end of 2022, despite the fact that billions of COVID-19 tests have been carried out and have become a regular feature of life for many people, there are actually no officially *approved* tests available in the US. All tests currently on sale are only available under an Emergency Use Authorization (EUA)[73], the Food and Drug Administration's (FDA) fast-track mechanism to by-pass normal levels of product scrutiny that determine approval. In the European Union, diagnostic devices are usually regulated under Regulation EU 2017/746[74], but - similarly to the EUA process in the US - suppliers seeking to sell diagnostic devices in the EU can apply for Medical Devices Regulation "Article 59" for derogation from the normal conformity assessment procedures.

Designed for situations like public health emergencies, an EUA requires less evidence and confers temporary permission to offer a product for sale. That's not to suggest that obtaining an EUA is worryingly easy - even in a pandemic rush to get tests to market, a streamlined EUA submission for commercial manufacturers runs to 200 pages and laboratory submissions require about 40 pages, compared to submissions in full approval documentation of about 2000 pages for commercial manufacturers which distribute tests[75] and about 1000 pages for laboratories.

Labs and Kits

As rapid tests for COVID-19 became available, the FDA at first cautiously only approved their use when overseen by a trained health care provider or requiring a prescription for self-testing. The thinking was that involving a physician would offer a chance to talk the user through the process, explaining any concerns around accuracy.

While much debate took place regarding the appropriateness of the speed of granting EUA to Over the Counter (OTC) consumer test kits, in the US the FDA, also being responsible for regulating the approval of assays to be used in laboratories carrying out tests, recognised that even the EUA process wasn't fast enough to meet the need. So, the FDA revised its guidance in an effort to expedite testing as the SARS-CoV-2 threat grew; as early as Feb 29th 2020, the FDA issued the (catchily titled) "*Policy for Diagnostic Tests in Laboratories Certified to Perform High Complexity Testing under CLIA[76] prior to Emergency Use Authorization for Coronavirus Disease-2019 during the Public Health Emergency*". This lab testing policy was released without the FDA's customary public comment phase and enabled manufacturers, for a reasonable period of time after validation and while they are preparing their EUA requests, to distribute their assays to certain labs for use in specimen testing. This approach could save precious weeks in developing testing capacity whilst commencing the EUA process.

In the context of a public health emergency involving pandemic infectious disease, it is critically important that tests are validated, because false results not only can negatively impact the individual patient but can also have a broad public health impact. False positive results for diagnostic tests, for example, can lead to unnecessary quarantine, wasted contact tracing and testing resources. False negative results can lead to lack of appropriate treatment for the individual and further spread of the disease[77].

In a pandemic situation, on the other hand, speed to market is critical, and some compromises on test performance may be acceptable if they can contribute to controlling an outbreak, but both regulators and the public will expect a minimum level of test integrity. In a sobering report published in Jan 2021, Pinto et al described the evaluation of 91 serological tests for SARS-CoV-2, with some tests returning incorrect results 90% of the time. The findings illustrate the challenge of balance between getting tests to market rapidly, whilst maintaining acceptable quality levels:

Sensitivity ranged from 27% to 100% for IgG, [and] from 10% to 100% for IgM. Approximately one-third (n=27) of the assays evaluated are now authorized by FDA for emergency use. The initial flood of serology assays entering the market with inadequate performance emphasized the need for independent evaluation of commercial SARS-CoV-2 antibody assays using performance evaluation panels to determine suitability for use under EUA. Two assays had EUAs revoked and were removed from the U.S. market based on inadequate performance.[78]

Scaling Priorities

In what may prove to be a useful dividend in the event of future pandemics, clear regulatory process challenges surfaced during the COVID-19 emergency. Although the EUA process was available, there were additional levels of granularity in the operational domain that had to be worked out. For example, in November 2021, the FDA further clarified its approach to maximise the wide scale availability of tests[79]:

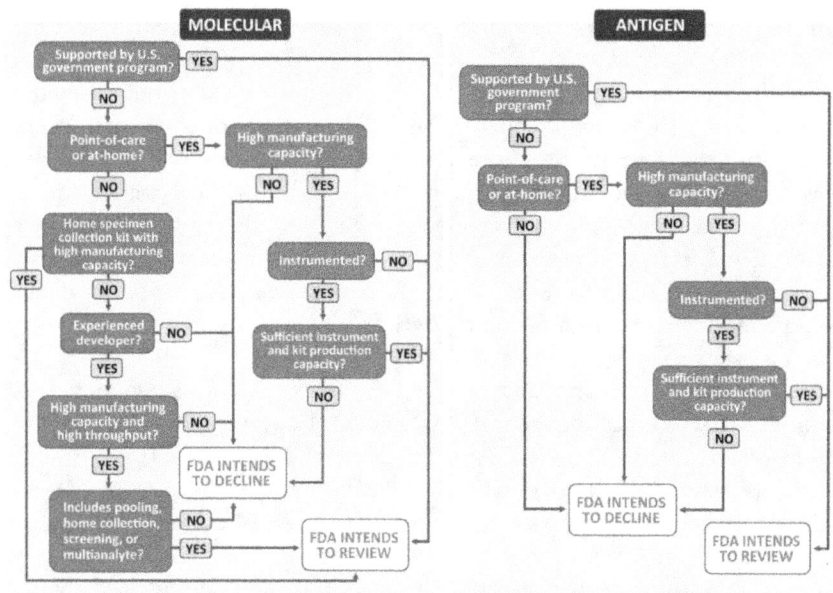

Figure 17: The FDA guidance flowchart for test manufacturers

Although with hindsight it makes sense, prior to the pandemic the FDA hadn't ever published criteria of how EUA applications would be prioritised. Faced with calls to quickly improve the availability of rapid tests, the FDA set the bar for submissions at the ability to demonstrate a manufacturing capacity of ≥500,000 tests per week within 3 months of authorization for POC or At Home tests. With many eager entrepreneurs offering their inventions to the FDA for EUA, it's also interesting to note the pragmatic negative response of the FDA to such submissions: FDA has received EUA requests for tests that require a new instrument to perform the test, but the instrument production capacity is such that the test developers would not be able to produce and distribute in a timely manner enough instruments to perform all the tests they are planning to offer. The addition of an instrument greatly increases the complexity of an EUA review. In addition, laboratories, including POC sites, are unlikely to purchase new instruments that will only be able to run a single test and will potentially not be able to run any tests after the pandemic.

After the Emergency

EUAs are temporary - so what happens when the 'emergency' is over? Given the magnitude of the COVID-19 Public Health Emergency (PHE), FDA recognizes that continued flexibility, while still providing necessary oversight, will be appropriate to facilitate an orderly and transparent transition back to normal operations. In December 2021, FDA issued its thinking for comment[80].

The FDA document requested feedback on the proposal that suppliers of devices with EUA would be given 180 days' notice of the intended termination of their EUA. Those that wished to continue selling the device beyond that time would need to apply through the normal market approval pathway (and could continue selling until an FDA decision on their market submission). Further, the FDA proposed that In vitro diagnostic devices that were distributed before the EUA termination date would not be recalled and could continue to be used for up to 2 years.

Although consumers may expect that their tests are being conducted using approved assays, another type of test, which places an additional burden on regulators, is increasingly widespread: lab-developed tests (LDTs)—assays that are created and used in the same facility, rather than being bought in from pharmaceutical companies. According to a 2021 Pew report,[81] labs often rely on LDTs in cases where an FDA-reviewed test is unavailable or needs modifications for use in a particular population. Interviewees said they may also run LDTs to reduce costs or improve the speed or efficiency of the testing process. LDTs are principally regulated under separate regulations known as Clinical Laboratory Improvement Amendments (CLIA). LDTs have not been required to meet FDA review standards; their number and the extent of their use is unknown. The regulatory loopholes around LDTs are likely to be addressed soon as the performance of tests is assessed post-pandemic.

Chapter 5: Sample Collection

"Proper specimen collection is the most important step in the laboratory diagnosis of infectious diseases. A specimen that is not collected correctly may lead to false or inconclusive test results"

CDC Guidelines[82]

The final area to focus on, before we talk about the mechanics of the tests themselves, is the key variable "ingredient" - the patient sample. Collecting an appropriate, high-quality sample is a key step in any diagnostic process. Whichever testing technology is used in the laboratory, the results are substantially dependent on the right specimen type, taken at the right time, appropriately stored and transported correctly.

A poorly collected sample gives the actual test less to work with, while an incorrect choice of sample site may nullify the test altogether - when choosing sampling methods or sites, it is important to align this with tests that have been validated for the method or specific type of clinical sample used. The same test may display different sensitivity when used with different samples. Understanding which samples a particular test has been designed to analyse, as well as the difference in analyte levels between collection sites is important. For example, even though they may look similar, a rapid test designed to work with a nasopharyngeal (NP) sample may perform differently with a saliva sample, while there may be higher levels of a virus present at different sites (nose/throat) during the course of an infection.

Although there is (rightly) a lot of focus on, and discussion of, the accuracy of each type of test, the majority of errors occur in the pre-analytical phase of viral diagnostics[83]. For all the focus on PCR tests during the COVID-19 pandemic as the "gold standard" of testing, it's important to note potential points of weakness in the process that might undermine the accuracy when the test is actually performed. If the sample is not collected and transported properly to the laboratory, its usefulness could be compromised before one even starts to worry about laboratory risks to accuracy. A PCR test carried out on an incorrectly collected or transported sample may offer no sensitivity benefit over a well-collected sample analysed by an inherently less sensitive test.

As we'll see in later chapters, each type of test can exhibit false positives or false negatives. Laboratory tests may be subject to contamination, but mistakes earlier in the process typically have a larger role to play in testing errors. There's particular concern in professional diagnostic circles around self-collection of samples by users with little awareness of sampling techniques. An incorrect choice of test, choice of sample site, choice of collection media or timing of collection relative to the disease stage are all likely to undermine the integrity of the result, regardless of the test type in question.

There are methods that can determine the quality of a sample, but these are employed after the fact. However, they can be useful, if available, to check the quality of a sample when the result doesn't match the clinical diagnosis or presentation. For example, one study[84] determined that human DNA levels, a stable molecular marker of sampling quality, were significantly lower in samples from 40 confirmed or suspected COVID-19 cases that yielded negative diagnostic test results (i.e., suspected false-negative test results) compared with a representative pool of 87 specimens submitted for COVID-19 testing. The results support suboptimal biological sampling as a contributor to false-negative COVID-19 test results and underscore the importance of proper training and technique in the collection of specimens.

Sampling Trade-offs

The increased concentration on alternative and high-volume diagnostic techniques driven by the COVID-19 pandemic has expanded research into better understanding of what options can be considered for collection - and understanding the trade-offs involved in this important phase of the testing process.

Sample collection involves many trade-offs - samples that are more invasive to collect are often demonstrably more accurate when analysed, but due to the complexity of collecting them, they are not obtained as often as more easily taken samples. Samples that are improperly collected or transported may not reach the test location (such as a laboratory) in a state that will yield a reliable result. This makes it important to reconsider the belief that a lab-processed test from a professionally collected sample is always preferable to at home testing; a poorly collected or transported sample could negate the perceived inherent reliability of the test and thus the treatment decisions arising from it.

Sample collection is the test stage most visible to the patient and is a key influence not only on the ultimate quality of the test but also on the viability of any testing programme. If the collection procedure is too uncomfortable for patients, their willingness to test will be adversely affected, leading to lower levels of testing.

Sampling Decisions

Breaking down the sampling part of the overall testing process, there are several important considerations including:

- What specimen is to be collected
- From what site is the specimen to be collected
- What medium is to be used to collect the sample
- Who will collect the sample
- Does the sample have to be transported before analysis
- Does the sample have to be treated in order to be tested

An understanding of the pathogenesis and epidemiology of the virus being sought will enable a professional to choose the ideal test type to use and specimen type to collect; a physician choosing a test will know what ones are available and consider the most pertinent factors affecting the sample choice from the list above. For domestic tests, these questions will be answered largely in advance as part of the test design and consumer packaging.

The Target Pathogen

It may seem obvious, but it's worth stating that where you may choose to collect your sample will be influenced by where the most easily detectable quantity of the pathogen or biomarker you're seeking will be. However, the best place to look may not always be known or obvious - if you don't know the pathogen you're looking for, it's hard to know where to start.

In the case of SARS-CoV-2, there wasn't accurate information available immediately as to which site would yield the most reliable testing results. Though many pathogens will be detectable in multiple sample types, some are more elusive: SARS-CoV-2 can be detected in faeces but not in urine, for example. As we'll discuss later in the section on Test Timing in Chapter 12, depending on the stage of the disease, the most appropriate sampling site may change. Likewise, as new variants emerge, the optimal sampling site may change.

Self-Collection

Traditionally, samples for testing were collected by a professional from the chosen site with appropriate collection equipment/instruments, before transportation to a laboratory for analysis, interpretation and subsequent communication of the result to the patient. The growing preference for at-home testing is a major influence on the sample collection process, introducing significant additional constraints. The widespread uptake of at-home testing requires that the procedure not be too invasive or error prone. The seemingly competing goals of attaining acceptable accuracy while reducing invasiveness are central to acceptance - from users on the one hand (who want quick and easy sampling) and from public health officials (who want results based on high quality samples) on the other.

Specimens & Sites

When endeavouring to understand what's going on at a sub microscopic level inside the human body, there are multiple collection sites that can yield viable samples for diagnostic testing. Among the most common sample types for testing are:

- Upper Respiratory
- Lower Respiratory
- Saliva
- Blood

Depending on the target, other sampling options can include urine, faeces, cerebrospinal fluid, biopsy tissue, vesicles/other skin lesions and amniotic fluid.

For SARS-CoV-2, researchers quickly compared the performance of tests carried out from a variety of sampling sites and sample types. They also looked at alternative bodily fluids to test for the presence of SARS-CoV-2, including tears, but without immediate success[85]. Initial guidance on diagnosing SARS-CoV-2 focused on lower respiratory samples collected from seriously ill patients in hospitals, but the focus soon moved to less invasive upper respiratory samples, such as various nasal/oral swabs.

Lower Respiratory Specimens

An early systematic review and meta-analysis of studies comparing respiratory sampling strategies for the detection of SARS-CoV-2, published in the Lancet in July 2020[86], concluded that *"Compared to nasopharyngeal swab sampling, sputum testing resulted in significantly higher rates of SARS-CoV-2 RNA detection while oropharyngeal swab testing had lower rates of viral RNA detection".*

The initial COVID-19 pandemic interest in lower respiratory samples was based on the high quality of these samples. However, the methods (sputum, tracheal aspirate and bronchoalveolar lavage - BAL) are quite invasive and uncomfortable for patients and only really indicated during severe cases. They are not feasible to scale to population-level testing.

Upper Respiratory Samples

Since the second half of 2020, the widely preferred sample for most laboratory testing of SARS-CoV-2 has been the Nasopharyngeal (NP) swab, taken by a trained professional that was then transported to a laboratory in a Viral Transport Medium - VTM - for processing in an RT-PCR test. In this section, we'll look at NP and other nasal/oral swabs that together have become the basis of virtually all testing for active SARS-CoV-2 infections.

A nasopharyngeal swab is a device used for collecting a sample of nasal secretions from the back of the nose and throat. This collection method is commonly used in suspected cases of many common ailments including whooping cough, diphtheria, influenza, and various types of diseases caused by coronaviruses, including SARS, MERS, and COVID-19.

Nasopharyngeal swabs are somewhat uncomfortable and are recommended to be carried out by a trained professional. They also pose a transmission risk for the tester that's higher than other methods, due to the likelihood that the insertion of the swab may provoke an exhalation response from the patient. As the pandemic progressed, therefore, researchers explored the viability of other, less invasive collection methods that could still provide a specimen suitable for RT-PCR processing.

Other nasal sites that aren't as deep as those for an NP swab, such as Mid Turbinate (MT) or a simple Anterior Nares (AN) swab are shown below, with more discussion on these options included in Appendix 2.

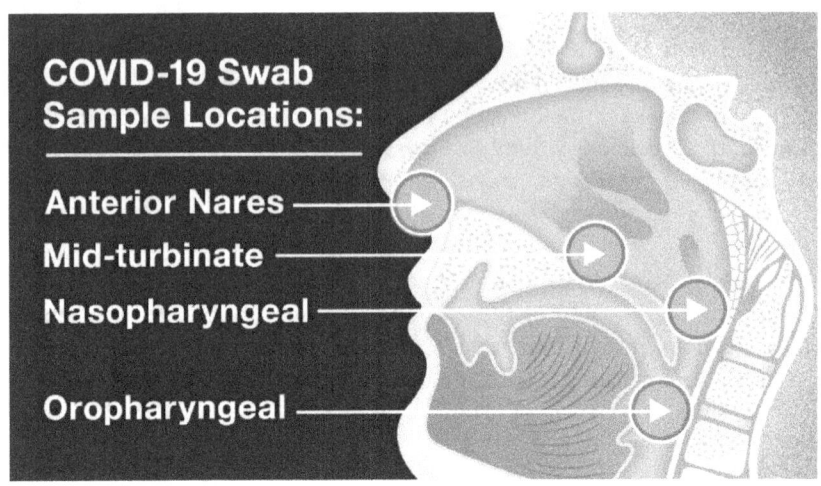

Figure 18: Nasal/Oral sample collection sites

Evolving Thinking

As we'll reference frequently, the COVID-19 pandemic has provided myriad examples of the testing trade-offs, and that's also true for the site choice and sampling type elements. Researchers have carried out detailed comparisons between simple nasal swabs versus deeper nasal options. As the scale of testing grew, so too did the opportunity to analyse differences in collection sites and techniques, providing potentially valuable insights for future testing practices, especially for common respiratory viruses, including influenza and RSV.

Although possibly specific to the behaviour of the SARS-CoV-2 virus, a dividend may be in greater awareness among healthcare workers of variations between sites and improvements in collection techniques. This remains an area in flux - almost all of the studies I've read on variations in sensitivity and specificity among collection sites caution that they are preliminary in nature and warrant further investigation. However, for a variety of upper respiratory infections going forward, even minor improvements in techniques will help reduce the number of false negative tests due to collection errors.

Oral Options

Moving (very slightly) away from the nose as the sampling site, there are also oral options. The options here are primarily swabbing or saliva collection, though some other less common approaches such as gargling are also briefly mentioned. An Oropharyngeal Swab takes an oral route to the pharynx.

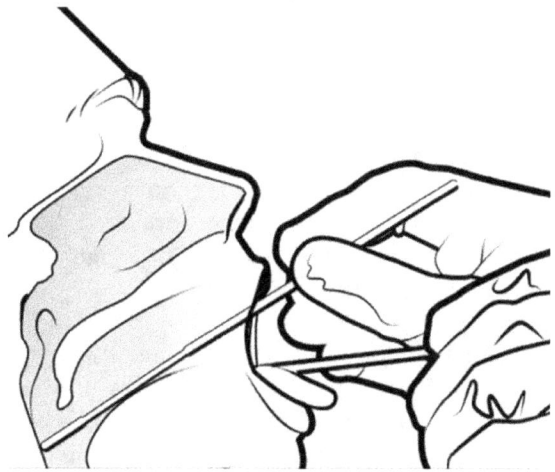
Figure 19: An Oropharyngeal swab. Source: CDC Image

Saliva

Compared to any form of nasal or oral swabbing, however minimally invasive, saliva can appear to be an attractive type of sample. Already widely deployed as a source of DNA for genetic/ancestry tests such as 23andMe, it involves no discomfort and doesn't require specialist swab availability. The sample quantity is also extremely easy to measure, while the quantity of material collected on a swab is difficult to assess. The key question regarding saliva is whether or not the analyte required is present in sufficient quantities and at a useful time in the course of the disease. The utility of saliva as a specimen varies across disease types and the presence of various enzymes and inhibitors in saliva can interfere with some testing processes.

It's also worth noting that saliva specimens, like nasal specimens, may be analysed using a variety of assay types and technologies that we'll discuss in later chapters. However, from a regulatory standpoint, most tests are approved for use with a specific specimen type - so while a test may be operating under EUA to analyse nasal swabs for the presence of SARS-CoV-2, the same assay may not be approved for use with saliva samples and it can't be assumed that the test will perform as expected on such samples.

A systematic review and meta-analysis[87] comparing saliva samples against NP swabs found sensitivity of 83.2% for saliva and 84.8% for NP, suggesting saliva could be an attractive alternative given the ease of collection and relative patient comfort.

In an interesting example of pandemic-related innovation,[88] researchers at the University of Illinois at Urbana-Champaign created a saliva-based test that received EUA from the FDA. The university scaled up the project to complete 15,000 tests per day in order to safely facilitate on-campus teaching.

Researchers are also assessing if high virus levels in saliva can be a significant indicator of the potential to develop a serious case of COVID-19[89]. Researchers at Yale found that patients who developed severe disease, were hospitalised, or died were more likely to have had high virus loads in their saliva tests, but not in their NP swabs.

There is a considerable amount of research into saliva testing for other diseases too, due to its unrivalled ease of collection. For example, a meta-analysis comparing the performance of saliva samples vs blood samples for HIV testing identified a sensitivity only about 2% lower in oral than in blood-based specimens[90].

Other Mouth Samples

Alongside investigations of saliva for covid-19 testing, researchers have also been considering additional options. In a study[91] comparing NP swabs with mouthwash samples and buccal (cheek) swabs, while 91.7% of NP tested positive, 63.1% of the mouthwash samples were positive, and just 42.4% of the buccal swabs. In a more promising study, a Canadian sample of nearly 1300 people found NP sensitivity of 97.9% and 89.6% for Spring Water Gargle (SWG)[92].

Combined Sites

Now that we've discussed the oral sampling options as well as nasal sites, it's time to revisit the topic of comparison - by comparing the combined sample from one non-invasive nasal and one oral source to the reference standard of NPs. A meta-analysis published in The Lancet in April 2021[93] found that Pooled AN and OP swabs performed extremely well.

Site	Sensitivity (Vs NP)
Nasal (AN)	86%
Saliva	85%
Throat swabs (OP)	68%
Pooled (AN) and (OP)	97%

However, the report noted that: *Throat swabs gave a much lower sensitivity and positive predictive value and should not be recommended.* Self-collection for pooled nasal and throat swabs and nasal swabs was not associated with any significant impairment of diagnostic accuracy. For all the three methods, self-collection of these clinical specimens did not associate with any significant impairment of diagnostic accuracy.

Similarly, a Canadian research project[94] found that a combined oropharyngeal/nares swab is a suitable alternative to NP swabs for the detection of SARS-CoV-2, with sensitivities of 91.7% and 94.4%, respectively. In a study of the usefulness of saliva swab specimens for the diagnosis of influenza compared with NP specimens[95], the agreement between saliva and NP swabs results was 97.6%, though viral loads in the NPs were higher.

Development Focus

Efforts to commercialise accurate tests based on various sampling approaches are gaining traction. As reported by the New England Journal of Medicine, applications to RADx-tech and RADx-ATP include multiple alternative sampling strategies for viral testing, not just traditional nasal swabs[96].

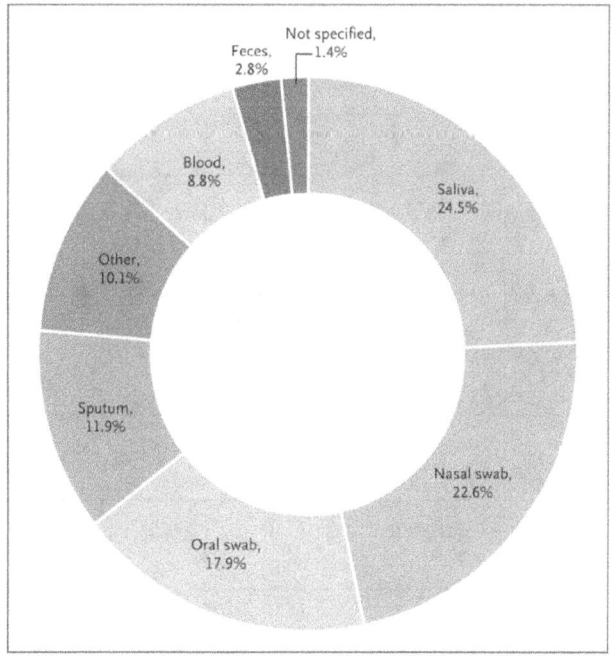

Figure 20: Breakdown of Sample Types submitted to RADx program

Summarising the sample types gives a table like this:

Specimen Type	Collection Method	Collected By
Upper Respiratory Samples		
Nasopharyngeal (NP) swab	A long swab inserted via the nose	Healthcare Professional (HCP)
Oropharyngeal (OP) swab	A long swab to the back of the throat	HCP
Nasal Mid-turbinate (NMT) swab	A short swab about 4cm into the nose	HCP or self-collected
Anterior Nares (AN) nasal swab	A short swab into the nostril	HCP or self-collected
Lower Respiratory Samples		
NP Aspirate	A saline solution passed through a tube inserted into the nose to the nasopharynx	HCP
Sputum	Patient coughs up deep sputum	HCP
Tracheal Aspirate	A saline solution via a catheter inserted into the mouth to the trachea	HCP
Bronchoalveolar Lavage (BAL)	A bronchoscope via the mouth into the lungs with saline solution	HCP
Blood Samples		
Whole Blood/Serum/Plasma	Venous blood draw	HCP
Capillary Blood	Fingerprick	Self-Collected

Self Collection vs Professional Collection

An area of debate and research in specimen collection is the impact, if any, of who collects the sample. Specifically, are self-collected samples comparable to those collected by trained HCPs? Given the importance of collecting a high-quality specimen for testing, it has been most often carried out by a trained health care professional. Consumer-collected samples are frequently considered less reliable (though not necessarily significantly inferior) than professionally administered sampling. But in changes that will likely define the future of much diagnostic testing, COVID-19 has led to increased levels of research into the viability of consumer collection as consumers turn to frequent, rapid/at home tests rather than attending professionally staffed facilities.

A team of German researchers found that self-collected nasal MT samples and professionally collected NP swabs yielded, in cases of high viral load[97], identical results. The self-collectors were observed, without intervention, having been given written and illustrated instructions to follow. Sampling technique errors that were noted included incorrect depth (too deep or too superficial), incorrect duration or intensity of swabbing and failure to swab both nostrils. However, 85% of participants indicated that they found self-swabbing easy to perform. Results of nasal sampling could potentially be further improved, if flocked swabs were used - more on that in the next section.

	MT (Self)	NP (Professional)
Sensitivity	84.4	88.9
Sensitivity (with high viral loads)	96.3	96.3
Specificity	99.2	99.2

In another study[98] comparing self-collection vs professional collection for COVID-19 some variations were found, with the sensitivities of self-collected OP/MT swab and saliva samples proving inferior to a HCP swab, but they could still be useful testing tools in the appropriate clinical settings:

Sample	Sensitivity
HCP Collected Swab	82.8%
Self-collected MT swab	75.1%
Self-collected Saliva	74.3%
Self-collected combined saliva and swab	86.5%

So, despite concerns about self-collection, when done with a reasonable level of instruction, the results don't diverge drastically from professionally collected MT samples. A 2011 study[99] comparing HCP-collected MT samples for influenza testing with self-collected swabs yielded 94.8% concordance, while a 2013 comparison[100] testing for group A streptococcus also yielded 94% agreement.

A Danish group of otolaryngologists (ear, nose and throat surgeons - ENT) has created a simulator and assessment to help further improve HCP techniques[101] for NP swabbing and I would expect to see additional training becoming common to maximise professional NP performance where it's used.

Instructions

Instruction in the proper technique for sample collection is vital. Nowadays, in locations where self-tests are widely available, it is generally assumed that most consumers have access to video guidance, which is a big improvement over written or illustrated instructions, previously the default instructional media for consumer medicine. Many of the self-tests I've tried come with extremely clear video-based instructions in an app.

In October 2020, the US FDA issued an advisory letter[102] to healthcare providers to ensure that clear instructions are given to patients self-collecting nasal samples, citing a concern that, in the absence of proper instructions, patients may not collect an adequate sample for testing, which may decrease the sensitivity of the test. The FDA recommended health care providers include visual (written or video) step-by-step instructions to patients self-collecting anterior nares (nasal) samples for SARS-CoV-2 testing. Concern over consumers' ability to complete the sampling procedure competently was a significant factor when considering regulatory approval for self-tests not requiring a prescription:

"Anterior nares [AN] specimens have numerous benefits as compared to other upper respiratory specimens such as nasopharyngeal [NP] specimens. They are less invasive and generally more comfortable for patients, they can be self-collected by adult patients, and they can decrease the risk of exposure to health care providers. There is scientific evidence that SARS-CoV-2 testing utilizing anterior nares specimens has a similar performance to testing that utilizes nasopharyngeal specimens, provided that a good quality anterior nares specimen is collected. Without clear instructions, however, patients who, in a health care setting, are self-collecting anterior nares (nasal) samples may not collect an adequate sample for testing, which may decrease the sensitivity of the test. Health care providers have a critical role in helping patients perform self-collection accurately".

The FDA recommends that instructions provided to patients should incorporate the following information:

"The entire tip of the swab (usually ½ to ¾ of an inch) should be placed inside the nose, and the side of the swab tip should be rubbed with moderate pressure against as much of the wall of the anterior nares region as possible, moving the tip through a large circular path inside the nose. At least four of these sweeping circles should be performed in each nostril using the same swab. This should take approximately 10-15 seconds per nostril. Simply twirling the swab against one part of the inside of the nose or leaving the swab in the nose for 10-15 seconds, is not proper technique and may result in an insufficient sample."

The further development of self-tests requires not only the ability of testers to secure a valid sample via instruction, but also to correctly *interpret* the test results - the end-to-end experience and integrity of self-testing is a critical concern as it expands as a diagnostic sector.

In an encouraging study[103], 94.4% of participants correctly understood the instructions for use, with 96.2% demonstrating the ability to correctly interpret test results. However, a note of caution is that about 15% needed verbal help to perform or interpret the test. It is vital that test manufacturers and regulators act to improve test design and instruction at every opportunity.

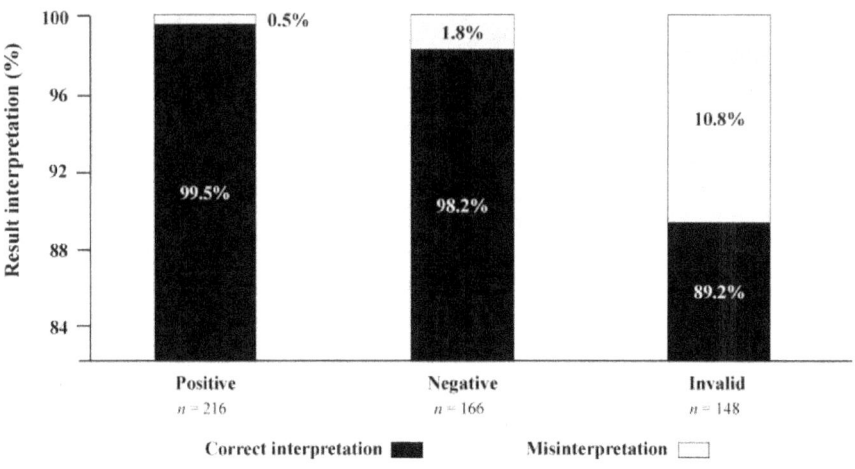

Figure 21: Public Understanding of Test Indications

One solution adopted to improve the quality of self-tests is the provision of live video-based proctoring, where a trained HCP watches the consumer taking the test and advises them of the need for any changes to their technique. This approach has been of particular interest where the result of the test is to be used for official purposes, such as travel, and thus requires increased integrity where the result is taken as proof required to comply with Public Health restrictions[104].

In an extreme example of a potential future direction of sample collection, a group of Korean researchers[105] has created a prototype of a robotic collection system to minimise exposure of healthcare professionals during sample collection.

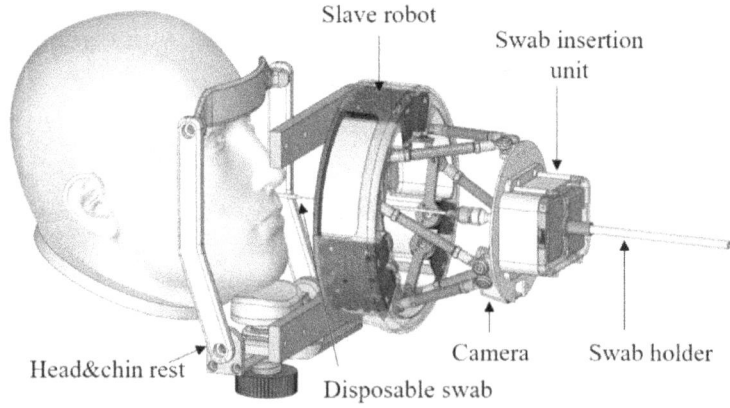

Figure 22: An automated swabbing machine to protect HCP from exposure during sample collection

Tears

In this discussion of sampling/sites, one bodily fluid mentioned briefly above was tears. A tears sample is usually relatively easily available so, if it is found to contain reliable biomarkers, it would be an attractive test option. Although not yet ready for commercial use, researchers[106] have shown promising progress in using tears to test for multiple conditions. Tears contain a variety of proteins and RNA from around the body, though in tiny amounts that make testing challenging. However, tears also tend to be less "contaminated" than samples such as nasal or saliva.

Location and Time to Result (TTR)

Having talked about which sample is to be collected and from where, the next major trade-offs to be discussed now are *where* the sample is to be tested and the *time* to a result (TTR). A crucial theme in all diagnostics is the time it takes to get the result so that appropriate action can be taken. The closer to the patient that the test takes place, the shorter the time to a result will be - tests that can be carried out at home typically give results in 30 minutes or less, while even laboratory tests that return results in less than an hour incur additional transport time getting the sample to the lab. And in cases where laboratories are busy or batch run tests to a schedule, delays can mount up.

Although an unusual event which placed exceptional pressure on testing capacity (especially early in the pandemic before alternatives were in place) the COVID-19 pandemic at times highlighted the challenge of scaling to population-level testing while still maintaining rapid results. A 2020 review of testing TTR in the US[107] showed a national average of 4 days, with only 37% of results returned within 2 days. Although a 2-day turnaround is perfectly reasonable for some diseases, when dealing with an infectious respiratory disease, faster results are of immense benefit for managing public health. And in cases where starting an antiviral treatment early provides better outcomes, TTR can alter the outcome significantly.

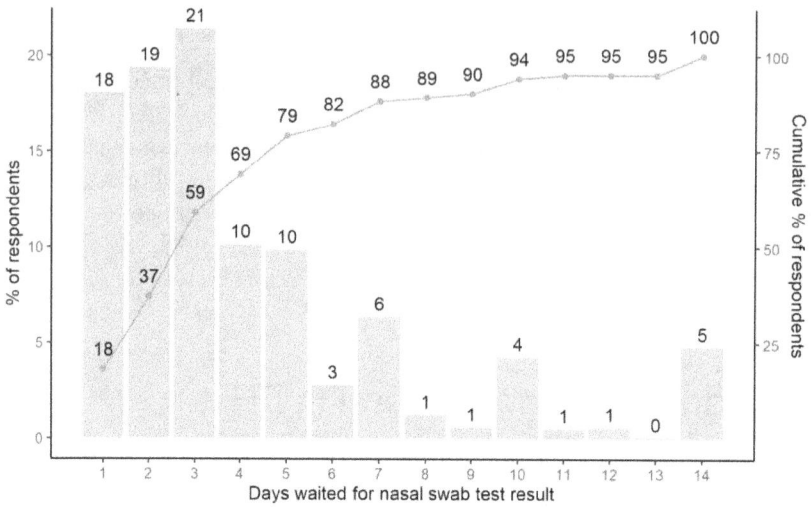

We find that the mean waiting time nationally was 4.1 days, and median waiting time 3 days. Only 37% of people received test results within 2 days, and 21% waited more than 5 days.

Figure 23: TTR study in the US in 2020

The key determinant in TTR has long been where the analysis of the sample has been carried out. This has been determined by the technology available at the various potential sites, as well as the challenges of collection that we've discussed. The collection of certain specimens to the desired standard may require special equipment and/or trained personnel. A blood draw is difficult to self-administer, as is an NP swab, whereas saliva or pin prick tests are readily self-administered. However, regardless of where the sample collection was carried out, the means to conduct tests, at least to reliable level, historically was firmly laboratory centric. Many companies started offering direct to consumer (DTC) tests with at-home collection, but samples were then sent to a laboratory for processing. While at-home collection could speed things up by removing the need to attend a location to have a sample taken, the transport delays ruled out instant results. Even the few home tests that did exist (e.g., Pregnancy) were usually confirmed with additional tests.

The last few decades have seen the emergence of a steady stream of Point of Care (POC) Tests; devices that offer laboratory-style tests in a clinic or doctor's office setting. These devices typically cost thousands of dollars but can carry out multiple tests. Though offering very limited throughput compared to laboratory-scale instruments (1-2 tests per hour vs hundreds or even thousands per hour), they are typically easy to use with minimal training and economically viable in affluent practices. We'll explore some of these in more detail in the upcoming Chapters but the key point for now is that, with the test taking place within the same appointment time/location as the sample collection, patients and their HCPs receive the result in minutes, not days.

Swabs

As with the collection site chosen, the actual instrument used to retrieve the specimen is important in determining the quantity and quality of the sample collected. In the illustration below, you can see the relative size of swabs for sample collecting, depending on the nasal site. The different types of tests, for which these swabs are intended, are covered in detail in Chapters 6 and 7.

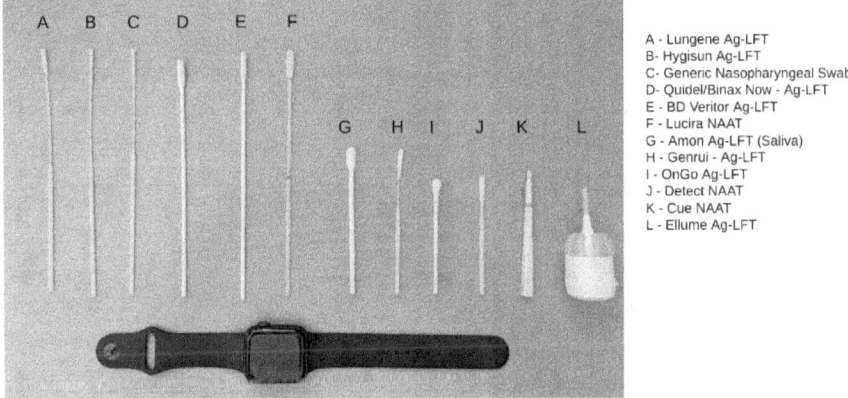

Figure 24: The variety of swabs supplied with consumer test kits (Apple Watch for Scale)

Visible liquid samples are relatively easy to manage - you can see if you've collected sufficient saliva or blood samples more easily than nasal secretions. In order to capture viable specimens from the nasal passage, the type of swab is particularly significant. There are multiple types available, made from varying materials intended to maximise both the contact with the target surface and the collection of the desired biological material while also facilitating the ability to release the material for analysis - swabs that collect material efficiently but then don't release the sample sufficiently for testing are not helpful.

Swab Composition

Most intranasal swabs use a "flocked" design with synthetic fibres such as nylon or rayon on a plastic shaft. It is important to use specifically designed swabs for collecting viral testing samples - wooden shafts can interfere with testing, and calcium alginate, a substance typically used for swab tips intended for use in wound care, can kill viruses.

A clear dividend of the pandemic will be a wider understanding of sample sites and collection techniques, as current inconsistencies in procedures are exposed. NP swabs are likely to remain prominent in HCP settings, where the additional accuracy is desired, the increased discomfort is tolerable, and a trained administrator with the appropriate equipment is available. What will change, though, is the ability to make informed decisions about the suitability of other testing methods, rather than defaulting to NP swabs in the belief that other methods are significantly or unacceptably inferior.

Breath Tests

Airborne or droplet transmission is, of course, a crucial means of spread for viruses, especially respiratory ones. So, it stands to reason that being able to analyse our breath may offer diagnostic promise. After all, breathalysers to look for the presence of alcohol have been in widespread use for decades. Consumer Devices such as Lumen and Marble are marketed as being able to analyse breath samples for metabolism purposes.

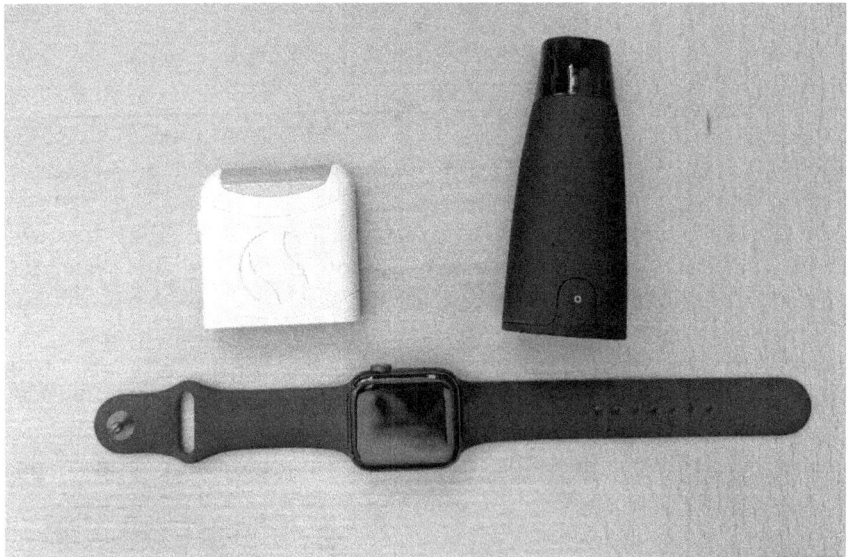

Figure 25: FoodMarble Aire Digestive tester[108] and Lumen Metabolic Analyser[109], (Apple Watch for Scale)

In future, will we all be breathing into a small device that can diagnose maladies? Perhaps not in the near term, but the possibility has taken a few steps closer to reality in the last two years. In April 2022, the US FDA granted its first EUA for a diagnostic test for SARS-CoV-2 that uses a breath sample instead of a nasal, oral or lower respiratory sample[110]. The suitcase-sized InspectIR COVID-19 Breathalyzer can provide results in just 3 minutes, using a technology known as gas chromatography mass-spectrometry (GC-MS), to identify volatile organic compounds (VOCs - not to be confused with Variants of Concern) associated with SARS-CoV-2 infection in exhaled breath. The FDA noted sensitivity of 91.2% and specificity of 99.3%. Although US approval for a breath testing device came late in pandemic, other countries have followed this route earlier - the Dutch Government, for example, used a device called the SpiroNose in early 2021[111].

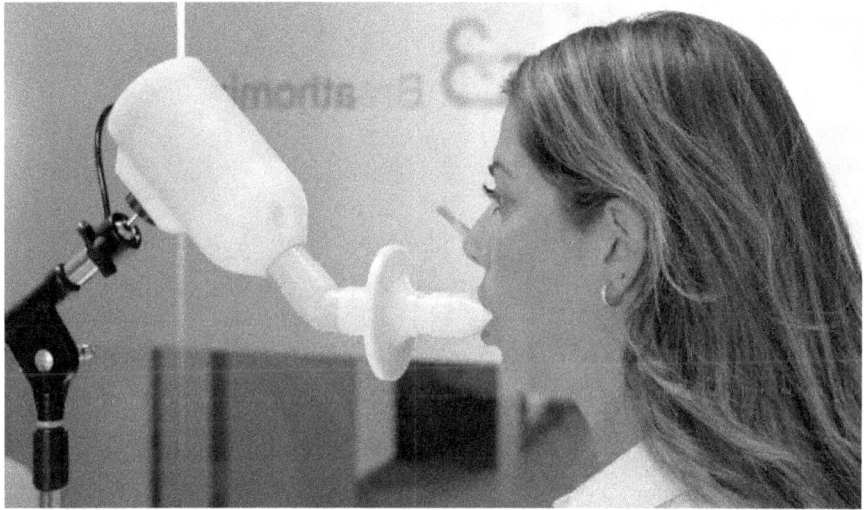

Figure 26: SpiroNose device

In Europe also, a Welsh firm, Imspex Diagnostics, has received the CE mark for its breath-based COVID-19 test, which is based on a combination of gas chromatography and ion mobility spectrometry in a POC-suitable device.

Scent Dogs for Covid

Not all diagnostic approaches to detecting SARS-CoV-2 rely on chemical or electronic sensors. Amongst the most effective detectors identified to date are canines! Of course, dogs are well known for their narcotics and explosive detection abilities, but a report shows that they can be trained to accurately identify the presence of SARS-CoV-2 in both symptomatic and asymptomatic individuals - overall, the dogs detected SARS-CoV-2 with 97 percent sensitivity and a specificity of 91 percent. For asymptomatic individuals, the dogs had a sensitivity of 100 percent and specificity of 94 percent[112].

Next, we move on to discuss how the sample is tested when it reaches the laboratory. As noted in Chapter 4, there are multiple types of test technologies available and we'll review these in the following three Chapters.

Chapter 6: Nucleic Acid Amplification Tests (NAAT)

Laboratory-based *Nucleic Acid Amplification Tests* (NAAT) are among the most powerful diagnostic tools ever developed. They operate by rapidly (typically in a matter of a couple of hours) amplifying genetic target material in a sample until it can be detected reliably. This allows for the identification of quantities of a pathogen that are too small to detect via other means or where alternative methods (such as cultures) are too slow to be of clinical benefit. Also referred to as *molecular* tests, this family of technologies has dramatically increased the accuracy, speed and flexibility of viral testing in the last few decades.

The most widely used form of NAAT is a technique known as *Polymerase Chain Reaction* (PCR), which has come to widespread global public attention since 2020 as the preeminent tool used to diagnose SARS-CoV-2 infections. In this section, we'll cover some background on the evolution of PCR and equivalent technologies, as we'll look at important recent developments that promise to broaden access to NAAT technologies, with their excellent accuracy and increasing speed. We'll also look at some of the challenges around NAAT that have emerged during the pandemic and discuss how they can be addressed.

The Emergence of PCR

In the 2 years after the initial identification of SARS-CoV-2, the world saw a vast number of "PCR" tests carried out to track the spread of the virus across the globe. It wasn't a term most people were familiar with, but as a technology, it directly contributed to our ability to quantify infections with a high degree of accuracy.

The result of a PCR test became the world-wide standard for counting cases of COVID-19. But although public awareness of PCR is at an all-time high, I'd be willing to bet that few people know what it stands for, let alone how it works. I think it's useful to try to understand a little bit about how it works in order to better trust in its results, which can have gigantic personal and policy implications.

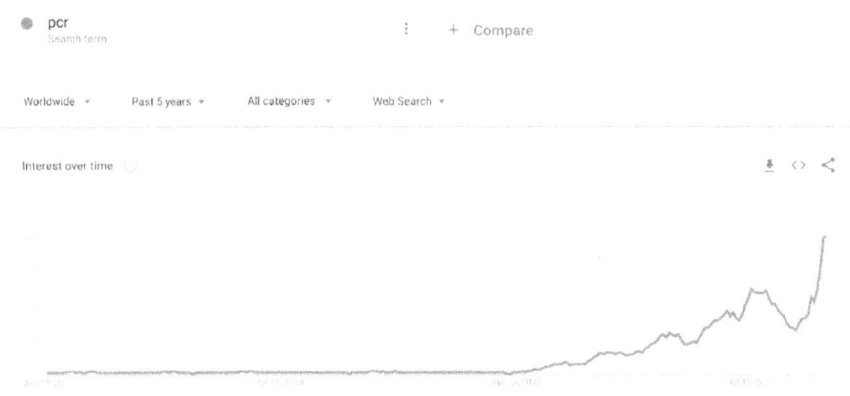

Figure 27: Google Searches for PCR before and during the COVID-19 pandemic

The invention of PCR was a seminal moment in diagnostic technology, revolutionising the speed at which the presence of microbes could be identified. PCR has a broad range of applications, including in research for infectious diseases, cancer, forensic analysis, and agricultural biotechnology. PCR emerged as a breakthrough technology in the mid-1980s following work by an American biochemist, Kary Mullis, who later shared the Nobel Prize in Chemistry in 1993 for his work[113].

Usually performed in a laboratory, PCR is a temperature controlled, enzyme-driven, biochemical process capable of rapidly amplifying a target DNA snippet into millions of copies which can then be detected, or even quantified. It enables a single copy of any gene sequence to be enzymatically amplified at least a million-fold within a few hours; thus, viral DNA extracted from a tiny sample can be amplified to the point where it can be readily identified.

One early application of PCR and its speedy operation was in the detection of mycobacterium tuberculosis (TB). Given the long delay in culture tests (greater than a week and sometimes a month) which rendered public health strategies on patient isolation difficult, the speed of PCR test results offered an opportunity to improve speed of care decisions significantly. PCR's effectiveness in detecting Chlamydia trachomatis has also seen it offer significantly faster results than previous tests, which can aid early treatment decisions. Other viral PCR assays, now routinely available, include those for herpes simplex virus, cytomegalovirus, Epstein-Barr virus, hepatitis viruses, and HIV[114].

Although widely understood as vital in the scientific community, I expect the new more general awareness of PCR and similar technologies will inspire even broader use in the coming years. While PCR is the most common type of NAAT and is the one we'll continue to focus on here, other methods such as Loop-mediated Isothermal Amplification (LAMP) will be mentioned also, due to its promise in creating Point of Care (POC) and even domestic NAAT solutions that offer "PCR-level" accuracy.

We talked, in the previous chapter, about the collection of the specimen to be tested. PCR tests are quite flexible in terms of sample types that can be used. For example, seven specimen types have been validated[115] and approved for use with a common SARS-CoV-2 assay from Thermofisher:

- Bronchoalveolar lavage (BAL)
- Mid-turbinate (MT) swabs
- Nasal (AN) swabs
- Nasopharyngeal (NP) swabs
- Nasopharyngeal aspirate (nasal aspirate)
- Oropharyngeal (OP) swabs
- Saliva collected with the Spectrum Solutions™ SpectrumDNA™ SDN

Before we describe the actual PCR process though, we need to talk about two earlier steps: (1) the design of the PCR assay - i.e., what is it looking for and, (2) in the case of RNA viruses (which includes SARS-CoV-2), the need to convert them before they can be used in PCR, which is a DNA-only test.

PCR Targets (Primers & Probes)

At the heart of PCR technology is the concept of primer - a primer is a fragment of DNA (oligonucleotides) used to detect the presence of a specific target DNA fragment within a sample - the primer is designed to attach to the target DNA, if present. During a PCR test, if the target DNA is present in the sample, the primers copy the targeted region. As they copy these regions, probes stuck to these new fragments release a visual signal which can be read as a positive result. If the target is not present in the sample, there is no signal, which is a negative result.

Designing the primer is critical to the accuracy of any PCR test. In order for PCR to work, the target sequence must be known in advance so that the primers can be designed to allow for the selective amplification of the target. Since the complete genetic sequence of SARS-CoV-2 (or novel coronavirus as it was known at the time) was shared to the Global Initiative on Sharing All Influenza Data (GISAID) platform on January 10, 2020, researchers around the world were able to begin designing probes that would become the key agents in PCR tests. In a dividend from the 2003 SARS outbreak, scientists were much better prepared to create assays for the new pathogen and had tests ready by February 2020, while it had taken 6 months in 2003.

The "RT" Part

As discussed in Chapter 2 about viruses, they come in two types: DNA and RNA. The PCR process is designed to work on DNA, so in order to work with RNA viruses, samples must first be converted to DNA. This conversion process is known as *Reverse Transcription* (RT) and is enabled by an enzyme called *Reverse Transcriptase* (not to be confused with the enzyme *Polymerase*, which accounts for the 'P' in PCR and is the key enzyme to copy DNA). So, for RNA targets (like SARS-CoV-2), the type of test used is described more properly as an RT-PCR rather than just PCR. For DNA viruses, the RT phase isn't required.

On a further potentially confusing technicality, an evolution of PCR technology is often referred to as Real Time PCR. This advance offers quantitative readings of an analyte while the test is still running, rather than having to wait until the PCR process is completely finished. This is commonly abbreviated to qPCR (for quantitative PCR) so the abbreviation *RT-qPCR* refers to Reverse Transcriptase Real Time PCR, which we'll discuss below in more detail, after first looking at the basic PCR process.

The PCR Process

Without going into too much technical detail about how PCR works, (the Mayo Clinic offers a good explanation[116] if you want to go deeper than here), the high-level process involves 3 key steps in a series of 'cycles':

1. *denaturation*, in which double-stranded DNA templates are heated to separate the strands;
2. *annealing*, in which short DNA molecules called primers bind to flanking regions of the target DNA;
3. *extension*, in which DNA polymerase extends the 3' end of each primer along the template strands.

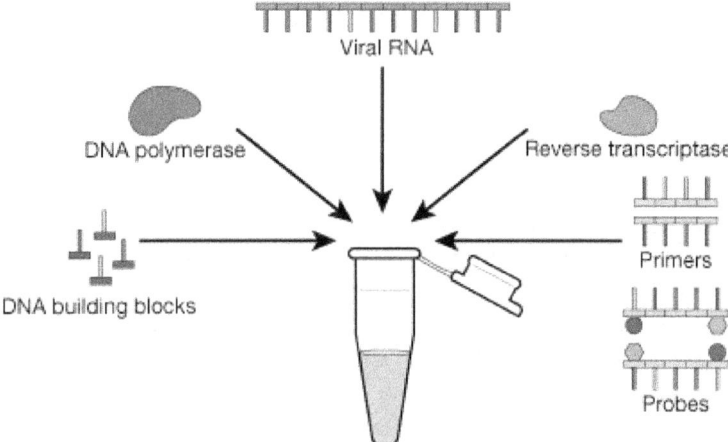

Figure 28: The Ingredients for an RT-PCR Test for an RNA Virus. Source: Mayo Clinic

These steps are repeated ("cycled") 25–40 times to exponentially produce exact copies of the target DNA. One of the reasons that PCR tests are typically laboratory based is the need for complex machines that can rapidly and accurately cycle samples which might be something like: 45°C for 15 min, 95°C for 10 min followed by 40 cycles of 95°C for 15 seconds and 60°C for 30 seconds. This means that a PCR test run time is rarely less than an hour, and more commonly 2-4 hours for a complete process from sample arrival to result.

The following figure shows the output from a PCR test to detect Malaria; the samples with higher concentrates require less cycles (see x axis) to show as positive:

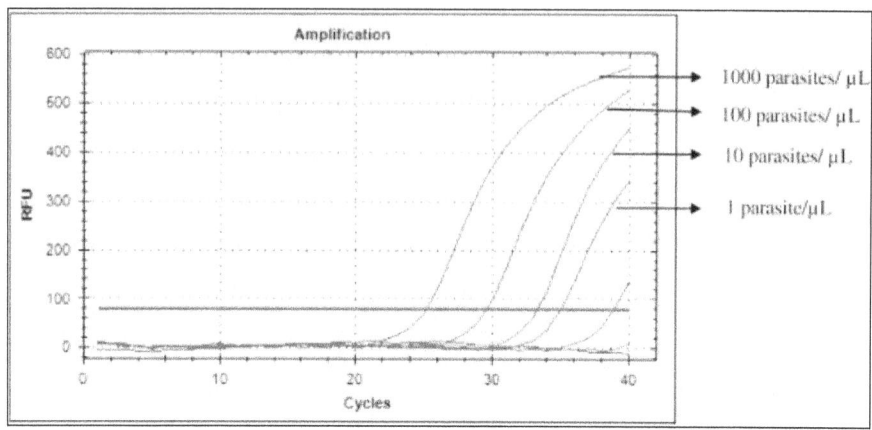

Figure 29: What a PCR Test result looks like. Source[117]:

The Real Time "Q" part

The original PCR process delivered a positive or negative result at the end of the test (now known as *Endpoint PCR*). In the further significant development of PCR technology known as Real Time Quantitative PCR or qPCR as mentioned above, scientists have developed the ability to determine a quantitative measurement while the test is still in progress. By adding a fluorescent source to the test, the increase in fluorescent output in each cycle can be measured. This quantitative data can be used to measure viral/pathogenic load either to inform treatment or to track relative changes in samples taken over time.

Some of the more technical aspects of PCR such as qPCR and the number of cycles in the test (*Cycle Threshold* - CT) may be more complex than most people will want to grasp but they are important in terms of measuring not just the presence of a target pathogen, but also quantifying it. This may be a clue to virulence, infectiousness and also help gauge whether treatments are working by showing a decrease in the quantity of virus present in a patient over time. qPCR can quickly get quite complex so here I'll just focus on the importance of being able to consider a quantitative result, rather than just a binary positive/negative. I'll include a link to a more detailed explanation of qPCR for anyone curious to dig deeper[118].

PCR CT value

Although PCR tests are widely regarded as the gold standard in detecting the presence of SARS-CoV-2, their use is not without controversy. While they are accepted as being extremely reliable, the main concern lies around their being *too* sensitive - thanks to the amplification, a PCR test may indicate a positive result even when levels of the virus were too low to be infectious.

Experts differ about what the "appropriate" number of cycles (CT) a PCR test should run - the lower the number required to detect the virus means the higher the viral load. So, if a PCR test only returns a positive after a large number of cycles, the quantity of virus present is relatively low. While different assays make direct comparisons between CT levels difficult, given the consequences of a PCR test, where a positive may lead to restrictions, standardisation may be required. This would prevent situations where different laboratories might classify a test that required 40 cycles as positive, the same as they would a test that showed positive after just 20 cycles, or that another lab which considered 35 as a cut-off for positivity would have labelled as negative.

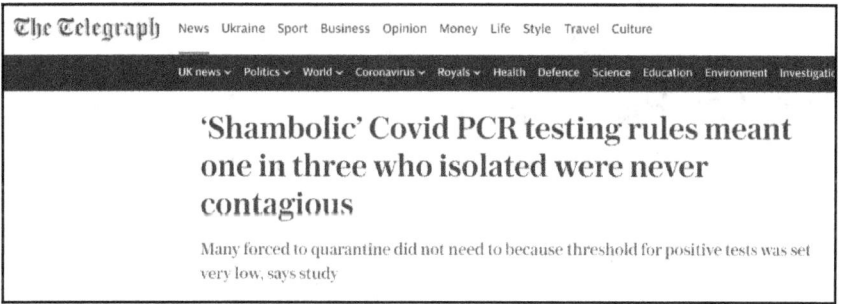

Figure 30: A Feb. 2022 headline reporting on concerns about PCR cycle thresholds[119]

RT-PCR Assays for SARS-CoV-2

Although it's common to refer to "a PCR test for COVID-19" as if it were a defined single entity, there are in fact hundreds of different RT-PCR assays for SARS-CoV-2 in use around the world. Neighbouring labs may run different PCR tests; different assays (primers) amplify and detect different regions of the SARS-CoV-2 genome. Different manufacturers have chosen different parts of the SARS-CoV-2 virus to search for as their targets. Some target one, two or more genes, including the nucleocapsid (N), envelope (E), and spike (S) genes, and regions in the first open reading frame (ORF1).

Searching for more than one target complicates the assay but reduces the possibility of a false negative test in the event that the target gene ends up being one that mutates and is no longer detectable - the odds of 3 target genes all mutating, before a test can be updated, are much lower.

The charts below show a summary of different PCR assays, reporting how many targets a test had (left) and which parts of the SARS-CoV-2 gene are targeted by the primers (right).

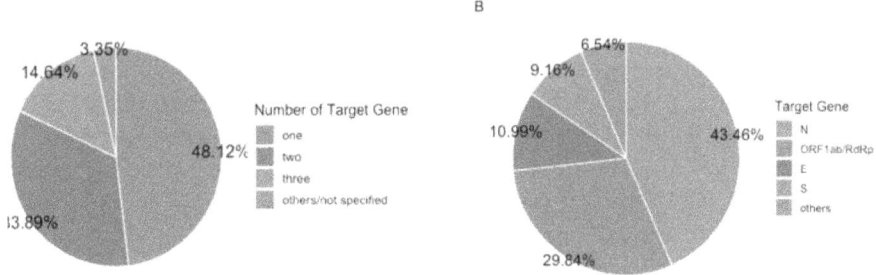

Figure 31: A study of EUA-approved SARS-CoV-2 assays[120]

Extending PCR Testing

The ability of PCR to work with a wide range of specimens and to amplify/detect DNA from bacteria and other microbes makes this kind of molecular diagnostic tool pivotal across a range of applications. And the additional PCR testing capacity, created to support population-level testing for SARS-CoV-2, may in the future provide affordable diagnostic capacity that was previously lacking. Below are some examples of how these advantages might benefit healthcare generally.

While PCR tests have come to prominence because of SARS-CoV-2, a respiratory disease, the ability to quickly and accurately identify the causative agent in non-respiratory diseases also offers significant health benefits. For example, although respiratory tract infections are the most common infectious diseases in the world, the second most prevalent category is gastrointestinal or enteric infections. Viral pathogens such as Norovirus, Astrovirus, Adenovirus and Rotavirus and bacterial causes such as Campylobacter, Salmonella, Clostridioides difficile among others, contribute to diarrheal deaths - the 2nd leading cause of death in under 5s worldwide - and to over $6 billion in hospitalisation costs annually in the US[121].

Increased PCR capacity may also contribute to efforts against HIV and Tuberculosis (TB). For example, PCR can be used to screen blood donations far more efficiently than the previous HIV tests that relied on antibody detection, while PCR testing is far faster than cultures for TB. It also allows for genetic analysis to determine antibiotic resistance, leading to more effective treatment decisions.

Multiplex Targets

During a pandemic, the population prevalence levels can make the presence of a certain pathogen more likely. However, there are many times when the HCP ordering a test is relatively unsure of what they are looking for, out of a range of possible causes. In cases where a respiratory infection is indicated but the etiological (causative) agent is unknown, a test that can identify the presence of any one of a number of potential pathogens is desirable. So, if a patient presents, a test that rules out SARS-CoV-2 may be somewhat useful; one that rules out SARS-CoV-2 but positively identifies Influenza is even better.

PCR assays can be designed to attempt to amplify multiple DNA targets in a single test - known as a multiplex assay. For example, in July 2020, the FDA granted an EUA for a CDC-designed multiplex assay to detect SARS-CoV-2 and two strains of Influenza[122] in a single test. The CDC Flu SC2 Multiplex Assay is a four-in-one assay that includes Primers and probes targeting SARS-CoV-2 and influenza viruses:

- Virus nucleocapsid (N) - gene for specific detection of SARS-CoV-2
- Matrix (M1) - gene for specific detection of influenza A virus
- Nonstructural 2 (NS2) - gene for specific detection of influenza B
- RNase P gene (RP) - serves as an internal control

Similarly, ThermoFisher[123] and Genesystem[124] offer a multiplex assay that adds respiratory syncytial virus (RSV) alongside SARS-CoV-2 and Influenza detection. A November 2021 report from researchers detailed a multiplex assay capable of detecting 14 different respiratory viruses (influenza A (3 strains) and B, parainfluenza 1–4 (PIV1-4), human metapneumovirus, adenovirus, human rhinovirus, RSV, and SARS-CoV-2) on a single PCR test in 45 minutes on a Genesystem POC PCR device[125].

Among the less visible, but still important, potential benefits of increased PCR awareness and capacity may be the opportunity to more quickly identify specific bacterial or viral strains that demonstrate antimicrobial resistance. Incumbent methodologies generally take 48-72 hours, which is usually too late to determine an initial treatment course, whereas PCR has shown great promise in a wide range of challenging areas[126]:

- methicillin-resistant Staphylococcus aureus (MRSA)
- vancomycin-resistant enterococci
- multidrug-resistant M. tuberculosis
- acyclovir-resistant herpesviruses

PCR Accuracy

Though seen as the gold-standard in testing, PCR is not infallible. Along with the concerns already mentioned about how the sample collection and transport can impact accuracy, there will be additional instances where a PCR test will return an unhelpful result:

Result Type	Potential Causes
False Positive	Contamination Poor Primer design Remnant RNA from prior infection
False Negative	Poor specimen collection RNA load below the limit of detection (esp. early in course of infection) Mutation evades primer target (see Variants Chapter for more)

Further discussion of inaccurate results is beyond the scope of this Chapter but this report[127] and its references provide a good starting point for anyone keen on further investigation.

PCR Costs

While the antigen tests we'll describe in the next chapter are relatively easy to cost, it's challenging to put an exact price on a PCR test. As they are typically run in laboratories, samples can be run in batches to spread costs of labour and overheads. In terms of the instruments required, there is a huge variety of machines available, with the key factors being number of sample wells, the level of automation and the speed of cycles. Some can only run a couple of samples at a time, but a typical machine is more likely to have around 96 or 384 wells. Cost ranges from a very basic small laboratory machine at $3k to a fully automated high capacity (over 1500 wells) qPCR machine around $100k[128].

Added to the fixed costs of the machinery and staff to operate them, the ingredients required (primers, probes and DNA nucleotides) typically cost about $10 per well.

NAAT Beyond PCR

Although PCR is the primary type of NAAT in use, there are a number of additional amplification methods that address some of the challenges of PCR, particularly focused on efforts to move PCR outside the lab by simplifying the process without sacrificing accuracy.

Despite the dramatic advances in time to result offered by PCR over older methods such as cultures, the runtime of a typical PCR of up to 3 hours remains "long", relative to the rapid tests available using other technologies (such as the Antigen tests we'll discuss in the next Chapter). While 3 hours may not be long in a laboratory, it is impractical in many POC settings, where an HCP ideally needs the result within the timeframe of the patient visit to a clinic or facility, as return visits may be impractical for patients due to work or other factors.

As mentioned, a key characteristic of PCR is the heating/cooling cycles. This process is extremely effective at amplifying DNA but leads to large/complex/expensive machines with significant power requirements and delays introduced by the need to heat/cool repeatedly. Achieving amplification at a constant temperature, without repeated temperature cycles, is known as *Isothermal* Nucleic Acid Amplification and has been an area of rapid development in recent years, accelerated by the diagnostic demands of SARS-CoV-2.

Isothermal Amplification Technologies

Multiple isothermal amplification technologies are either already available or being developed. These tests run at a constant temperature and this removal of the traditional need for heat/cool cycling is a key factor in the promise of tests that offer PCR-level accuracy outside laboratory environments. In this section, we'll briefly describe the leading emerging isothermal technology, Loop-mediated isothermal amplification (LAMP). Among the other technologies under development in this area are:

- Nicking endonuclease amplification reaction (NEAR)
- Strand displacement amplification (SDA)
- Transcription mediated amplification (TMA)
- Helicase-dependent amplification (HDA)

- Nucleic acid sequence-based amplification (NASBA)
- Recombinase Polymerase Amplification (RPA)
- Multiple Cross Displacement Amplification (MCDA)

For a detailed but accessible overview of these and other emerging isothermal amplification technologies, refer to this review[129], while a more technical explanation of these methods is available here[130].

LAMP

As shown in the graph below, scientific interest in LAMP has grown rapidly in the last two decades as the search for an isothermal alternative to PCR accelerated. LAMP devices operate at a static temperature of 60-65°C and use multiple primers that enable faster amplification of DNA than PCR. LAMP runtime is usually about half that of PCR, with many tests offering results in 30-40 minutes. For a detailed technical explanation of the operation of LAMP, refer to this article[131].

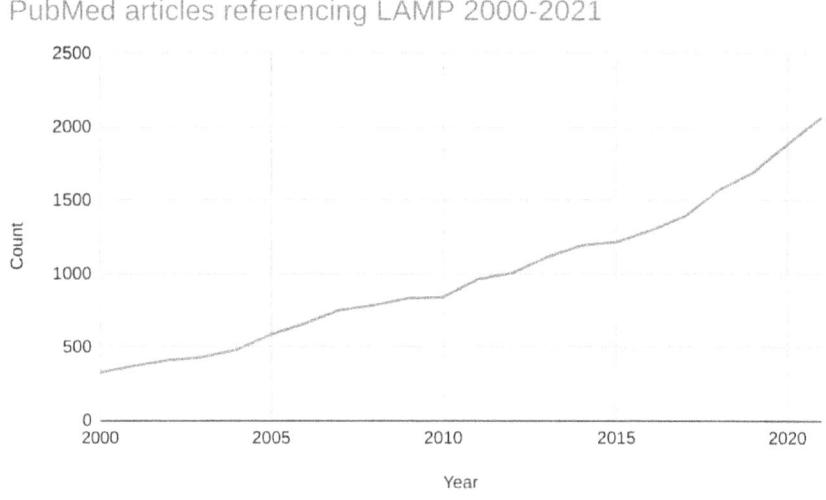

Figure 32: Growing interest in LAMP

As well as faster run times than PCR, the other key promise of the technology is the creation of smaller, simpler, cheaper machines enabling far wider access to laboratory-quality diagnostic results. We'll return to this exciting development in Chapter 9.

According to a 2021 study[132], there were already nine FDA-EUA approved diagnostic devices utilizing RT-LAMP techniques. These devices have a significantly reduced runtime of ~38 min on average, while maintaining a high specificity, with the minimum being 91.7% and a sensitivity of 98% in clinical evaluations.

Next Steps for NAAT

Molecular testing techniques will remain at the forefront of global viral diagnostics for the foreseeable future, thanks to their accuracy, capacity, speed and potential for further development and miniaturisation. As we'll see in Chapter 9, these technologies are rapidly bringing laboratory-quality results closer to patients, while advances in laboratory-based tests continue to expand the utility of PCR and related technologies.

Chapter 7: Antigen Tests (Ag-RDT)

While laboratory-based NAATs (primarily RT-PCR) were the definitive means of detecting SARS-CoV-2 infections, the low cost, self-administered Rapid Antigen Test will be an enduring memory of the COVID-19 pandemic for many people. Unlike the wait for laboratory results, the rapid tests on simple nasal or saliva specimens can tell you in less than 15 minutes if you're COVID-19 positive. The population-level use of these tests represents the largest self-diagnostic exercise in human history.

Unlike PCR tests, the wider public was already somewhat aware of these types of tests (if not by the name Lateral Flow) - since the 1980s, the home pregnancy test has used the same technology that was repurposed for home COVID-19 testing. Official advice to use antigen tests led to unprecedented demand for them.

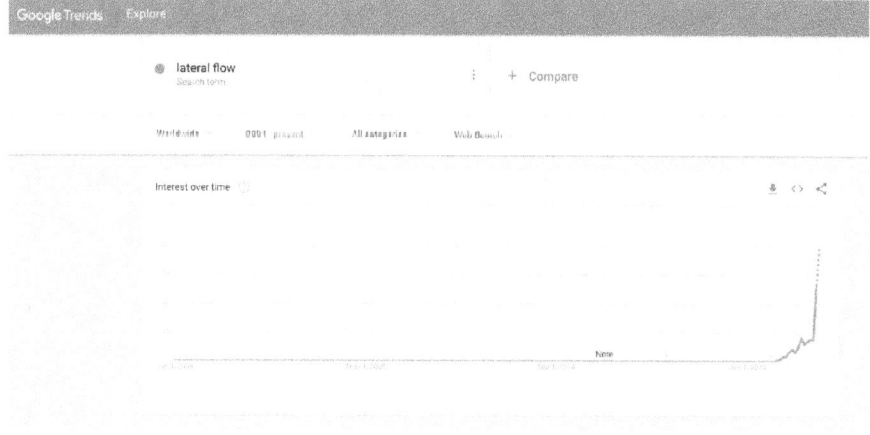

Figure 33: Google Searches for Lateral Flow

Before we dive into this Chapter, just a note on terminology. Multiple different names are typically applied in media and popular coverage of rapid immunochromatographic tests for antigens. I'll refer to them here broadly as Ag-RDTs or Antigen Rapid Detection Tests. Less technically, they may be known as Rapid Antigen Tests (RATs) or, in many countries, they are widely referred to as Lateral Flow Tests (LFTs). However, LFT more correctly refers to the type of technology used, rather than the type of assay being conducted - as we'll see in Chapter 8, antibody tests can also adopt lateral flow technology - so an LFT can be an antigen or an antibody test, depending on what it's being used to detect. In this section, we'll explore the lateral flow principles that underlie both most home antigen tests and the antibody tests we'll talk about in the next Chapter.

Antigen detection tests can be laboratory-based (using technologies such as enzyme-linked immunosorbent assay - ELISA) or intended for use in clinical or domestic settings (using rapid technologies such as LFT). Given the promise of LFTs to bring wider access to testing, we'll focus on those here. For anyone seeking more information on laboratory-based antigen tests, a good starting point for current thinking is Kyosei et al on developing an ELISA test for SARS-CoV-2 antigen detection[133].

Antigens and Antibodies

In order to better understand how rapid tests based on lateral flow technology operate, we need firstly to describe briefly antigens and antibodies as they are the key players in these widely used immunochromatographic tests.

- An *antigen* is any molecule that stimulates an immune system response, specifically the production of an antibody. Antigens are usually proteins but may also be lipids, polysaccharides or nucleic acids. Each antigen has distinct surface features, or *epitopes*, which are crucial to the interplay between them and our antibodies. In the case of SARS-CoV-2, the virus has several antigens, including its nucleocapsid (N) phosphoprotein (the most abundant protein in SARS-CoV-2) and spike (S) glycoprotein.

- An *antibody* (or *immunoglobulin*) is a Y-shaped protein produced by the B cells of the immune system in response to the presence of an antigen. The antibody is designed to attach or bind (via a *paratope*) to an epitope on the antigen - this binding is the basis of immunochromatographic tests. Once bound, the antibody may then neutralise the antigen, or mark it for elimination by another part of the immune system.

Lateral Flow Tests (LFTs)

The antigen tests most people are familiar with are implemented using Lateral Flow (LF) Technology. This is an inexpensive technique that uses paper-based devices to detect analytes and display a visible indication of a positive result. Since they were first created in the late 1980s, a vast array of LF immunoassays have been created for diagnosing various conditions, with a global market worth over $7bn pre-pandemic[134].

At first glance, LFTs offer a highly compelling proposition - low cost, laboratory-free results in less than 30 minutes, often with user-collected samples. Among the rapid LF tests for human use are viral targets such as Influenza and RSV, STDs, TB and hepatitis but also hormones, narcotics, inflammation and sepsis markers, and cardiac markers such as troponin. There are even LFTs with multiplex capability to detect multiple analytes in a single device. But questions about the accuracy of LFTs, especially regarding the timing of the test, have led to hesitancy to use them widely in some jurisdictions during the COVID-19 pandemic.

We'll discuss LFT in more detail below but if you're interested in a comprehensive review, including a list of 45 different analyte types, and discussion of more complex designs, including hybrid nucleic acid lateral flow immunoassays that combine PCR amplicons and LFTs, refer to this open access 2008 article, "Lateral flow (immuno)assay: its strengths, weaknesses, opportunities and threats. A literature survey"[135].

Samples

Starting with the sample types, LFTs are often quite flexible in the samples accepted. Depending on the target analyte, the most common types are saliva, diluted upper respiratory samples and blood/serum. Urine and sweat can also be used by some tests. For SARS-CoV-2, early LFT designs were approved for use on nasal swabs, either AN or MT, as discussed in Chapter 5. However, several manufacturers also produced saliva-based tests.

A key phase in performing an LFT is the preparation of the sample in an extraction buffer; this fluid is crucial to move the sample along the pads described below, but also usually contains preservatives and chemicals for cell *lysis* (breaking open cells to improve access to the antigens).

LFT Design

An LFT is made up of a sample pad, a conjugate pad, a nitrocellulose strip that contains test and control lines, and an absorbent wicking pad. The components are housed in a casing to make them easier to handle and minimise the chances of contamination.

Nanoparticle-labelled antibodies to the target antigen are sprayed onto the pad. So, in the case of an LFT for SARS-CoV-2, antibodies to the target S or N proteins would be used. Interestingly, many LFTs include gold as part of the reaction chemistry to show a colour change on a positive test. Before you get too excited though, the nanoparticles in this colloidal gold are <40nm in size. Alternative approaches, such as that from Fujifilm[136], also use silver, but again in minute quantities.

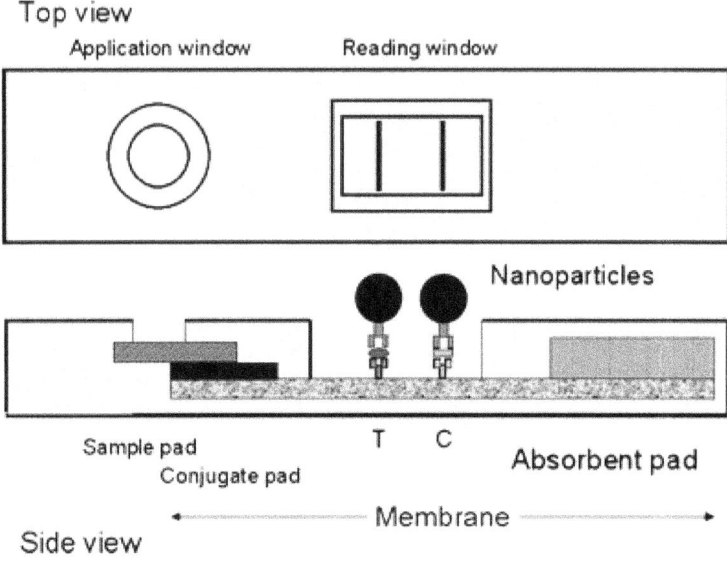

Figure 34: Image showing top and side view of a typical LFT

In an LFT for SARS-CoV-2, a patient sample (usually two or three drops) is applied to a test strip. The sample moves along the paper, via capillary action, where two lines have been placed on the strip: a line of SARS-CoV-2-antigen-specific antibodies that have been conjugated with luminescent indicators and a control line to confirm that the sample has successfully traversed the test line (especially important in the event of a negative test). If SARS-CoV-2 antigens are present in the sample, they will bind with the antibodies on the test strip and then be seen as a coloured line.

Sizes and shapes

Although the cartridge mechanism is among the most common, other formats exist, including a growing interest in form factors that eliminate the need for environmentally undesirable single-use plastic casings. As you can see below, though LFTs typically look quite similar, there are some different formats such as "pen" designs that have an integrated swab. The range of LFTs I assembled below ranged in cost from around $4 to $35 per test.

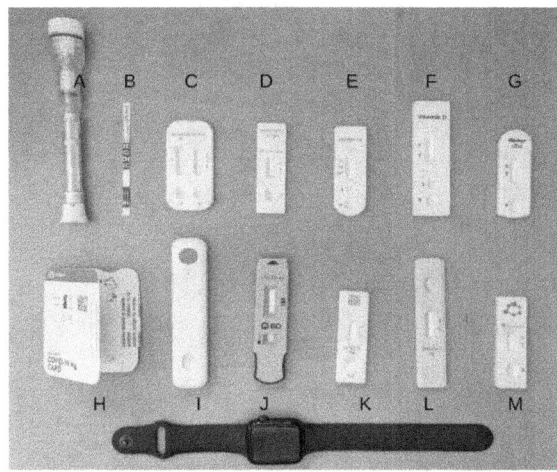

A - Rapid Response® Pen Ag-LFT (Saliva)
B - Quidel Ag-LFT
C - Multiplex Influenza/SARS-CoV-2
D- Anbio - Ag-LFT
E - IgG/IgM Antibody test Ig-LFT
F - Vitamin D LFT
G - Troponin LFT
H - Binax Now - Ag-LFT
I - Ellume Ag-LFT
J - BD Veritor Ag-LFT
K - OnGo Ag-LFT
L - Genrui Ag-LFT
M - AmonMed Ag-LFT (Saliva)

Figure 35: Variety of LFTs (including SARS-CoV-2, Ag, Ig; Vitamin D and Troponin examples) with Apple Watch for Scale

Reading Devices: Quantitative Results

Although best known for binary (positive/negative) results, LFTs can be quantitative in some cases. When used in conjunction with a reader device, some LFTs can interpret the intensity of the response, to quantify the given analyte against a calibrated value. Further development of this technology with dedicated reader devices or even smartphones could drastically extend the use of LFTs where more granular results are useful. Researchers are continuing to explore ways to improve the readout of LFTs. Along with the colloidal gold mentioned earlier, fluorescent markers and electrochemical are among the techniques under review[137]. BD Veritor offers a POC reader device called BD Veritor Plus (shown below) at a cost of approx $330[138], to systematize the reading of LFT results[139]. Diagnostics makers such as Lumos[140] and Quidel also offer readers for LFTs while several researchers have proposed smartphone-based systems[141] with affordable 3D-printed components that offer potential in Resource Limited Settings (RLS) and Low- and Middle-Income Countries (LMIC).

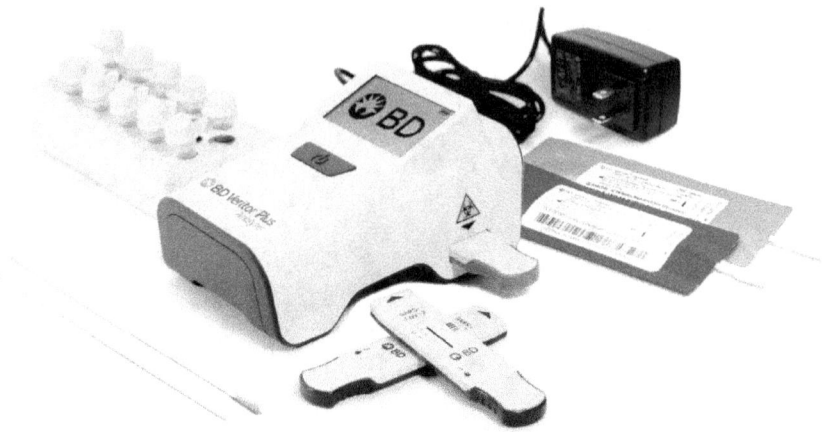

Figure 36: POC BD Veritor Plus Device and 2 LFT cartridges. Source: BD

In one study, for digital immunoassay antigen tests, the sensitivity was 78.3% and the specificity was 97.6%. When technicians visually analysed the antigen test results, the sensitivity was 71.6% and the specificity was 99.2%. The increase in false positives suggests the device detected slight, non-specific colour changes, which resulted in an increase in false positives[142]

A popular LFT widely used during the COVID-10 pandemic, produced by Ellume, uses fluorescence to improve the readability of test results - see device labelled "I" in Figure 35 above.

Suitability Debate

Despite their low cost, speed and convenience, LFTs are generally regarded as inferior to NAATs when it comes to accuracy, with the potential for false negatives to give dangerous reassurance. Proponents of LFTs argue that serial use of LFTs can overcome inherent weaknesses in sensitivity and that the cost and especially speed, compared to laboratory tests are critical to achieving widespread testing.

Antigen tests don't amplify their targets the way NAATs do, so they are inherently less sensitive - and that's before accounting for the fact that the sample is diluted in the buffer to enable the specimen to flow along the test strips. On the positive side, they are cheap to manufacture in volume and provide an alternative in the event of reagent shortages that hampered PCR testing during the COVID-19 pandemic.

Ease of Use

Even setting aside accuracy debates, ease of use concerns have slowed the rollout of LFTs in some jurisdictions during the COVID-19 pandemic. Initially, regulators in the US only allowed the use of some tests when prescribed by a physician, before later permitting their use at home via Over The Counter (OTC) sales at pharmacies. US authorities later followed the lead of the UK and other countries in making quantities of tests freely available to the public.

Due to initial concerns about how the public, largely unfamiliar with swabbing and home testing, would use tests, some suppliers offered remote supervision. For example, early users of the Abbott BinaxNOW test were required to download the NAVICA app and follow instructions via a video call with a remote proctor. Several of the tests that I've tried replaced live video calls with video tutorials and step-by-step instructions in an app, including timers to help ensure good sampling technique. As discussed above, various LFT vendors have tried to minimise the steps required by users in terms of sample preparation, by adjusting the test design and have included the option to interpret the result by a smartphone to address uncertainties, especially in the case of faint lines.

Accuracy in Context

There have been numerous studies comparing rapid antigen LFTs and laboratory-based NAATs. However, these studies are not always easy to interpret, as we know from previous chapters that factors other than just the type of test, such as sample site, collection technique and specimen processing, as well as the pathogenesis phase of the infection, impact the result.

It's also important to note that the next steps after the test result are relevant when considering what is acceptable accuracy for a test. The nature of SARS-CoV-2 "treatment" has highlighted another regulatory challenge; diagnostic testing is typically regulated on the assumption that a result may lead to medical treatment for the individual taking the test. The potential for any medical treatment to cause harm has always led to a conservative approach to test appraisals, with a very high accuracy threshold being required, often higher than that of rapid tests. However, the regulatory regime wasn't designed for a scenario where the test result isn't focused primarily on the person taking the test - in the case of SARS-CoV-2 testing, the resulting non-pharmaceutical "treatment" was isolation, which is, in fact, aimed at protecting other members of society from infection, in the absence of a pharmaceutical/medical treatment.

A Cochrane review[143] concluded that Rapid antigen (lateral flow) tests are better at identifying COVID-19 infection in people with symptoms than in those with none, although the diagnostic accuracy of different brands of tests varies widely. The European Centre for Disease Prevention and Control (ECDC) concluded that Rapid Antigen Detection Tests (RADTs) are less sensitive than NAATs, especially in asymptomatic patients, but are sensitive enough to detect cases with high viral load, early in the course of infection in pre-symptomatic and early symptomatic cases up to five days from symptom onset[144].

Among all the reviews I've read, the general conclusion seems to be that a well-collected sample for an LFT test conducted at a time of relatively high viral load is likely to be extremely reliable. Given the widespread coverage/concern about LFTs being better at detecting higher viral loads, you may be surprised to learn that in the past, some LFT designs were prone to false results in the presence of very high concentrations of an antigen analyte. This is known as the Hook Effect[145] but the good news is that it typically no longer affects modern tests that are designed with an awareness of the issue.

NAATs are likely to be able to pick up an infection somewhat earlier and somewhat later in the course of infection, compared to an LFT. But it's hard to ignore the speed of LFTs compared to laboratory tests, as long as users understand that false negatives are not entirely rare and act accordingly. In August 2022, the FDA issued updated advice to the public on serial testing with LFTs: *If you plan to use at-home COVID-19 antigen tests, have several tests on hand so you can test more than once*[146]. We'll return to the topic of test timing in Chapter 12.

LFTs beyond COVID-19

Although LFTs have become the dominant consumer testing mechanic during COVID-19, prior coronavirus outbreaks (SARS-CoV-1 and MERS) didn't utilise rapid antigen testing: given the relatively small scale of the 2012 MERS outbreak, an LFT antigen test for MERS-CoV wasn't developed, but researchers did create an ELISA antigen test to offset the cost of the pervasive RT-PCR testing.

For non-coronaviruses, multiple antigen tests have been available since the 1990s for pathogens such as RSV and Influenza. However, accuracy concerns had limited their adoption. Studies that took place prior to the widespread interest in the topic caused by COVID-19 found that with rapid antigen tests for RSV, sensitivity in adults was as low as 29%[147].

A 2011 study regarding rapid antigen tests for Influenza during the H1N1 outbreak found overall sensitivity and specificity estimates of the tests were just 51% and 98%[148]. Another 2017 meta-analysis[149] of multiple accuracy studies of existing Rapid Influenza Detection Tests (RIDTs) found that 3 RIDTs consistently provided sensitivities and specificities >70%.

A potential side-effect of the global focus on COVID-19 is likely to be a renewed and lasting awareness of Influenza and other non-COVID-19 respiratory viruses (often referred to as *ILI* - Influenza Like Illnesses). While there were substantial annual seasonal healthcare efforts targeting reducing ILI-harms, many people weren't acutely aware of the toll of ILI.

The CDC official guidance for physicians regarding rapid influenza testing suggests there is still substantial work to be done to improve on the performance of these assays: *However, RIDTs have limited sensitivity to detect influenza viruses in respiratory specimens compared to RT-PCR or viral culture and negative RIDT test results should be interpreted with caution given the potential for false negative results, especially during peak influenza activity in a community.*[150]

Amid rising concern about the poor performance of some rapid tests for Influenza, the US FDA reclassified them from class I to class II medical devices in 2017. This imposes additional controls on test manufacturers. Improving accuracy of influenza detection can not only improve infection control, but reduce unnecessary overuse of antibiotics:

Accurate influenza diagnosis can also prevent the overuse of unnecessary antibiotics. From 2005 to 2006, 59% of ambulatory visits for acute respiratory tract infections in the United States resulted in an antibiotic prescription, even though the majority are caused by viruses (1). Antibiotics increase patients' risks for Clostridium difficile and antibiotic-resistant infections and cause an array of side effects, together accounting for 1 out of every 5 adverse drug event visits to emergency departments[151].

With the eventual availability of higher quality Influenza diagnostic tests, it is likely that people interacting with higher-risk groups in the future may be more inclined to take a test before meeting vulnerable people. Although, at a population level, flu doesn't pose a significant threat to younger age groups, it can have very serious consequences in certain cohorts.

I would be optimistic that COVID-19-derived improvements in diagnostic technologies will see much improved accuracy in the next generation of rapid/POC influenza testing. Another likely trend will be the incorporation of multiplex assays into a single test to help distinguish among ILI cases. In mid-2022, CorDx received the first CE-mark approval for a combined COVID-19, influenza and RSV LFT[152].

Antigen Test Costs

In addition to the speed of result and ability to use at home for on-demand testing, a further advantage of antigen testing is the relatively affordable nature of the tests. Despite the fact that, at time of writing, twin packs of tests in the US typically retail for $18-25, the cost of production is closer to $2.50 per test. In many European countries, tests are available for about $5 each, with many public health authorities providing some kits free to close contacts of positive cases, in order to encourage detection and isolation. While these prices compare favourably with collect-at-home/mail-to-lab tests (from $35 on Amazon.com) or at home molecular tests from c.$50 per test (see Chapter 9), there may still be price barriers to frequent testing. A survey by Harvard University and Hart Research Associates in January 2021[153] found that 79% said they would test themselves regularly if an at-home test cost $1, while only 33% indicated they would frequently test if the price was $25.

Environmental Impacts

As is often the case with convenient, disposable products, there are concerns about the environmental impact of their widespread use. Now that the immediate need to produce LFTs urgently has largely been met, researchers are turning their attention to approaches that would reduce the environmental impacts: for example, Intelligent Fingerprinting offers a test strip without the standard plastic housing[154], while Birmingham Biotech has announced plans to launch an LFT with 75% less plastic than current models[155].

Studies have shown that laboratory tests also produce plastic pollution: an RT-PCR generates 37.27 g of plastic residues per sample and 97% of the plastic residues from diagnostic tests for coronavirus are incinerated due to their hazardous nature[156]. Some degree of plastic use may remain inevitable for the foreseeable future - and justifiable both on the basis of overall benefits to health and the importance of disposability to avoid contamination. However, if testing levels remain elevated into the future, there will be an imperative to look for ways to reduce the harmful environmental impacts of large-scale testing.

Chapter 8: Antibody Testing (Ig-RDT)

While both NAAT and Antigen testing, discussed in the previous two Chapters, are aimed at detecting people who are currently infected with a pathogen (direct tests), antibody testing instead looks for signs of the body's response to a pathogen (indirect tests), in the form of antibodies, rather than the current presence of a pathogen itself - the presence of antibodies indicates that a person has been previously exposed to a pathogen or has a subclinical current infection.

It is important to note the difference between antibody and antigen tests - so, while antigen tests use antibodies to find antigens, antibody tests use antigens to detect antibodies. (Note: Antibody tests are sometimes referred to as serological tests - serology more technically refers to the study of blood serum but is frequently used interchangeably to refer to antibody testing).

Although this Chapter is primarily about antibody tests, antibodies are only a part of our overall immune system response. We'll end the chapter with a quick review of tests for the other components of our immune system.

Antibody Basics

In order to discuss the pros and cons of Antibody testing and how it can contribute to improving healthcare post-pandemic, we need to start with a little detail of how antibodies work, without getting too far into the intricacies of the entire immune system. This will help in the discussion of test timing, test targets and potential uses. Note that antibody response can vary across individuals, especially in those who are immunocompromised, but we'll focus here on the most common typical responses.

As mentioned in the previous chapter, Antibodies (Ab) - also referred to as immunoglobulins (Ig) - are proteins produced by special white blood cells (called B cells) in your body which provide defence against antigens, such as bacteria or viruses. Antibodies are found in the plasma element of our blood - human blood is about 45% red/white blood cells and platelets and 55% plasma (water, clotting factors, CO_2, Hormones, Minerals, Glucose and other Proteins).

In what's sometimes described using a plug and socket analogy, each antibody acts like a socket (more technically a *paratope*) into which the plug (*epitope*) of the antigen binds. In the case of the SARS-CoV-2 virus, an antibody can attach to the Spike (S) protein thus stopping it from binding to a cell and infecting it. We'll come back later to the importance of which specific part of the virus the antibodies target.

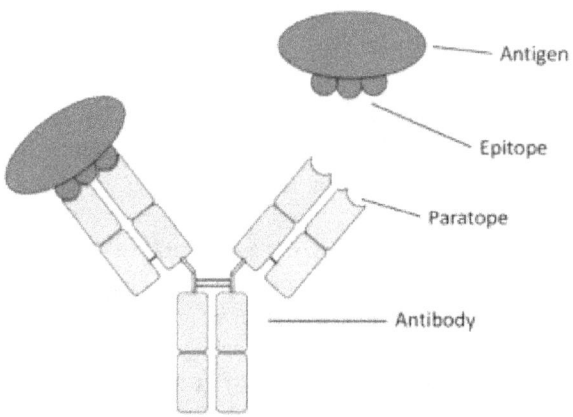

Figure 37: Antibodies, Paratopes & Epitopes. Source[157]

Crucially from a testing perspective, without symptoms, the presence of antibodies against SARS-CoV-2 in serum, plasma or venous blood samples demonstrates recent or previous SARS-CoV-2 infection, rather than an active/acute infection.

Types of Antibodies (IgM, IgG and IgA)

Our bodies produce several different types of antibodies that play different roles in our defence over time:

- The first line of defence when our bodies detect an invader is Immunoglobulin M or *IgM*. These initial antibodies are usually short-lived and replaced or supplemented by more effective antibodies after a few days.
- The most common type of antibody that provides a strong defence is Immunoglobulin G or *IgG*. It accounts for about 75% of your body's antibodies. While there are subclasses (*isotopes*) of IgG called IgG 1-4, I'll refer more generally to IgG here. Other antibodies, called *IgD* and *IgE*, are beyond the scope of this book as they are not used in diagnostics.

- The final type of antibodies relevant here are Immunoglobulin A or *IgA* antibodies. They are found in the mucous membranes of the lungs, sinuses, stomach, and intestines, so are only relevant for certain types of infection. In respiratory tract infections, they provide a locally derived mucosal immune response and thus can be hard to detect in serum samples due to their localised nature.

In the case of SARS-CoV-2 infection, IgM and IgA typically respond first, usually about 3-4 days after symptoms develop, in what's known in immunology as *seroconversion* - the development of specific antibodies in the blood as a result of infection or immunization.

IgG usually responds a few days later (5-6 days), though it can be simultaneous with IgM in some people. IgA and IgM then tend to abate over time as IgG has more success binding to the SARS-CoV-2 spike (S) protein[158]. IgM, therefore, is seen as an indicator of more recently acquired infection while IgG antibodies appear towards the end of the active infection and can persist for months to years following infection. For example, one study[159] showed an IgM peak at 15–21 days while IgG peaked between 22–39 days. Due to the shorter lifespan of IgA and IgM, IgG is the recommended antibody analyte for testing, according to the Infectious Diseases Society of America (IDSA)[160].

In an example of how insights gained from previous challenges can inform future responses, researchers working on understanding SARS-CoV-1, (the etiological agent behind the 2003 SARS epidemic) learned that the initial immune response of IgM antibodies was short-lived and replaced by more durable IgG antibodies as part of a secondary immune response within days/weeks[161]. This insight was a useful starting hypothesis for early investigations into our immune response to SARS-CoV-2.

From a diagnostic perspective, the reason it's important to differentiate between the types of Ig is because different tests will target detection of different Igs. In this US report[162] looking at the EUA-approved serological assays, they span equally across all four types (IgG only, IgM only, IgG and IgM, or total antibodies (IgG, IgM, and IgA)), providing greater options and flexibility for the healthcare providers to choose from. The report shows (left chart) that few tests target only the presence of IgM, while the majority have been designed to look for antibodies to the S(pike) antigen (right chart).

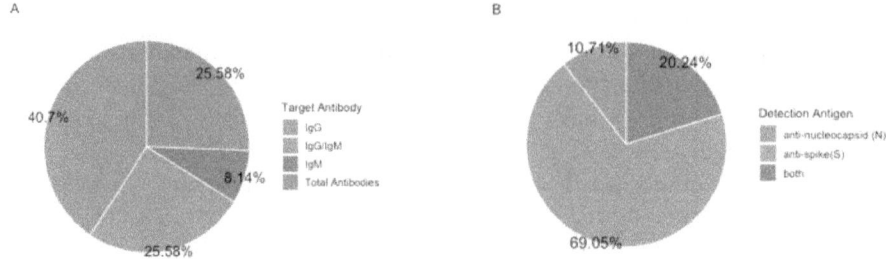

Figure 38: (L) EUA antibody tests by target antibody and (R) by detection antigen used

Detection Antigens

In order to detect the presence of disease-specific antibodies, these tests use particular antigens which may vary across tests from different manufacturers. Again, taking SARS-CoV-2 as our example, you'll recall it has a number of potential antigen targets for our antibodies - and although there is a variation in the target viral protein our antibodies choose to target, the ones of interest are the two most plentiful in a SARS-CoV-2 virion, the N and S antigens. As the protein on the surface of the virus, the S is highly likely to generate an antibody response first.

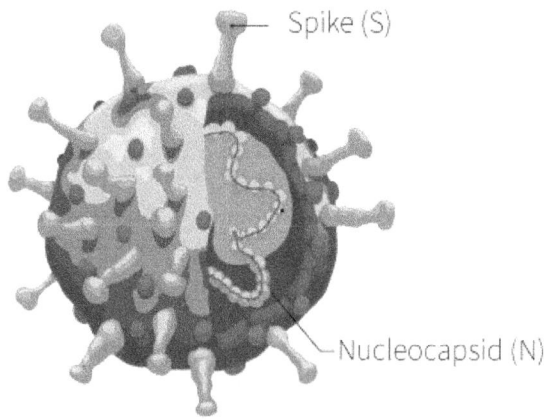

Figure 39: SARS-CoV-2 S and N antigens are most used to identify antibodies[163]

In designing diagnostics, there's a need to ensure that the target is specific and not also associated with another virus. In the case of SARS-CoV-2, there is, unsurprisingly, a large overlap with SARS-CoV-1. The S protein, though, is more specific to SARS-CoV02; the N protein homology (similarity) between SARS-CoV-2 and SARSCoV-1 is 90 percent, compared with the S protein (77%). In particular, the S1 subunit homology, including the receptor binding domain (RBD), is less (66%). S1 contains the immunologically crucial RBD, which is the key target of neutralizing antibodies. In practice, the lack of prevalence of SARS-CoV-1 now means the detection of a target protein is currently almost certainly indicative of SARS-CoV-2.

Most concerns regarding SARS-CoV-2 serologic assay specificity revolve around the potential for cross-reactivity with antibodies to the commonly circulating alpha- (NL63 and 229E) and beta- (OC43 and HKU1) coronaviruses (CoVs). Prior seroprevalence studies indicate that over 90% of adults aged 50 and older have antibodies to all four common circulating CoVs; therefore, the potential for cross-reactivity in SARS-CoV-2 serologic assays is significant[164]. However, further analysis has now shown there is no cross-reactivity of SARS-CoV-2 with human plasma positive for IgG antibodies against NL63, 229E, OC43, and HKU1. However, a strong cross-reactivity was observed between SARS-CoV–positive human plasma and SARS-CoV-2[165].

Vaccines and Antibodies

The development of vaccines relating to Covid-19 (there were 10 approved at last count, with at least another 10 in various stages of trials[166]) is outside the scope of this book and worthy of a large book of its own, but the relevant point for this discussion is that the antibodies we're talking about may be naturally produced either by an organic exposure to SARS-CoV-2 or induced by a vaccine-mediated exposure, or by a vaccine-directed mRNA instruction.

Based on existing understanding of Coronaviruses, most vaccine researchers chose the S protein as the target for vaccine-induced antibody defences to SARS-CoV-2. Thus, the presence of N-targeting antibodies shows evidence of a prior infection to which you developed natural immunity rather than vaccine-derived immunity[167]. The US CDC has produced this quick guide regarding vaccination status[168], to assist in interpreting antibody tests, based on their antigenic targets:

Interpretation of anti-S and anti-N antibody results based on vaccination status

Vaccination status	Anti-S antibody	Anti-N antibody	Interpretation*
Vaccinated	+	+	Vaccinated and previously infected
Vaccinated	+	−	Vaccinated and not previously infected
Unvaccinated	+	+	Not vaccinated and previously infected
Unvaccinated	−	−	Not previously vaccinated or infected

Figure 40: Antigenic Targets of Antibodies by Vaccination Status. Source: CDC

More on Timing & Seroconversion

I mentioned briefly above, in the section about Antibody types, how the different Ig serve different functions as the immune response to a pathogen evolves (*immunopathogenesis* is the term for development of a disease/immune response).

It's vital, therefore, to understand the timing vs function of diagnostic testing, as our bodies respond differently over time - it takes our bodies some time from first exposure to a virus to respond, but in time, the detectable response fades. As we've seen, the response typically happens in two phases: an initial generic response (IgM) and then a more targeted response (IgG).

Data suggests that in the case of SARS-CoV-2, the IgM antibody response peaks around 15-20 days after infection, followed by the IgG antibody peak at around 20-25 days. IgM levels may be too low to detect until at least 5 days post onset of symptoms (POS), but seroconversion occurs in over 80% of patients by day 10[169].

In an area of study known as *antibody kinetics*, researchers have seen large variations in response between individuals, but also over time in each individual. To further complicate the interpretation of antibody tests, there are instances where some patients show an IgG response at the same time as IgM or even before it. This plot shows the distribution across a study of 208 samples[170]. Although this graph illustrates the relatively consistent and rapid response of IgM and IgA, it also shows significant outliers of early and delayed IgG response.

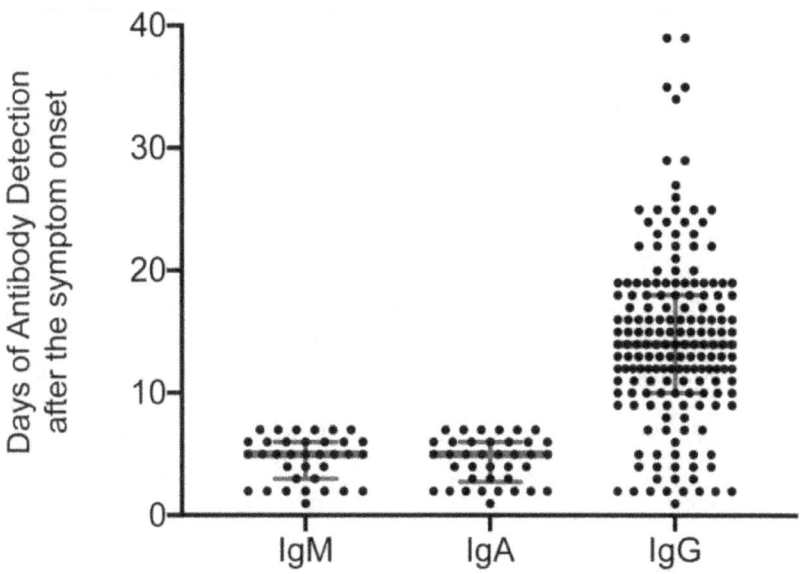

Figure 41: Typical timing of different antibody responses POS

For SARS-CoV-2 infection, the timing of seroconversion appears to be similar to, or slightly earlier than, SARS-CoV-1 infection. Seroconversion in most cases of COVID-19 occurs during the second week of symptoms.

Waning/Longevity

A key interest area for antibody tests is the longevity of antibodies. Although it's hard to establish the strength of immunity over time, the continued presence of antibodies may give important clues to the chances of reinfection. Of particular interest is what's known as *Anamnestic Reaction* - the renewed rapid production of an antibody following second or later contact with the provoking antigen or with a (closely) related variant.

However, it's not yet clear what level of protection antibodies to SARS-CoV-2 may confer against further reinfection or transmission, so diagnostic tests for the presence of antibodies are not recommended as a means to support the use of "immunity passports" as has been suggested in some countries. Data from a recent study showed that antibody levels begin to wane after two months. This could mean that the window for which antibody testing can identify people who have been infected is relatively short, and therefore antibody test results will need to be interpreted with caution.[171]

Diagnostic Dividend of SARS-CoV-1

Turning again to research on other coronaviruses for clues on how future immune responses to SARS-CoV-2 may play out, there may be insights from a 2011 study[172] that followed up on recovered patients from the 2003 SARS epidemic:

Six years post-infection, specific IgG Ab to SARS-CoV became undetectable in 21 of the 23 former patients. No SARS-CoV Ag-specific memory B cell response was detected in either 23 former SARS patients or 22 close contacts of SARS patients. Memory T cell responses to a pool of SARS-CoV S peptides were identified in 14 of 23 (60.9%) recovered SARS patients. SARS-specific IgG Ab may eventually vanish, and peripheral memory B cell responses are undetectable in recovered SARS patients. In contrast, specific T cell anamnestic responses can be maintained for at least 6 y. Whether the T cell anamnestic response is adequate to protect a person from reinfection requires further investigation. These findings have applications in preparation for the possible re-emergence of SARS.

In a large meta-review of scientific literature on antibody immunity to coronaviruses[173], researchers noted that protection after coronaviruses (primarily mild endemic human coronaviruses (HCoVs)), may last for only 1 or 2 years. It's clear that, despite our experience with other coronaviruses, we're still very early in the process of understanding how our relationship with SARS-CoV-2 will develop, a topic we'll return to in the section on Variants in Chapter 12. Meantime, now that we've discussed antibodies, let's review the tests used to detect them in more detail.

Antibody Tests

As with the current infection/direct detection test types described in the previous Chapters, antibody tests can be carried out in central labs (following hospital or at-home sample collection), at point of care, or at home. Laboratory tests tend to use ELISA (Enzyme-Linked Immunosorbent Assay), while point of care (POC) and at-home tests are primarily based on lateral flow technology similar to those discussed in the previous Chapter, though portable ELISA machines are available. NAAT technologies are not typically involved in antibody testing. By mid-2021, over 80 serological tests for SARS-CoV-2 had already received US FDA EUA-approval[174].

Specimens and Collection

The standard specimens used for serological testing include serum, plasma, or whole blood. In practice, saliva or sputum can also be tested for the presence of antibodies. Serum and plasma samples require an additional centrifuge extraction step, which makes them less suitable for POC or domestic testing. For at-home antibody tests, a fingerprick blood sample is sufficient, while venous blood is usually preferred in a clinical or hospital collection due to its lower potential for contamination versus capillary samples.

Types of Serological Testing

Once a sample has been collected, a number of test types can be used. There are four major types of serologic testing: lateral flow assays (LFA), chemiluminescent assays (CLIA - but not to be confused with the Clinical Laboratory Improvements Amendments regulatory framework of the same initials!), enzyme-linked immunosorbent assays (ELISA), and neutralization assays.

The following graph from a review of Covid-19 antibody tests shows the split in approaches by different vendors. Researchers found that ELISA produced the most sensitive results, though performance across all types of test varies based on the type of antibody (IgG/IgM) and antigen (N/S) utilized in the assay. Where mail-in diagnostics are offered based on at-home collection, the samples are typically processed using ELISA or CLIA assays.

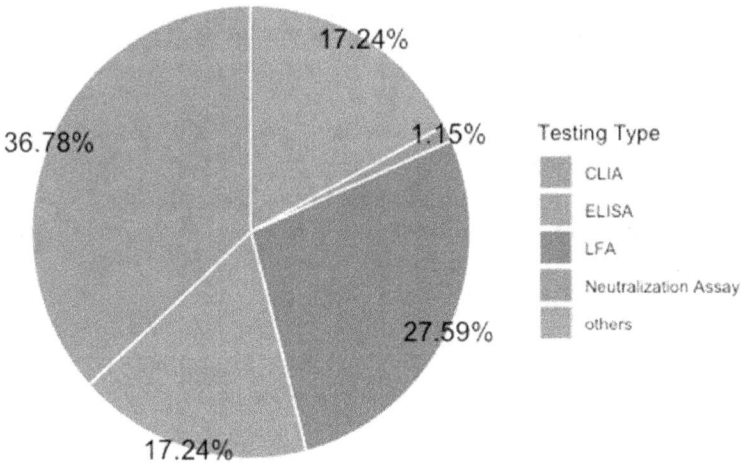

Figure 42: Testing Technologies used in Antibody Tests for SARS-CoV-2. Source[175].

Laboratory Antibody Tests

Enzyme-linked immunosorbent assays (ELISA) and chemiluminescent immunoassay (CLIA) are common laboratory platforms that can measure IgG and IgM antibody titres (concentration). Unlike the LFT-based tests, these lab tests can return quantitative results rather than just binary positive/negatives. While qualitative LFTs typically deliver results in less than 30 minutes, more advanced laboratory quantitative processes take longer: CLIA tends to take 1-2 hours while ELISA takes up to 5 hours, and a newer variant of ELISA, Microsphere Immunoassay (MIA) can take up to 8 hours. Similar to the pros and cons of laboratory-based NAAT techniques, these laboratory-based tests offer excellent accuracy, throughput and multiplexing, while requiring transport to the laboratory, trained personnel and expensive equipment.

Neutralization assays can take several days but have the added benefit of testing whether the antibodies can effectively inhibit a virus, rather than just identifying their presence. However, due to their use of live virus samples, they can only be conducted at BioSafety Level 3 (BSL3) facilities.

Lateral Flow Immunoassay

Essentially the mirror of the antigen tests described in the previous chapter, rapid antibody tests use the same lateral flow technology but use an immobilized viral antigen in place of the antibodies used to trigger the reaction described in Chapter 7.

Lateral flow tests for antibodies have received significantly less interest than lateral flow antigen tests, as people are typically more concerned with testing for a current infection than a prior one. Antibody tests have not been made widely available for consumer use - as at April 2022, for example, Walgreens.com offered consumers a choice of 5 rapid antigen tests (BinaxNow, OnGo, Quickview, Intelliswab and Flowflex), with no antibody self-tests on sale. For my own research, I was able to purchase a box of 10 IgG/IgM Lateral Flow tests online from a medical supplies firm for an approx. cost of €6.50 per test.

While most antibody testing is traditionally done using ELISA techniques in a lab, the portability, speed and low cost of lateral flow testing for antibodies makes it attractive where quantification is not important. Applying emerging microfluidic techniques, a Hong Kong research team published a paper detailing a 20-70 minute SARS-CoV-2 antibody test, which also offers a quantitative result[176]. Although driven by SARS-CoV-2, the researchers note the potential to apply the approach to potential usage with other scenarios such as biomarkers for cancer, Alzheimer's and prostate specific antigens (PSA)[177].

Beyond Blood

I mentioned earlier how serology testing can often be used to refer to all antibody testing rather than the stricter definition of blood-based tests. While most antibody testing is conducted on blood samples, there is growing interest in the use of urine tests for antibody detection.

According to a report published in Science Advances[178], researchers found SARS-CoV-2 antibodies in patient urine samples with 94% sensitivity and 100% specificity with the urine-based ELISA test. Although not widely studied or reported, urine-based diagnostic tests that detect antibodies have been suggested as a possible non-invasive alternative to diagnose several conditions, such as dengue, Helicobacter pylori infection, hepatitis A and C, human immunodeficiency virus, strongyloidiasis, schistosomiasis, paragonimiasis, and leishmaniasis.

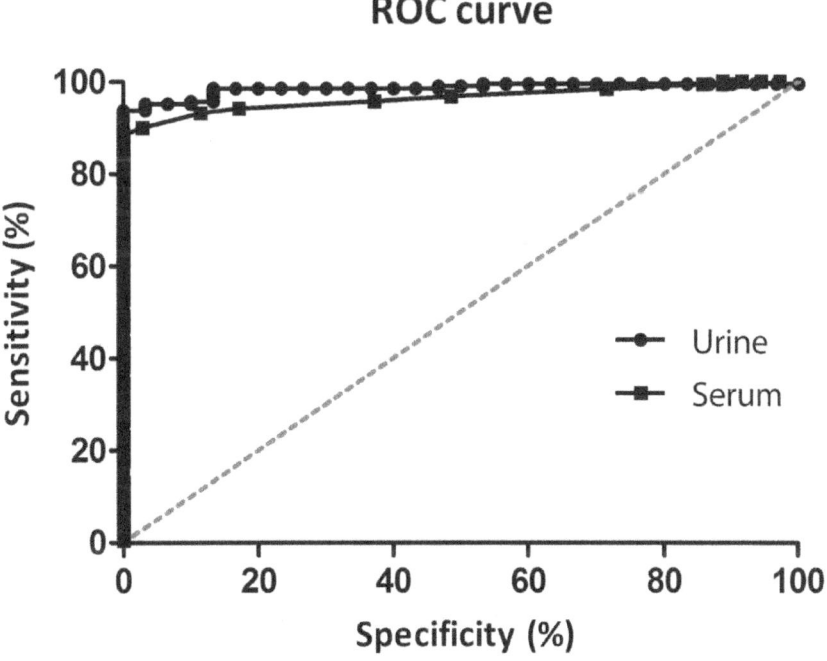

Figure 43: ROC curve for comparative diagnostic performance of urine- and serum-based ELISA for COVID-19

Assessing Antibody Tests

Though not a part of the testing regime for active infections, antibody tests are still useful to help track the spread of a disease retrospectively, to help quantify those who had asymptomatic infections, identify those who may need to be prioritized for vaccinations (due to low levels of antibodies), and highlight potential donors for convalescent plasma therapy (due to high levels of antibodies).

In an example of how antibody testing can inform public health policy and statistics, a report published by the Irish Blood Transfusion Service[179] showed that, across a random selection of blood donor plasma samples from donations received between February and September 2020 (n = 8509), seroprevalence was between 2.5–3.5%. The donor seroprevalence rate was higher than that reported by direct methods, confirming a higher rate of infection in the community than was diagnosed using PCR testing, which shows that not all cases were diagnosed/reported, even at the height of community testing.

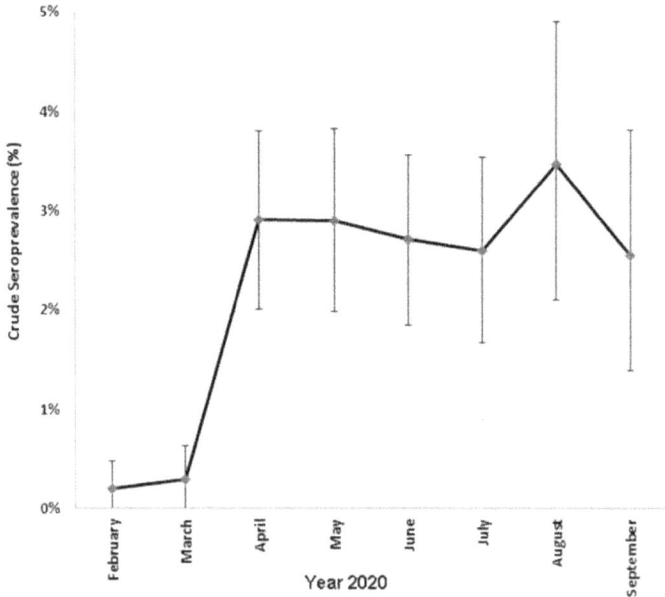

Figure 44: SARS-CoV-2 antibody detection in blood donations received between February 2020 and September 2020. Error bars represent 95% confidence intervals.

As with other types of tests, there are variations in the effectiveness of different assays and a need for regulatory oversight. Due to the lack of reliance on these tests for acute treatment or non-pharmaceutical intervention policy decisions, serological tests have often been at the back of the queue for regulatory approval during the exceptional times of the pandemic public health emergency[180].

Test Accuracy

On the topic of regulatory approval, in the early rush to get tests for SARS-CoV-2 scaled, the US FDA allowed voluntary submission for EUA of serologic assays, meaning the EUA process could be by-passed. However, this was rescinded in July 2020[181] and test manufacturers were required to follow the EUA process. Again, this is likely to be an area of learning for dealing with future outbreaks and how to balance regulatory oversight with the rapid availability of novel tests. As early tests were developed in April 2020, the UK government was forced to admit that none of the 17.5m antibody tests it ordered were accurate enough to be used[182].

In a comparison of 10 commercially available serological assays[183] (1 x CLIA, 2 x ELISA and 7 x LFTs), researchers found sensitivity ranges from 60.9% to 87.3% and specificities from 82% to 100%. However, illustrating the importance of timing of tests, sensitivities rose to over 95% in samples more than 20 days post onset of symptoms - when patients were far more likely to have seroconverted.

A slightly perverse diagnostic dividend from the Covid-19 pandemic may be an increased awareness of when *not* to trust tests. Some marketing claims for direct-to-consumer antibody tests may exceed the certainty of research into its applicability - there is no definitive level or threshold of antibodies, in a positive result for the presence of antibodies, that is known to provide protection. So, while the determination that someone is seropositive indicates a degree of immune response or protection, it doesn't guarantee total protection[184].

Beyond Antibodies: Cell-Mediated Immunity

"Emerging studies suggest that all or a majority of people with COVID-19 develop a strong and broad T cell response, both CD4 and CD8, and some have a memory phenotype, which bodes well for potential longer-term immunity. Understanding the roles of different subsets of T cells in protection or pathogenesis is crucial for preventing and treating COVID-19"

Center for Evidence Based Medicine[185]

While the focus of immunological testing for SARS-CoV-2 has been on antibody responses, a dividend from previous coronavirus research is the insight that other elements of the immune system are likely to be involved, not just antibodies. When faced with a pathogen, our immune response is often multi-pronged, where the humoral (antibody) response is complemented by cell-mediated immunity; our antibody-producing *B cells* efforts are supported by *T cells* (T-Lymphocytes), which recognise and destroy infected cells. As with antibodies, an exhaustive discussion of cell-mediated immunity is beyond the scope of this book, but here we'll highlight some basic principles and recent advances in the field that are likely to form the basis of on-going research relating to Covid-19 and beyond, and the diagnostic advances that will play a crucial role in better understanding immunity.

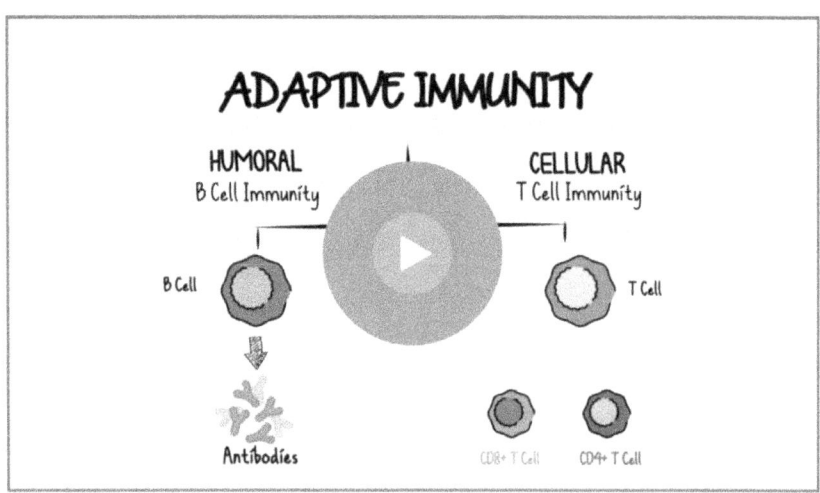

Figure 45: Combined Immune System Response. Source: https://www.tspotcovid.com

T-Cells and Immunity Memory

A growing body of evidence points to a key role for SARS-CoV-2-specific T-cell responses in COVID-19 disease resolution and modulation of disease severity. Milder cases of acute COVID-19 were associated with coordinated antibody, CD4+ and CD8+ T-cell responses, whereas severe cases correlated with a lack of coordination of cellular and antibody responses and delayed kinetics of adaptive responses[186].

Although they may not prevent people from becoming infected with SARS-CoV-2, T-cells may reduce the duration and severity of their illness. The importance of T-cells in fighting SARS-CoV-1 and establishing immune memory has also been well documented and discussed in a number of pre-COVID-19 papers[187]. Two types in particular are important - *CD4+* T cells which help B cells to produce antibodies and *CD8+* T cells which help to kill virus-infected cells. These cells have been important mediators of infection in other coronavirus diseases, which fact also seems to be relevant for SARS-CoV-2 so far - emphasising that continuing research is a crucial part of pandemic preparedness.

As discussed in the earlier section covering antibody longevity, there is intense interest in understanding the duration of immunity which infection and/or vaccination confers. This information will be crucial in determining future patient care, public health policies and therapeutic development directions. Our efforts to better understand the immunity situation for SARS-CoV-2 require not just a focus on antibodies but on the complete response of our broader immune system.

Compared to antibodies, T cells are primed to recognise more protein snippets from viruses, which makes them more resilient in the face of new variants. T cell responses also remain in the body for longer - antibodies are unlikely to be detectable 1 year after infection, whereas people who had SARS during the 2003 outbreak, still had T cell responses to the virus 17 years later[188]. And if someone encounters antigens from the pathogen again – either as a result of infection, or additional vaccine doses, these existing T cells will be backed up by fresh T cells generated from memory T cells. It's also worth noting that, while seroprevalence testing has been mooted as an important public health tool to identify people with immunity who may have been asymptomatic, some people appear to respond to SARS-CoV-2 exposure or infection by mounting a T cell response without an antibody response. The recurring suggestion that Vitamin D is useful against Covid-19 stems from research suggesting an important role for Vitamin D in supporting T-Cells[189].

Testing for T-Cells

T-cells are harder to detect than antibodies, and there aren't many widely available tests to detect them, even in laboratory settings. One available T-cell test is the T-SPOT ELISA assay used for tuberculosis and cytomegalovirus testing, which has been adapted to detect SARS-CoV-2 cases[190]. A clinic in the UK was offering consumers this test for £195 with a two-day time to result from when the blood sample was taken[191].

Pharma giant Roche has received CE approval for its laboratory blood test that measures the secretion of interferon-gamma, a cytokine produced by T cells that indicates an immune response[192]. The T-Cell test is intended to be used alongside antibody tests to better understand the combined response of our immune system, though the understanding of the correlation to protection from severe disease is still far from complete.

However, as the research effort into understanding Covid-19 continues, already a growing number of T-Cell diagnostics should be commercially available shortly. Researchers at Duke-NUS Medical School, together with collaborators from the National Center for Infectious Diseases (NCID) and Singapore General Hospital (SGH) have created a test to measure T-cell response by detecting *cytokines* (short chains of amino acids) released by T-Cells in response to the presence of SARS-CoV-2 proteins[193]. In March 2021, the US FDA issued an EUA for a next generation sequencing based (NGS) test, known as T-Detect[194], to aid in identifying individuals with an adaptive T cell immune response to SARS-CoV-2. According to the T-Detect website as of April 2022, the test costs $150 plus sample collection fee ($60-$140) and can detect prior COVID-19 infection for up to 10 months with 90% sensitivity[195]. While the T-Detect is an at-home collection test and takes up to a week, a much simpler skin-based test for SARS-CoV-2 T-cells using a technique known as delayed-type hypersensitivity (DTH), currently widely deployed for TB testing, is under development[196].

Ongoing Research

Advances in NAAT and Antigen tests for detecting active SARS-CoV-2 infections mean that future diagnostic directions will likely focus on increasing access to these tests and ensuring their continued accuracy against variants. But much work remains to be done in the area of diagnosing and understanding immune response to infection, including potential future protection. Researchers have yet to understand how the presence of antibodies relates to protection from reinfection. Despite the appeal of an antibody test as a measure of vaccine effectiveness, the interplay with T-cells means antibodies alone are not a complete indicator.

In its National Strategy for Serology report[197], the Johns Hopkins Center for Health Security identified the following significant gaps in understanding:

1. Correlates of immunity: It remains unclear if antibodies detected by serological tests are virus-neutralizing and what this means for protection from reinfection. We also do not know the amount of antibody needed for protection, or how important other parts of the immune system are, such as cell-mediated immunity (T-cells) for protection against COVID-19.
2. Length of immunity after infection: It is not known how long antibodies last in patients recovered from COVID-19, and how long those persisting antibodies remain effective. It is not known if SARS-CoV-2 infection elicits immune memory, which provides long-term protection.
3. Cross-reactivity of patient antibodies: The COVID-19 serology tests are meant only to detect patient antibodies specific to SARS-CoV-2, but there are many circulating coronaviruses to which patients may have pre-existing antibodies. It remains unclear if patients who have had other coronavirus infections could have antibodies that test positive on COVID-19 serology tests, and which parts of the SARS-CoV-2 virus should be used in serology tests to ensure that the patient antibodies detected are specific to that virus.

Chapter 9: Honey, I Shrunk the Lab

In late 2020, as a consumer, it was impossible to purchase a Nucleic Acid Amplification Test (NAAT) for home use - they simply didn't exist. By the end of 2021 however, I had 3 such devices on my kitchen table, promising laboratory-grade testing in around 30 minutes. This may be the ultimate diagnostic dividend of the COVID-19 pandemic - the emphasis on miniaturised, high quality diagnostic solutions enabling POC and even domestic testing.

Improving access to fast, easy to use testing, without compromising on accuracy, is the holy grail of patient-level testing. Laboratories, with their high throughput, will remain vitally important, but extending high quality testing to more people has the (hyperbolic sounding but real) potential to drastically alter global healthcare for the better.

From Lab to POC and Domestic Testing

Decades of developments in bioanalytical laboratory techniques have enabled increased accuracy and speed in the identification of pathogens. Combined with concomitant breakthroughs in diagnostic imaging, physicians have never before enjoyed such abilities to see inside patients, right down to the molecular level. But, as empowering as these new diagnostic tools have been, they frequently require large, complex and expensive machines, confined to centralised, specialist facilities where they are operated by skilled staff, meaning access to the insights they provide is limited and all too frequently restricted only to those able to pay for them.

In recent decades, smaller and more affordable instruments have seen laboratory-level assays move closer to patients at point of care (POC), significantly reducing waiting times. The advances from the COVID19 pandemic-led investment in testing technologies will see this trend both continue and accelerate and even perhaps lead to the personal ownership of domestic molecular testing devices capable of running an assortment of assays.

From Lab to POC

Moving testing capability closer to patients invariably speeds up the time to result (TTR) by eliminating travel and/or transport time. Recent years have seen important advances in the miniaturisation and automation of tests to enable desktop-sized machines, at a cost within the reach of some clinics, to provide testing at point of care.

There are multiple definitions of what constitutes a POC but for my purposes here, I'm referring to any test that can be carried out in a clinic-type setting, without sending a sample to a lab for processing. These tests may require medical training and (relatively) expensive equipment but provide HCPs with rapid results that may lead to a change in patient management.

Laboratory testing, which tends to be highly accurate and facilitates processing of large batches of tests efficiently, is vitally important and will remain a crucial part of diagnostics for the foreseeable future. When tests are required at population-scale for screening or diagnosis, every fraction of a percent improvement in accuracy counts in terms of numbers but also, of course, in terms of the importance of the result to the individuals concerned; we mustn't forget that behind each sample is a person who is likely to be nervous about their result and dependent on its accuracy for treatment or guidance.

However, in situations where access to a laboratory test is difficult, or where the delay in getting a sample to a lab is materially important to the choice of intervention, POC testing is a vital tool in the diagnostic armoury. While early attempts at creating POC testing often resulted in assays that were significantly less reliable than lab-based tests[198], the last 20 years or so has seen a huge investment in developing both POC devices and Consumer Self-Test (CST) devices. Many available POC tests now offer acceptable reliability and can be used either by HCPs or even consumers themselves.

Key trends include:

- Emergence of isothermal NAAT
- Miniaturisation of devices
- Expansion of test types available outside the lab
- PC and Smartphones as interface

And that's before you include the potential of the newer technologies such as microfluidics, CRISPR and even NGS to have an impact on the POC/CST segments, as we'll discuss in Chapter 11.

In 2014, the WHO Sexually Transmitted Diseases Diagnostics Initiative (SDI) developed the ASSURED criteria to describe the ideal characteristics of POC tests required to tackle the burden of curable bacterial infections (e.g., syphilis, chlamydia and gonorrhoea in LMICs):

A = Affordable
S = Sensitive
S = Specific
U = User-friendly (simple to perform in a few steps with minimal training)
R = Robust and rapid (results available in less than 30 min)
E = Equipment-free
D = Deliverable to those who need them

Researchers working on POC have recently proposed extending the ASSURED framework to add "-SQVM"[199], showing the growing ambition and capabilities envisaged for POC tests:

- Self-testing - suitability for unsupervised or minimally supervised personal use
- Quantifiable - provide quantified not just qualitative (pos/neg) results
- Viability of pathogen - determine if pathogen is viable
- Multiplex - detect Multiple pathogens

The breadth of medical conditions that POC can be applied to with these kinds of capabilities is almost unlimited. Aside from viral diagnostics that we're focused on here, POC testing is already a massively important market - millions of tests are regularly carried out either in clinic settings or even in people's own homes. And, although the infectious disease element of this market is our focus here, any improvements in diagnostic technologies are likely to be widely applicable and offer great hope to people all over the world in helping to tackle other diseases and conditions.

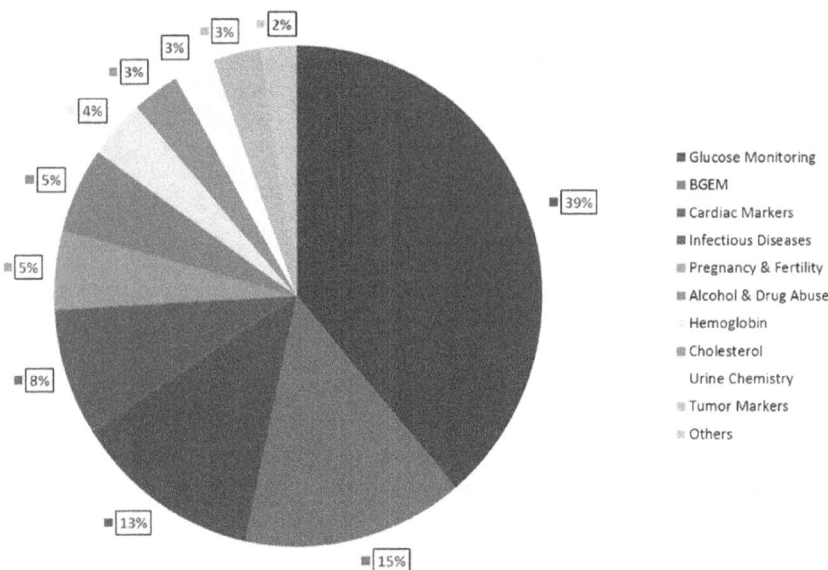

Figure 46: 2018: In Vitro Diagnostics: Technologies and Global Markets[200]

NAAT Outside the Lab

As we saw in Chapter 6, for the majority of its time in use in diagnostics, PCR technology has been confined to laboratories. The complexity of thermocycling machines made reducing their size challenging and concerns over potential contamination in uncontrolled environments further reduced interest in expanding their use outside the lab. It must be remembered too, that POC-based machines will not provide the throughput required for large-scale testing, which will likely remain tied to laboratories or similar dedicated facilities. However, technological and methodological advances in recent years have seen the emergence of devices for use closer to the patient, offering improvement possibilities in situations where point of care diagnostics is highly desirable.

Desktop-sized PCR machines that can operate outside a lab have existed for about a decade - MiniPCR[201] was founded in 2013 to create a PCR thermocycler small enough for science educational use in schools (from about $650). A more extreme example is Biomeme's portable qPCR device, Franklin,[202] that costs $10,000 but offers multiplex capabilities in a device weighing just 1kg (2.2lbs), is controlled by a smartphone app and is battery powered for fully remote operations.

The urgent need for increased testing, as the severity of SARS-CoV-2 became apparent in early 2020, led to a flurry of attempts to adapt existing technologies to reduce the dependence on lab-based PCR testing. Among the first existing POC machines to be repurposed for COVID detection were the Abbott ID NOW[203] and the Cepheid GeneXpert. The GeneXpert, originally developed to detect biothreat agents, has successfully crossed over to clinical diagnostic applications and is already quite widely used for tuberculosis and HIV testing, especially in low- and middle-income countries. Several studies of the Abbott ID Now SARS-CoV-2 test have shown results comparable to PCR except in cases of very low viral load[204].

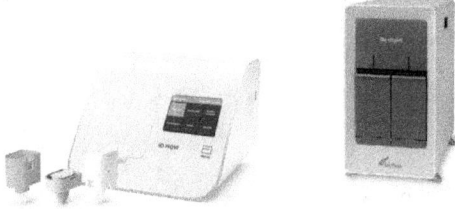

Figure 47: Abbott & Cephid POC NAAT Devices

Machine	Abbott ID Now	Cephid GeneExpert Xpress
Launched	2014	2017
Technology	NEAR	RT-PCR
Cost (Machine/Assays)	$5,000/$40	$11,500/$15
Machine Weight	6.6lbs/3kg	18lbs/8kg
Assays available (Respiratory)	Influenza Strep RSV SARS-CoV-2 (EUA)	Influenza Strep RSV SARS-CoV-2 (EUA)
Runtime (mins)	5(+) to 13(-)	36
Capacity (per run)	1	2/4/16
Specimen Types	Nasal Nasopharyngeal Throat	Nasal Nasopharyngeal Nasal wash/aspirates

The increased awareness of POC testing may see at least some devolution of testing to smaller centres, including perhaps workplaces or primary care centres. As molecular diagnostics capabilities become more available to local settings, HCPs will have powerful new tools to speed diagnosis, which is especially encouraging in the case of infectious diseases, where outcomes are frequently directly associated with time to pathogen identification.

POC PCR diagnostics may, over time, revolutionise clinical care. PCR technology offers great potential in the arena of infectious disease. A universally reliable infectious disease diagnostic system could become a fundamental tool in the evolving diagnostic armamentarium of the 21st century clinician. For front-line acute care physicians, or physicians working in disaster settings, a quick, universal PCR assay, or panels of PCR assays targeting categories of pathogens involved in specific syndromes such as meningitis, pneumonia, or sepsis, would allow for rapid triage and early, aggressive, targeted therapy[205].

The two examples above are of "benchtop"- sized machines, but they aren't readily portable. San Jose-based Visby Medical had earlier developed a handheld rapid PCR test for sexually transmitted infections (Chlamydia, Gonorrhoea and Trichomoniasis, which have the same symptoms, but their treatment requires three different antibiotics). The company started work on a rapid SARS-CoV-2 test with funding from the National Institute of Health's (NIH) program for diagnostics which allowed the firm to scale from producing 100 devices per week to 9,000 per week.

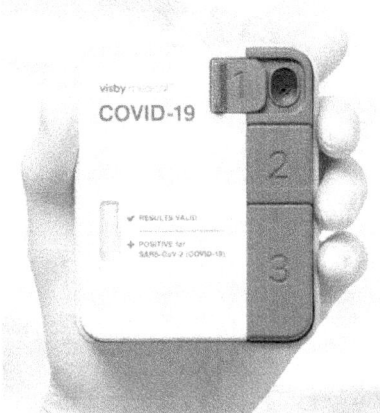

Figure 48: A Visby handheld NAAT for SARS-CoV-2

The device received EUA point-of-care authorisation for use in CLIA-waived locations but, despite its small size and ease of use, it is not (at this time) approved for home use. It produces results in about 30 minutes, and it is a single-use device. One study[206] into its accuracy reported 95% sensitivity and 100% specificity.

From POC to Home - Diagnostic Devices

Recent years have seen a dramatic shift in the availability of health and well-being devices targeted at consumers, largely supported by the growth in smartphone and wireless technologies. Although usually described as "non-medical" to avoid closer regulatory scrutiny, consumers are encouraged to buy fitness trackers, heart rate monitors, blood pressure devices and myriad other gadgets to quantify their well-being. COVID-19 saw a huge increase in interest in home-use oximeters to measure blood oxygen levels and it's likely that the home health gadget trend will continue, consumers having seen what's possible with at-home, technology-supported care. Alongside the obvious benefits of relieving pressure on hospital resources, the appropriate use of at-home care can have additional benefits in reducing nosocomial (hospital-acquired) infections. We'll discuss this class of devices in more detail in the next Chapter, but here I want to discuss devices that are designed to bring laboratory grade diagnostics to domestic settings.

Joining the consumer devices mentioned is a growing list of domestic diagnostic solutions that are clearly perceived as "medical" rather than just well-being gadgets - the claims of laboratory grade test results at home that we'll discuss in this Chapter signal the next generation of home healthcare, building on trends I described in my 2015 book, "Your Phone Can Save Your Life".

Design for Consumers

To be effective, devices intended for use outside of medical facilities have several critical design requirements when operated by non-trained staff. Even when these criteria are met, there may still be a risk of misuse or misinterpretation, especially by the "worried well". Widening of access to high quality testing is not just a matter of miniaturising laboratory equipment and making it affordable/easy to use. As consumer-targeted devices proliferate, their use will need to be supported by wider education about when testing is useful and when there are no medical grounds for it. Not all possible tests will make sense in a domestic setting and/or, in some cases, would be unlikely to be useful without an HCP to interpret them.

Testing should be done only for good reason and with an informed understanding of what the test result means, so there is justified concern in the healthcare sector that unbridled availability of direct-to-consumer test offerings will lead to an inefficient or even unsustainable increase in demand for HCP consultations where direct-to-consumer (DTC) testing doesn't include adequate context and follow-up. Although not an at home test, similar concerns might well apply to at home collection services such as Numan[207], that offer free testing if nothing unusual is found, which could be interpreted as encouraging over-testing.

Where their use is justified, consumer-use devices should be designed to:

- Require minimal user involvement
- Be able to analyse easily-obtained direct samples (samples that require little to no preparation/pre-processing)
- Safeguard against incorrect use
- Be easy to interpret correctly
- Be cost effective

These criteria mean that devices described above that were designed for POC-use, such as at clinics, are likely to be unsuitable for domestic use, where the potential for user error is higher.

Any home diagnostic device meeting these criteria, where the user is likely also the person being tested, will be designed to work with samples that can be obtained safely in a domestic setting with a minimal level of invasiveness. For example, a device that relies on nasopharyngeal swabs is much less suited to home use than one which processes MT or nasal swabs. Practically, the biological fluids that can be obtained minimally invasively at home, by the patients themselves, are blood (finger-prick, not venous), nasal secretions, urine, saliva, and sweat.

Regulators tend to set high standards for "medical-grade" devices intended for unsupervised consumer use, although it varies by jurisdiction. The development of a new diagnostic device is very expensive; a study has identified that in 2010 the average cost to bring a diagnostic device (that requires FDA 510(k) approval[208]) from concept to market into the US is more than $30 million, the major part of the cost being associated with the regulatory clearance of the device[209]. However, the high cost of entry has proven little of a deterrent to the plethora of firms seeking a piece of the highly lucrative well-being market.

Is that a Lab in your Living Room?

Prior to the COVID-19 pandemic, there was little consumer appetite for domestic testing devices for infectious diseases. Since then, however, PCR tests have become a familiar concept to consumers, and the importance and benefits of testing have been etched in consumers' minds.

I mentioned at the start of this Chapter that I now have 3 devices (Cue, Detect & Circle) capable of nucleic acid amplification testing at home. These devices feel like consumer electronics products, not medical devices. Clearly, they have been designed to fit discreetly into a modern home alongside Google Home or Amazon Alexa devices. (I have no relationship with any of these firms, am not recommending any device over another and I purchased publicly-available devices personally to evaluate them). There may be other devices available by the time you read this, but these represented the state of the art available in 2022.

Cue

Cue Health was the first firm to gain FDA EUA for an at-home molecular testing device that didn't require a prescription[210]. The device itself is very compact and takes cartridges that contain the test assay into which you insert the sample. Cue promises that multiple types of tests will be available in time, but only SARS-CoV-2 tests are available currently.

The Cue device uses isothermal amplification and is controlled via a Smartphone app. Trumpeting concordance between the Cue test and the reference laboratory tests of 97.8%[211], the device returns results in about 20 minutes.

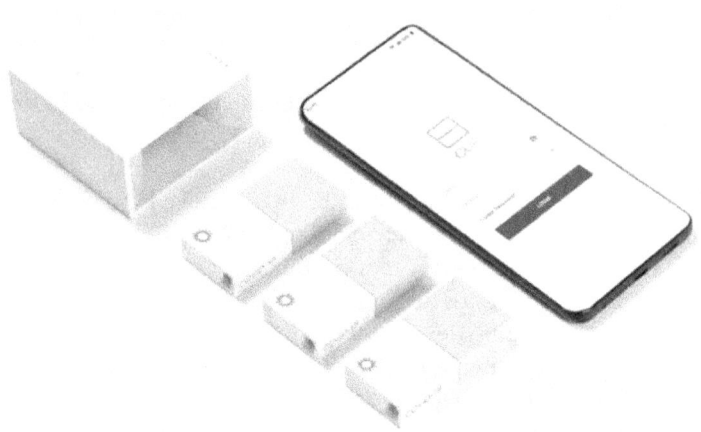

Figure 49: Cue Reader device and 3 test cartridges

Cue is a prime example of a device that received a tremendous boost from the COVID-19 testing focus. The firm was founded during the H1N1 (swine flu) outbreak in spring of 2009, so Cue was already developing its technology before the pandemic - in 2018 it was awarded $30m in funding from the U.S. Department of Health and Human Services' (HHS) Biomedical Advanced Research and Development Authority (BARDA) for the development of Influenza and Multiplex Respiratory Pathogen diagnostic cartridges[212]. These have yet to launch but a key selling point for the Cue device is its ability to test for virtually any analyte once a cartridge is produced for it. The crucial challenge for Cue post-COVID will be its ability to deliver relevant, affordable and accurate tests. Cue also offers enterprise packages that enable up to 6 devices to run from a single smartphone, while pooled testing is promised for later release in low-prevalence settings.

Beyond COVID-19, Cue Health says it's working on a number of tests that can be completed using saliva, urine and blood samples and nasal swabs. Those diagnostic tests will cover things like respiratory health, sexual health and determining risk of chronic illnesses such as heart disease.

At $249 for the test reader and $195 for 3 COVID-19 test cartridges, Cue is substantially more expensive than most rapid antigen LFTs but, as well as offering enhanced accuracy, it is very simple to use with no fluid handling required - the user inserts the swab directly into the cartridge. More detailed information about the Cue, including its cross-reactivity and other information, is available on the FDA site in a free to download 122-page document[213].

Reflecting the extent of interest in the domestic and corporate diagnostic opportunity, Cue Health went public in late 2021 at a valuation of $2.9bn, numbering Google and the NBA among its users. Before going public, Cue had shipped 115,000 readers, had capacity to manufacture over 15 million test cartridges per annum[214]. Cue clearly believes that personal access to diagnostics is a potentially lucrative area. According to the company's S-1 filing[215] with the SEC prior to its public listing, its mission is "to enable personalized, proactive and informed healthcare that empowers people to live their healthiest lives". The summary continues: *"We are now witnessing what we believe is the beginning of a transformational shift as consumers take control of their own health…We further believe that healthcare is finally ripe for a digital transformation and that it will begin with diagnostics, since approximately 70% of all clinical decisions are made utilizing diagnostic data"*.

The filing illustrates 11 different cartridges and refers in detail to the following planned tests, with the caveat they may not all come to fruition. *"Five additional Test Kits in late-stage technical development (influenza A/B, or flu, respiratory syncytial virus, or RSV, fertility, pregnancy and inflammation) for which we expect to begin submitting for FDA authorization or clearance in the second half of 2022. Our additional planned care offerings include tests in the categories of respiratory health, sexual health, cardiac and metabolic health, women's health, men's health, and chronic disease management."* The filing includes simulated images of tests for Testosterone, RSV and Haemoglobin A1C (Blood Sugar) while the following intended test menu is included:

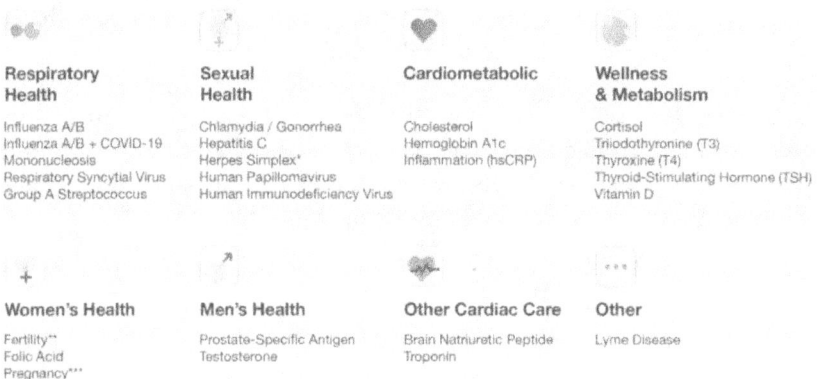

Figure 50: Cue Future Testing Menu

The Cue filing also provided further detail provided about sample types and development status:

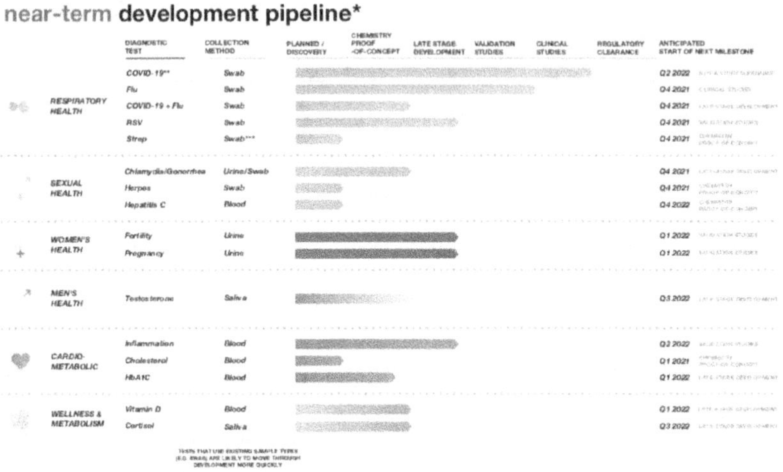

near-term development pipeline*

	DIAGNOSTIC TEST	COLLECTION METHOD	PLANNED / DISCOVERY	CHEMISTRY PROOF-OF-CONCEPT	LATE STAGE DEVELOPMENT	VALIDATION STUDIES	CLINICAL STUDIES	REGULATORY CLEARANCE	ANTICIPATED START OF NEXT MILESTONE
RESPIRATORY HEALTH	COVID-19**	Swab							Q2 2022
	Flu	Swab							Q4 2021
	COVID-19 + Flu	Swab							Q4 2021
	RSV	Swab							Q4 2021
	Strep	Swab***							Q4 2021
SEXUAL HEALTH	Chlamydia/Gonorrhea	Urine/Swab							Q4 2021
	Herpes	Swab							Q4 2021
	Hepatitis C	Blood							Q4 2022
WOMEN'S HEALTH	Fertility	Urine							Q1 2022
	Pregnancy	Urine							Q1 2022
MEN'S HEALTH	Testosterone	Saliva							Q3 2022
CARDIO-METABOLIC	Inflammation	Blood							Q3 2022
	Cholesterol	Blood							Q1 2021
	HbA1C	Blood							Q1 2022
WELLNESS & METABOLISM	Vitamin D	Blood							Q1 2022
	Cortisol	Saliva							Q3 2022

Figure 51: Cue Development Timeline

Detect

A company named Detect launched its home NAAT test device in December 2021, shortly after Cue. The Detect system consists of a reusable reader device (much more affordable than Cue at just $39) and single-use test cartridges ($49 for a single COVID-19 test). Results are available in just under an hour, and claimed to be 97.3% accurate, with no false positives. While Cue doesn't specify the exact isothermal technology used, Detect is clear that it uses RT-LAMP and lateral flow to read the result.

The Detect reader device is compact and simply designed, with just a small entry slot for the cartridge. The user needs to combine their sample with the supplied test tube, then insert it in the Detect hub to process; the Detect app provides step by step instructions for the whole procedure.

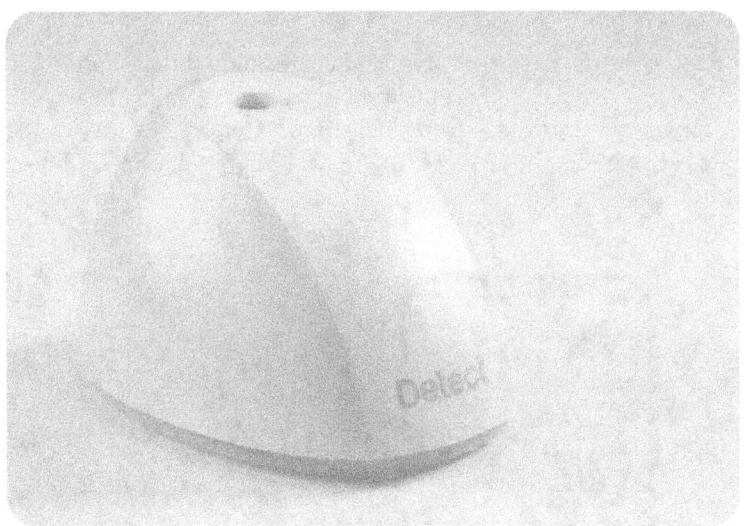

Figure 52: Detect Reader Device

When the test is complete, the app notifies you that your sample is ready to read. Although Detect hasn't shared as much detail as Cue, it has revealed plans to extend testing into STIs, additional respiratory tests and others as yet unannounced. Detect's decision to hire an ex-Google and Facebook executive as CEO shows that it's thinking of Detect as a consumer electronics device as much as a medical diagnostic device. This seems in line with an accelerating trend that has seen brands such as Apple and Amazon invest heavily in health tech in recent years. It's increasingly clear too that the nascent/burgeoning consumerisation of medical technology has been greatly accelerated by COVID-19, at least for the well-off. We'll talk more in the next Chapter about consumer health technology and its growing role in well-being, as well as its general acceptance by consumers.

Circle

Although Cue was the first device to receive EUA in the US, the first home test device I was actually able to try was the Circle Health Pod[216] from Hong Kong. Built on technology from Oxford University, the Pod uses Isothermal NAAT. Circle claims 98.4% accuracy. As with Cue and Detect, it consists of a reader device (c. $130) and test cartridges (c $30 for a single test cartridge). Taking the test requires a nasal swab, following step by step instructions in the app, inserting the swab into the cartridge and putting the cartridge into the device. After about 30 minutes, the device and the app indicate the result. Thanks to the positive/negative/invalid indicator lights on the test device itself, the tests can be completed without the app.

As with the two other devices from Cue and Detect, Circle currently only provides COVID-19 cartridges but claims to have Influenza and STI assays in development. Unlike the cartridges from Detect and Cue, Circle advises the storage of their cartridges at 4-8 degrees, so I have a five pack of tests sitting in my refrigerator!

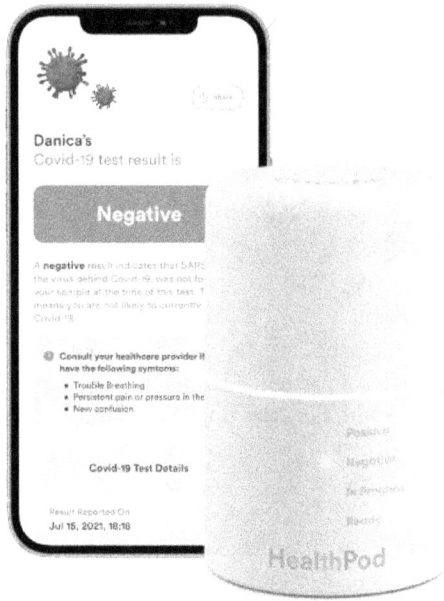

Figure 53: Circle's HealthPod device

The 3 devices described above are of particular longer-term interest as they are comprised of reusable devices with the promise of multiple types of test. Taking a different approach, a firm called Lucira used the COVID-19 pandemic and EUA process to bring a single-use NAAT device to market.

Lucira

Based on work already underway to develop a more accurate Influenza test using LAMP isothermal technology, Lucira received EUA clearance in November 2020 for its SARS-CoV-2 assay, initially requiring a prescription, but that stipulation was subsequently been removed and it's available for OTC sale or direct from the company website. (I bought mine direct from Amazon).

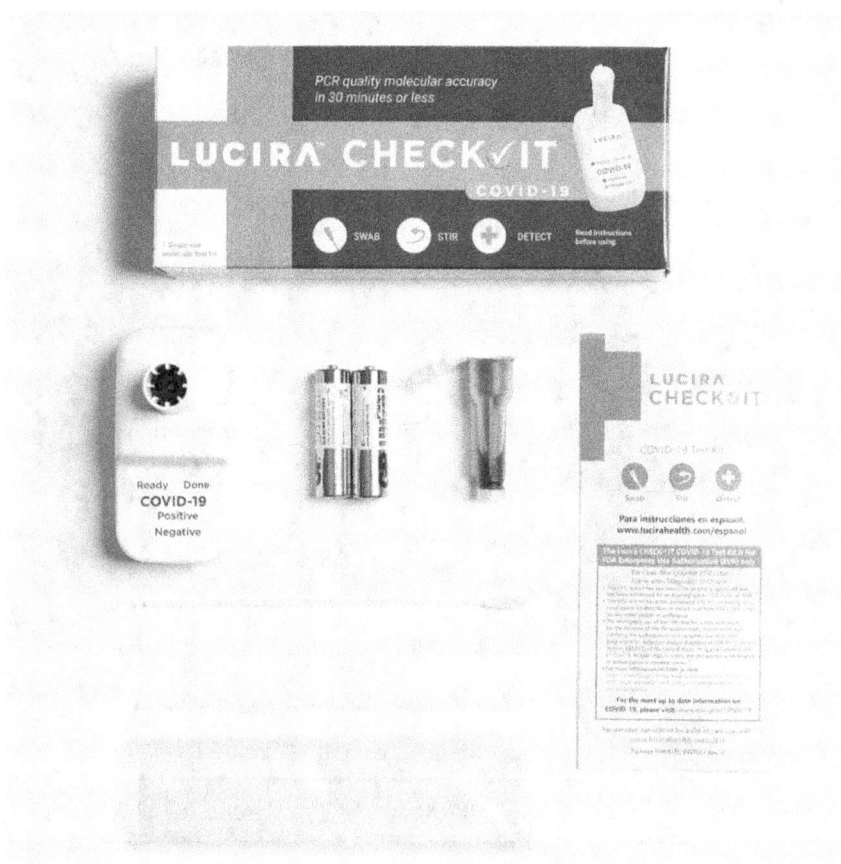

Figure 54: The Lucira COVID-19 Kit

Each single-use test kit costs $75 and can indicate a positive result in as little as 11 minutes, or a negative result within 30 minutes. Lucira's accuracy was 98% when compared to laboratory PCR results with PCR cycle thresholds lower than 37.5. Each test kit contains the test device, two AA batteries, sample vial, swab and instructions.

In May 2022, Lucira announced that a version of the test offering a combined COVID-19 and Influenza test had received CE marking and would be launched in Europe in Q3 2022[217], pointing towards the emergence of multiplex domestic tests becoming more normal in the years ahead.

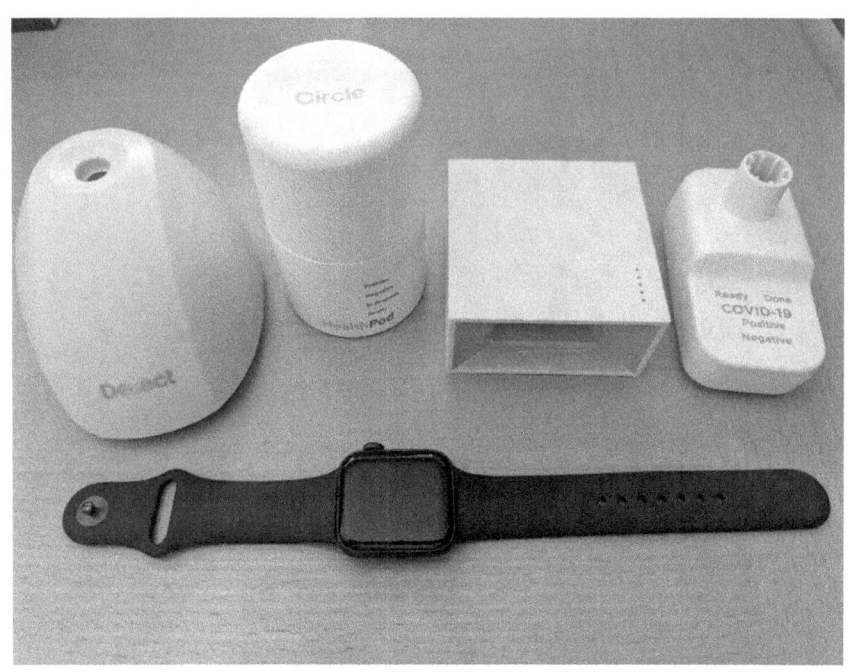

Figure 55: Domestic NAAT reader devices: From L to R: Detect, Circle, Cue Reusable Readers and the single use Lucira device. With an Apple Watch for Scale

Domestic NAAT for SARS-COV-2 Summary

Device	Cue	Detect	Circle	Lucira
Launched	2021	2021	2021	2020
Technology	Isothermal/ LFIA	Isothermal	Isothermal	Colorimetric LAMP
Form Factor	Reader/ Cartridge	Reader/ Cartridge	Reader/ Cartridge	All-in-One
Cost (Reader/ Assays)	$249/$65	$39/$49	$130/$30	$75
Reader Weight	146g	91g	98g	99g (inc. batteries)

Device	Cue	Detect	Circle	Lucira
Assays available (May 2022)	SARS-CoV-2 (EUA)	SARS-CoV-2 (EUA)	SARS-CoV-2 (EUA)	SARS-CoV-2 (EUA)
Runtime (mins)	20	65	30	11(+)/30(-)
Capacity (per run)	1 (Pooled TBC)	1	1	1
Specimen Types	Nasal Others TBC	Nasal Others TBC	Nasal	Nasal

As we've seen with examples in this section, several companies were already working, over the last few years, on miniaturising technologies traditionally used in the lab and adapting them for consumer use. However, there was little commercial imperative with no proven appetite for moderately expensive domestic testing capabilities among generally healthy people. The pandemic changed that. Suddenly, testing capabilities were top of the daily news, funding was available from Governments to speed devices to market and regulators offered shortcut approvals.

The POC technology platforms developed this year should quickly be translated to the detection of new pathogens, once the sequence of the new pathogens is known.

Point-of-care testing will reduce many technical and operational challenges associated with laboratory-based testing but will create others; for example, more patients tested will lead to more requiring treatment, while quality assurance will become more distributed. Since testing is only as useful as the action taken on (assured) results, treatment capacities will require adaptation and some form of clinical-grade spot checks on quality of test results may be needed.

More Molecular

While I've examined some of the leading domestic NAAT solutions coming onto the market, excitingly, there are far too many new entrants in the space of portable and personal molecular diagnostics to list them all here. The

COVID-19 pandemic has spurred multiple new entrants to speed up the deployment of technologies that have been years in the pipeline but lacked a commercial incentive. Here are a few examples:

- Startups such as Imperial College London spinout, ProtonDx is commercialising a LAMP device, Dragonfly[218], to offer a 30-minute multiplex assay covering SARS-CoV-2, influenza A/B, respiratory syncytial virus, and human rhinovirus in a POC device. Although currently requiring expert sample preparation, a self-contained test is in development.

- Another example garnering attention at the time of writing is a POC solution from Domus Diagnostics[219]. This start-up has developed an instrument-free proprietary laminate card using RT-LAMP to test (initially) for SARS-CoV-2, targeting a test price of less than $5. The intended evolution of the approach is to adapt it for other infectious diseases including pathogens like strep A and strep B, influenza A and B, tuberculosis, and chlamydia and gonorrhoea[220].

- A female-health focused, molecular diagnostics start-up founded by two PhDs from Dartmouth college, Nanopath[221], secured $10m in funding to support the development and commercialisation of their 15 minute, amplification-free, desktop biosensing platform, starting with women's pelvic and gynaecologic infections.

- As a final example for now, Rover Diagnostics[222] claims to have created a POC PCR test offering results in approximately 25 minutes, from a device costing just $1,500 and around $5 per assay[223]. The solution is based on a microfluidic technique to enhance PCR, called plasmonic nanoparticle thermal cycling[224].

Written in 2013, the book To Catch A Virus, concluded with the belief that it might "one day" be possible to have a hand held molecular test in our fight with viruses. SARS-CoV-2, for all its ills, has given us exactly that, with many more devices to come. It's a breakthrough that, when applied to more viruses and made more affordable through increased scale, unlocks a new era in the fight against viruses - what we do with it is up to us.

Chapter 10: Wearables: Sensors as Diagnostics?

All of the diagnostics discussed in this book to date rely on chemical reactions or specialist instruments to identify and/or quantify viral pathogens. But research interest has been growing in what role non-invasive measurement techniques, such as wearable sensors, might play in alerting us to illness. Consumers can now purchase an array of wearable devices that offer to track their vital signs and other biomarkers continuously. In this Chapter, we'll examine the role they've played in COVID-19 diagnostics and what we can take from this period for future learnings regarding digital disease tracking.

For clarity, perhaps an important starting point here is to state that wearable technologies cannot generally *diagnose* COVID-19 or other illnesses in the same way as the diagnostic testing techniques we've discussed thus far. What they may be able to do, is provide an early warning of some form of illness, based on non-specific indicators and thereby prompt an asymptomatic or presymptomatic person to perform one of the actual diagnostic tests we've discussed to identify the culprit.

Diagnostics to Wellness

Home-use domestic diagnostic devices have been growing in popularity for specific cases. One example is wearable, patch-format continuous glucose monitors (CGM) from companies including Abbott and Dexcom. These minimally invasive devices can monitor blood sugar levels in interstitial fluids and transmit them to a companion smartphone app. Further patches or temporary tattoo products are being researched to continuously monitor various chemical levels which, in certain cases, may be preferable to periodic measurements via techniques such as rapid LFTs:

Several biomarkers related to diseases (e.g., cancer, HIV, intestinal infections, cystic fibrosis, and schizophrenia, etc.) could be detected in sweat, tears, and saliva. It should be noted, however, that the concentration of several biomarkers in sweat, saliva, tears, and breath might be correlated with pathological conditions, but normal and pathological levels have not been established yet. After establishing these levels, eDiagnostic wearable devices could cover many diagnostic needs[225].

Recent years have seen a trend towards health-related features in more general-purpose devices, with consumer electronics firms showing increasing interest in the well-being space. Most people are familiar with wearable technology for well-being in its simplest form - step tracking - popularised by brands such as Google's Fitbit or smartwatches such as the Apple Watch. The technology has moved on rapidly and many middle and up-market wearable devices are now capable of sophisticated tracking of biomarkers such as temperature, blood oxygen levels (Spo2), heart rate (HR), resting heart rate (RHR) and heart rate variability (HRV), in a range of form factors from watches and fitness bands to rings. A basic device with HR monitoring may cost from only $25, while a top of the range device with sensors for HRV and temperature might run to $400. Here, I'll refer to them generically as trackers unless discussing specific examples.

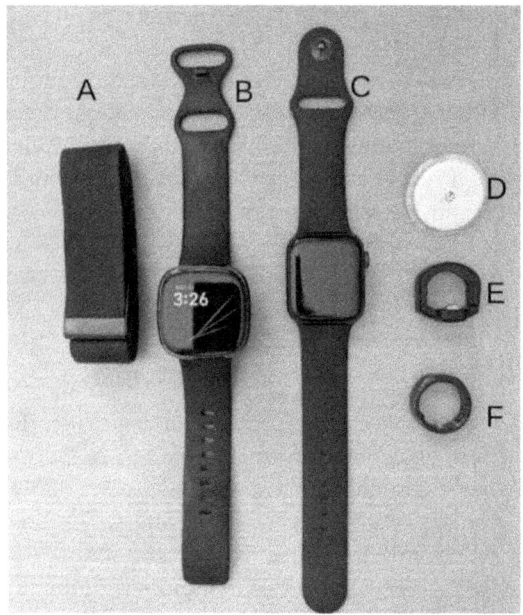

A - WHOOP 4.0
B - Fitbit Sense
C - Apple Watch Series 5
D - Abbot Libre CGM
E - Circul+
F - Oura Gen 3

Figure 56: Some Wearable Sensors

According to 2020 Pew Research, about 20% of the US population has a Smartwatch or Tracker[226]. The report doesn't go into detail about what type of sensors the devices have, but it's reasonable to assume that the majority offer the ability to track HR and RHR, with a significant proportion capable of HRV and Spo2 measurement. Temperature is probably the least common type of sensor to date, as typically it has been exclusive to higher-end devices.

Cost and accessibility are key considerations when discussing whether these devices can play a significant role in public health. And, at present, there's a clear selection bias in the types of people who are attracted to these devices - as one report from wearable maker Whoop noted, its (athletically-inclined) customers are typically healthier than average people. So, there's a likelihood that these devices are primarily worn by the people least likely to need them for health monitoring.

Prior to COVID-19, there was a growing number of fitness/well-being devices targeted at consumers, largely focused on quantifying training/exercise activities and reporting cardio metrics intended to reflect progress/effectiveness of fitness regimes. As the focus grew on identifying asymptomatic COVID-19 cases, several device manufacturers turned their attention to understanding if these gadgets could provide any relevant insights. Trackers provide an interesting medical research case study - instead of the normal challenge of recruiting participants and collecting data frequently, there are millions of people voluntarily wearing these sensors 24/7, collecting myriad data points, potentially making it difficult to identify useful data.

How It Works

We've started previous Chapters with a discussion of specimen types and testing methodologies. In the case of wearables, however, the inputs will largely be sensor readings, not bodily fluids and the interpretation process will refer to algorithms that sift through and interpret the data rather than chemical reactions.

At their simplest, trackers used to consist primarily of an accelerometer to measure steps (movement), some memory to store data, a battery to power the device and Bluetooth to send the data to a smartphone. However, a modern health-focused wearable such as a Whoop 4.0 band contains 5 LEDS with green, red, and infrared light, while the latest Oura ring contains 7 thermometers. The miniaturisation of powerful sensors means that these devices are now capable of far more detailed tracking than just movement.

Given the variety of tracker types available, there isn't room here to describe all of the possible technologies involved. From a technical point of view, in terms of measuring biomarkers, I'll discuss perhaps the primary one that makes modern wearables so powerful - Photoplethysmography (PPG) - and which enables most of the key cardiovascular measurements.

PPG

A combination of LEDs and photodetectors offers a low cost and simple means of non-invasively monitoring pulse rates and some elements of blood composition. A PPG sensor measures changes in light intensity reflected back through the skin. The changes in light intensity are associated with small variations in the blood through the cardiac cycle. Modern green LEDs, compared to infrared light[227], are especially sensitive for both oxyhaemoglobin (oxygenated blood) and deoxyhaemoglobin (blood without oxygen present).

PPG detection can be achieved at multiple sites around the body. Fingertip sensors are used in hospital settings where normal body movement may not be available. However, in consumer settings, the preferred sites tend to be fingers or wrists due to practicality for all-day wearing, while earlobes may suit some devices such as earphones or earbuds, worn during sports training or sleep. In an example slightly outside the scope of our focus here on viral diagnostics, a potentially very interesting development is the use of PPG, in devices now coming to market, that enable continuous Blood Pressure monitoring on a wristband.

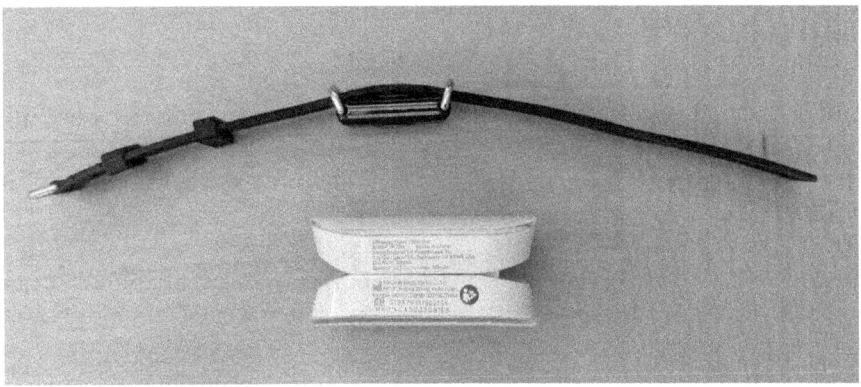

Figure 57: An Aktiia[228] PPG Continuous Blood Pressure strap (top) and a fingertip Pulse Oximeter (bottom)

For a more detailed technical description of PPG, refer to this 2018 article in the International Journal of Biosensors & Bioelectronics[229].

PPG technology underlies many of the important parameters measured by trackers:

- HR/RH
- HRV
- SPo2

Heart Rate (HR) & Resting Heart Rate (RHR)

HR is a staple output of almost all so-called fitness trackers. While chest-worn bands are typically more accurate than wrist devices, the convenience of watches or bands means they are far more popular for consumer use. Using PPG, the HR (measured in beats per minute or bpm) is determined by the volumetric change of blood - i.e., measuring how much blood passes through the spot illuminated by the LEDs as the heart beats.

Between individuals, there's a wide range of values for what constitutes a normal heart rate, and it varies based on an individual's activity levels - for example you'd expect it will be higher when walking compared to sitting, though many other factors will influence it, including age and medications[230]. Of more diagnostic value is your Resting Heart Rate (RHR) - your typical HR when at rest in a normal temperature without recent strenuous activity. Research looking at individual daily RHRs over two years found that each person has a relatively consistent RHR, for them, that fluctuates by a median of only 3 bpm weekly[231].

As a metric, RHR is useful for monitoring your overall fitness levels and cardiac health - a lower resting heart rate is usually a positive sign - in general, when your HR decreases, it means that each beat is more effective. Women's RHR tends to be about 3pm higher than males of equivalent age - a detailed 10-year study of average RHR for all age groups from the US DHHS is available on the CDC website[232]. While averages are useful in general comparisons, a healthy baseline reading is essential for individual diagnostic applications.

Heart Rate Variability (HRV)

A more advanced metric measured using PPG technology, but not found on all trackers, is Heart Rate Variability (HRV). HRV refers to the small changes in the time intervals between heart beats - known as the interbeat intervals (IBIs) or RR intervals.

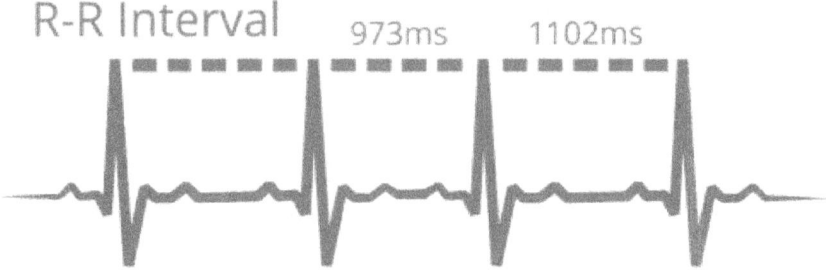

Figure 58: RR Intervals. Source:[233]

HRV is determined by the interplay between the parasympathetic and sympathetic nervous systems and follows a 24-hour circadian pattern. HRV changes significantly with age and is also influenced by gender, diet and stress. HRV is a complex field and not just the simple number presented by most fitness trackers, though a decrease in this average value may be sufficient to signal potential infection or other adverse influence - for example, one study explored lowered HRV as an indicator of the onset of sepsis[234]. For a more complete discussion of HRV, refer to this article[235] or, for non-technical explanation, this link[236] is quite accessible.

SPo2

The widespread availability of PPG means that today, a simple $50 pulse oximetry device can test arterial oxygen saturation in a quick, simple, non-invasive, affordable way, whereas previously this required an intra-arterial needle puncture and a laboratory test, known as an arterial blood gas (ABG) test.

Pulse oximetry is a PPG-powered technique used to measure the oxygen level (oxygen saturation) of the blood. Unlike the other PPG measures discussed above relating to cardiac function, in this case the purpose is to determine if the oxygen level in your blood is sufficient. Heavily oxygenated blood absorbs more infrared light, which is measured using the PPG sensors; the reading is given as a % and a value of less than 92% would usually be a cause for concern, meriting further investigation.

There are many stories, from the COVID-19 pandemic, of the importance of these devices to enable remote monitoring of patients to determine if their condition was at risk of deteriorating to the point of requiring hospitalisation. At times of peak hospital demand, this enabled at-home supervision of patients who otherwise would have required admission for observation[237,238].

Although affordable pulse oximeters offer a non-invasive method for monitoring blood oxygen saturation, further work needs to be done urgently to address differences in performance of the devices by skin type. As shown in multiple reports[239], including this 2022 study[240], many pulse oximeters have not been adequately calibrated and tested across a diverse range of skin colours.

Respiratory Rate

Your respiratory rate, or the number of breaths you take per minute, is expected to be between 12 and 20 for typical adults while at rest. An increase in this rate may be a sign of illness as it indicates your body is struggling to supply sufficient oxygen. For adults, an elevated respiratory rate would usually be considered to be more than 20 RPM, though it would need to be assessed relative to an individual's normal rate where known. Rapid breathing is more technically known as *tachypnea*; to most people it would feel like the sensation of shortness of breath.

Sensors use a variety of techniques to measure respiratory rate but most commonly *Respiratory Sinus Arrhythmia* - monitoring the fact that your heart rate increases when you inhale and decreases when you exhale. While respiratory rate monitoring can be included in fitness trackers, there are some dedicated respiratory rate monitors.

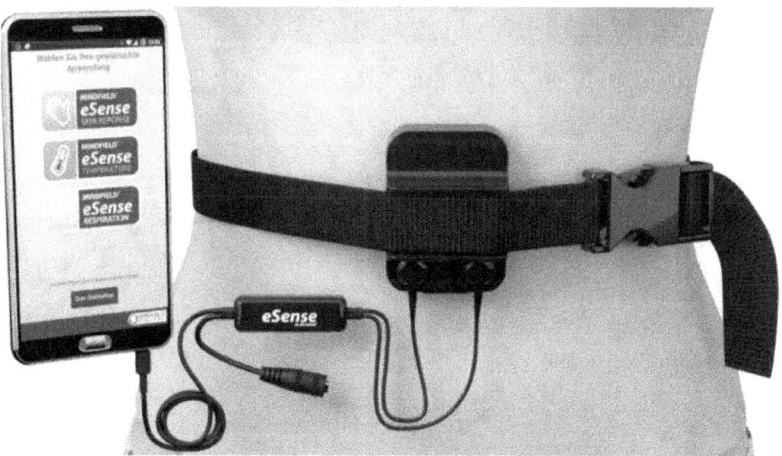

Figure 59: the Mindfield eSense Respiration sensor offers dedicated respiratory rate tracking[241]

As noted earlier, a change in respiration rate is not a diagnosis of SARS-CoV-2 or any other infection. However, it *can* indicate an infection - which could be COVID-19, Influenza or another respiratory infection e.g., RSV. although increased respiratory rate is more common with COVID-19 than other ILI. It could also indicate stress, dehydration or non-medical etiologies such as drugs, caffeine or even poor air quality due to pollution.

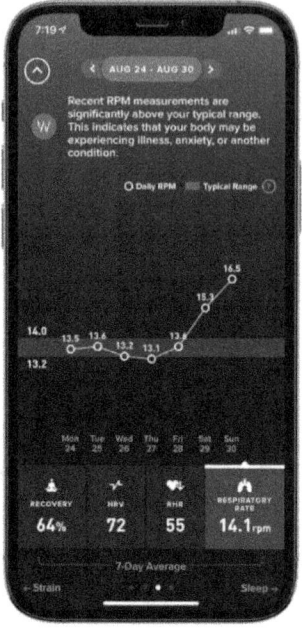

Figure 60: An example WHOOP report showing an increase in respiration per minute that might indicate illness. Source: WHOOP

Temperature

From the beginning of the COVID-19 pandemic, fever or elevated core body temperature was one of the major symptoms of infection. Although there was widespread use of temperature checks for admission to various locations, this "snapshot" checking of temperature at a point in time only isn't as potentially useful as continuous monitoring.

While some tracking devices include temperature sensors, there are dedicated wearable temperature sensors that can be used where the exposure risk for viral infections is elevated. For example, the TempTraq patch is being trialled for frontline healthcare workers at the University Hospitals Cleveland Medical Center. Each patch lasts for 72 hours and enables the hospital to remotely monitor staff for signs of elevated temperature[242]. A 2017 study from Stanford University, using a variety of wearable devices, noted correlations between detected increases in temperature/HR/RHR and illnesses confirmed by external gold-standard testing devices[243].

Although not a wearable device, studies conducted by smart thermometer maker, Kinsa, showed elevated levels of fever in areas with high incidences of COVID-19[244].

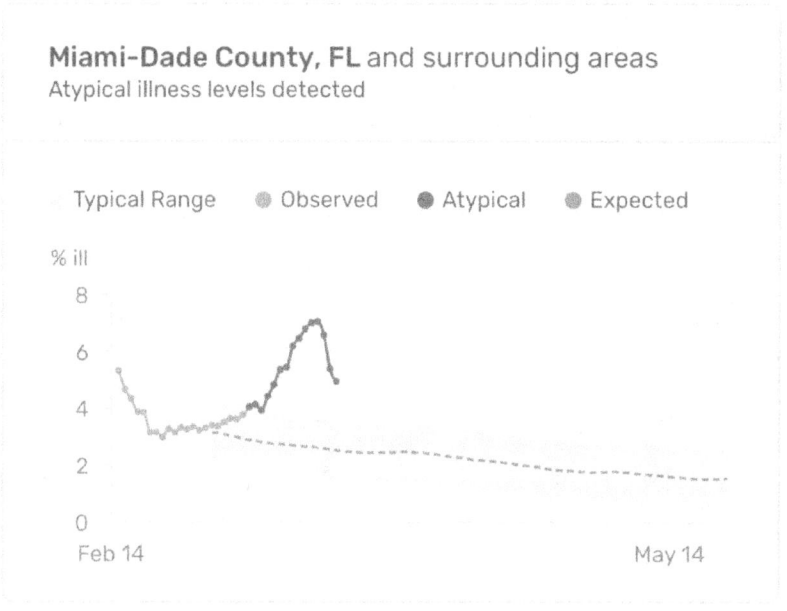

Figure 61 - Kinsa data showing unexpected increase in tracked incidences of fever as COVID-19 emerged in 2020

The accuracy of skin temperature tracking can be impacted by the monitoring site, exercise and environmental factors. So, on its own, skin temperature tracking may be of limited value but, when combined with changes in RHR and HRV data, can be an additional supporting indicator.

As noted in the study regarding HR, individual context is also important when dealing with temperature. A tracking device's sensitivity to detect small, but meaningful, changes in body temperature may be limited without contextual information, such as baseline variability in circadian body temperature, phase in menstrual cycle and other temperature-modulating biological rhythms.

For COVID-19 infections, though frequent, elevated temperature is not as common a symptom as often believed - one study of NYC hospital admissions showed just 31% had a fever at time of admission. A greater percentage (43.1%) of individuals had a heart rate of >100 bpm[245], which emphasises the added value of combining vital sign monitoring and not over-relying on a single reading.

Early Warnings: Trackers

A key benefit of trackers is that users wear them continuously, allowing the app associated with the tracker to analyse biomarkers non-invasively and establish a normal/baseline for comparison purposes. Even when a user may be unaware of any deviation from normal, the algorithms in the app can spot even minor variations that may indicate a potential concern.

The individual personal element of trackers is very important. Take, for example, heart rate as an indicator. There is a wide natural variation between people which makes an absolute number less useful - if my resting heart rate (RHR) is typically 65 and my brother's is normally 55, the difference isn't indicative of an infection. However, if mine suddenly rises to 75, this may be an early sign of my body's reaction to an invader. Changes in resting heart rates are a reasonably reliable indicator of a potential problem:

Doctors have long known that a higher resting heart rate -- the number of times each minute the heart beats while a person is sitting or sleeping -- can be a sign that the body's immune system is ramping up for a fight. For example, research has shown that young men with fevers had increases in their resting heart rate of about 8.5 beats per minute (bpm) for about every 2-degree Fahrenheit increase in body temperature[246].

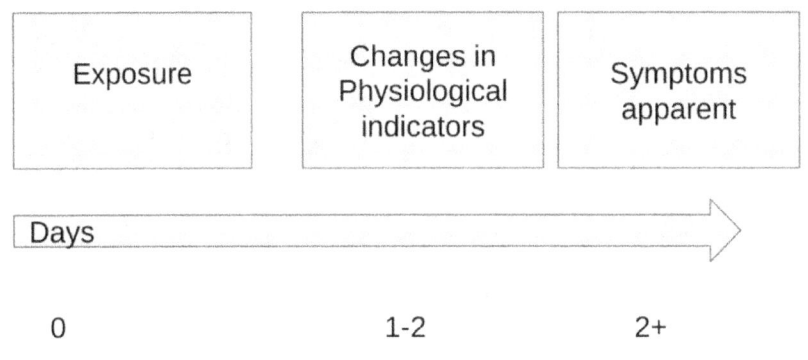

Figure 62: Trackers can notice changes before onset of symptoms

So, while a change in resting heart rate may be nothing untoward - perhaps a bad night's sleep - if a person can't easily explain it, there may be a basis for further investigation. Depending on the pathogenesis of a given disease, the vital signs monitored by trackers may or may not be relevant. In the case of COVID-19, fever is a fairly common early symptom and thus trackers that monitor body temperature could highlight increases before the user is aware they have pyrexia (fever). For someone who has a confirmed case of COVID-19 (or other respiratory ailment), those trackers that include SPo2 monitors may warn of a deteriorating condition, again before the user is fully aware themselves - Silent hypoxemia (below-normal level of oxygen in your blood is another sign of infection and evidence impending deterioration[247].)

Wearable Parameter Summary

Here's a quick summary table of some of the devices mentioned in this Chapter.

Device:	**Fitbit Sense**	**Whoop 4**	Oura 3	Circul+
Form Factor	Watch	Band	Ring	Ring
Price	€249	€288 (annual membership inc free device)	€314	$299
Temperature	Y	Y	Y	Y
HR/RHR	Y	Y	Y	Y
Respiratory	Y	Y	Y	N
SPo2	Y	Y	Y	Y
HRV	Y	Y	Y	Y
Other	EDA, ECG			ECG, BP

Diagnosing the Sensors

In this section, we'll outline some recent research into the viability of trackers for detecting illness ahead of symptom onset or user awareness, with a particular emphasis on studies into the use of wearables in finding presymptomatic COVID-19 cases.

Interest in the utility of trackers for illness detection predates COVID-19 but (a recurring theme in this book), interest in the space has accelerated rapidly with the advent of the pandemic. It also aligns with the greater availability of capable wearable devices in the decades since prior epidemics. Before we talk about Covid, though, let's review some earlier studies. The more recent improvement in wearables' sensor capabilities means it's not useful to look back too far - even the difference between parameters measured in a 2016 study[248] and more recent studies show meaningful advances in the technologies in a 4-5 year timeframe.

Influenza Studies

Recognising that there were no presymptomatic screening methods to identify individuals infected with a respiratory virus, so as to prevent disease spread and to predict its trajectory, a 2018 Challenge study[249] (i.e., where volunteers are knowingly infected) inoculated 31 participants with influenza (H1N1) and 18 participants with rhinovirus. Models trained using data on wearable devices were able to distinguish between infection and non-infection with 92% accuracy for H1N1 and 88% accuracy for rhinovirus. Participants in the H1N1 challenge study wore the E4 wristband (Empatica Inc, a $1500 research-focused wearable rather than a consumer device) for 1 day before and 11 days after the inoculation (on the morning of day 2), before clinical discharge. The E4 wristband measures heart rate, skin temperature, electrodermal activity (EDA), and movement. The research benefit of a challenge study is that the exact time of exposure is known, unlike retrospective studies that search the data for indicators after symptoms appear or a diagnostic test confirms infection.

Another 2019[250] study evaluated whether wearable sensor data could improve influenza surveillance at the state level and examined de-identified data of 47,249 users in the top five states who wore a Fitbit consistently during the study period, including more than 13·3 million total RHR and sleep measures. The conclusion was that the Fitbit data significantly improved Influenza Like Illness (ILI) predictions in all five states: *Week-to-week changes in the proportion of Fitbit users with abnormal data were associated with week-to-week changes in ILI rates in most cases.*

COVID-19 Studies

The emergence of COVID-19 has super-charged investment and research into technologies, both novel and existing, that can be applied to identifying respiratory illnesses. Again, it's important to emphasize here that no tracker can (yet) differentiate COVID-19 indicators or symptoms - the research for now needs to address the ability to detect any signs that *might* relate to a COVID-19 infection, but which on diagnostic analysis, may be confirmed to be another condition with similar presentation, such as Influenza or RSV. Myriad studies have been set up since the emergence of COVID-19 that may yield invaluable insights into the pros and cons of wearable sensors in seeking infection indicators that are not otherwise apparent. In this section, I'll highlight extracts published to date from a number of major studies.

DETECT Study

The Scripps Research Institute launched an app-based research project named DETECT[251] (Digital Engagement and Tracking for Early Control and Treatment), where individuals share their sensor data, self-reported symptoms, diagnoses and electronic health record data with researchers. The aim was to track both individual and population-level viral illnesses, which in many cases were then confirmed by laboratory tests as COVID-19. Although a number of wearables devices were eligible for the study, the majority (78.4%) were from market leader Fitbit. At 62% female, the 30,529 cohort was not nationally representative, though there were participants from all US States.

TemPredict

The TemPredict study by UCSF in March of 2020[252] used the Oura Ring to capture continuous physiological data (HR/HRV), including peripheral temperature. The study was expanded from 50 initial users to over 65,000 following a $5m research award[253], though the composition - 66% Male, 81% White/Caucasian - highlights questions of access to technology. The study supports the hypothesis that wearable sensors can detect illnesses in the absence of symptom recognition, as the majority of participants exhibited temperature anomalies prior to symptom reports.

In another variation of testing with Oura Ring users a study[254], looking at whether the response detected by an Oura ring correlated with the strength of antibodies generated by vaccination, found that on the night immediately following the second mRNA injection (Moderna-NIAID and Pfizer-BioNTech) increases in dermal temperature deviation and resting heart rate, as well as decreases in heart rate variability and deep sleep, were each statistically significantly correlated with greater antibody responses.

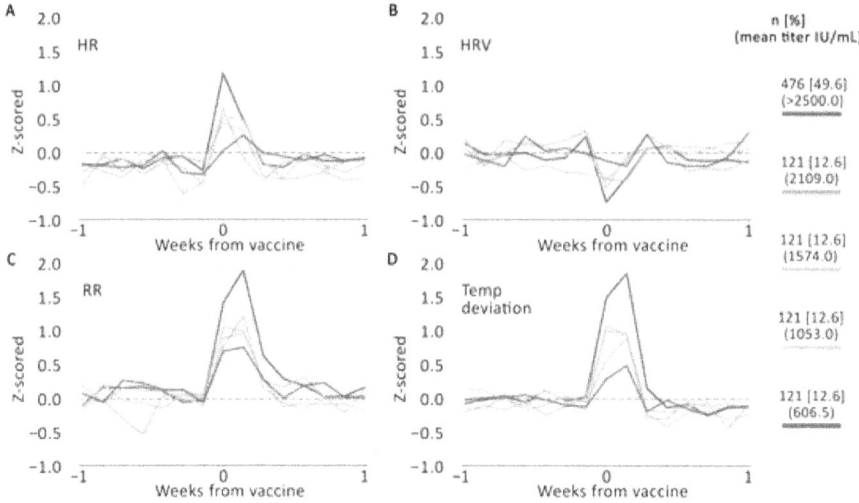

Figure 63: Indicators (HR, RR, HRV and Temperature) before and after vaccination

Mount Sinai/Warrior Watch

A Mount Sinai[255] study of 297 staff found that subtle changes in a participant's heart rate variability (HRV) measured by an Apple Watch were able to signal the onset of COVID-19 up to seven days before the individual was diagnosed via a PCR test.

Significant changes in the HRV (or more precisely the standard deviation of RR Intervals - SDNN) were observed in participants during the 7 days prior to and the 7 days after a diagnosis of COVID-19 when compared to uninfected participants. Focusing on one particular HRV parameter, there was a significant difference between the amplitude of the standard deviation of the interbeat interval of normal sinus beats (SDNN) between uninfected participants (5.31 milliseconds) compared to individuals during the 7-day period prior to a COVID-19 diagnosis (0.29 milliseconds) and participants during the 7 days after a COVID-19 diagnosis (1.22 milliseconds).

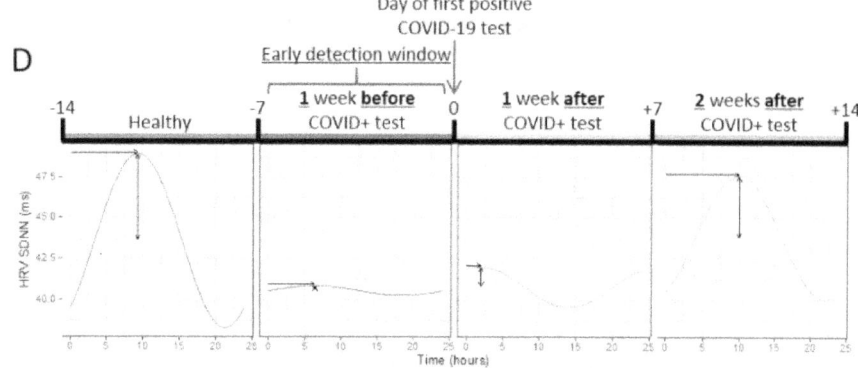

Figure 64: changes in HRV values observed in the study

Additionally, the researchers found that, 7 to 14 days after diagnosis with COVID-19, the HRV pattern began to normalize. The study was published as a peer-reviewed article in February 2021[256] with the conclusion:

In summary, we demonstrated a relationship between longitudinally collected HRV acquired from a commonly used wearable device and SARS-CoV-2 infection. These preliminary results support the further evaluation of HRV as a biomarker of SARS-CoV-2 infection by remote sensing. Although further study is needed, our findings may enable the identification of SARS-CoV-2 infection during the presymptomatic period, in asymptomatic carriers, and prior to diagnosis by a SARS-CoV-2 nasal swab PCR test. These findings warrant further evaluation of this approach to track and identify COVID-19 infections and possibly other types of infection.

Miscellaneous Studies

A further study, a preprint report at time of this writing, describes a real-time smartwatch-based (primarily Fitbit and Apple Watch) alerting system for the detection of aberrant physiological and activity signals (e.g., RHR) associated with early infection onset at the individual level. With a cohort of 3,246 participants, the study found that alerts were generated for pre-symptomatic and asymptomatic COVID-19 infections in 78% of cases, and pre-symptomatic signals were observed a median of three days prior to symptom onset[257].

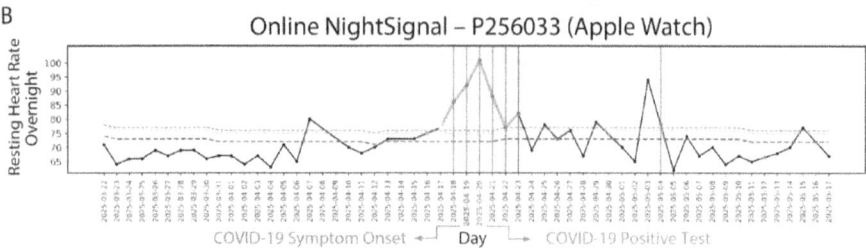

Figure 65: Example of an Alert triggered 2 days before onset of symptoms based on RHR

Another study, published in late 2020 by wearable maker Whoop, identified 20% of presymptomatic COVID-19-infected individuals two days before symptom onset on the basis of changes in respiratory rate detected by the wearable. The study concludes: *the findings indicate that the early stages of the infection may have a detectable signature that could help identify individuals who should self-isolate and seek testing. Future investigations should examine the performance of respiratory rate-based algorithms to classify infection among larger and more diverse cohorts.*[258]

Covid-Red

COVID-RED, an EU project[259] that is part of the EU Innovative Medicines Initiative, was designed to use a wearable device (A €160 bracelet named "Ava"[260] measuring respiration rate, pulse rate, skin temperature, and heart rate variability, originally designed to support fertility tracking) for the purpose of early detection and monitoring of COVID-19. The project aims to recruit 20,000 people in the Netherlands and will compare the wearable biometric data and user-reports with serology and PCR results.

Also in Europe, the Robert Koch Institute (a key German Public Health organisation) created an app[261] to collect user data from a variety of wearable technology sources - Apple Health, Amazfit, Fitbit, Garmin, Google Fit, Huawei Health, Oura, Polar, Samsung Health and Withings devices were all supported. The app was downloaded over 500,000 times and helped researchers correlate HR data with reported symptoms.

Finally for this section, I'll mention another report[262] showing promising findings of detectable changes in monitored signs before user-reported symptom onset. The graph below shows summary findings, including respiration rate, heart rate, 2 HRV submetrics (root mean square of successive differences or RMSSD and shannon entropy), from a Fitbit Data study of 2745 (self-selecting) individuals, as a function of day, where day 0 represents the start of symptoms. This study also shows a 2-3 week recovery to normal readings.

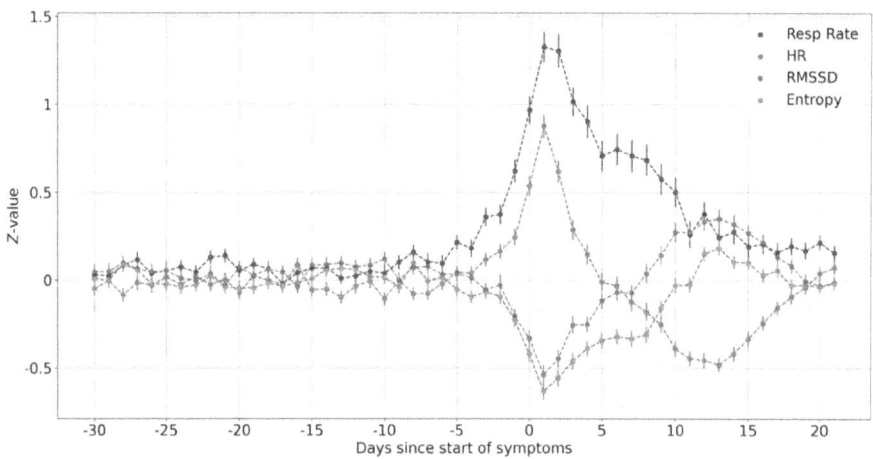

Figure 66: HRV Changes before symptom onset

Accuracy and Regulation

While most of the studies clearly show some promise in being able to point to a potential infection, based on changes in physiological markers, concerns remain over the accuracy of sensors. Also, as with the tests we described earlier, there may be user error - failure to wear the device correctly can adversely affect results. To avoid complex regulatory requirements, many device manufacturers take care not to classify their products as suitable for medical use. Some manufacturers do submit their products for FDA approval (e.g., Withings with its Scanwatch that measures HR, RHR, RR, SPo2 and ECG), while even some high-end manufacturers opt to rely on marketing messaging to position their products as non-medical but clearly of interest to well-being enthusiasts and athletes. As an example, Whoop provides the following warning:

The products and services of WHOOP are not medical devices, are not intended to diagnose COVID-19, the flu or any other disease, and should not be used as a substitute for professional medical advice, diagnosis or treatment. All content available through the products and services of WHOOP is for general informational purposes only.[263]

As well as addressing concerns about the fundamental accuracy of consumer devices, there is likely to be increased regulatory scrutiny too of issues that have come to light during the COVID-19 pandemic, such as the accuracy of PPG measurements being affected by skin colour[264].

Personally, I can attest that my Fitbit (Sense) and Oura Ring (Gen 3) both reacted to vital signs changes after my COVID vaccine doses - as I experienced normal brief side effects - and returned to baseline as the symptoms subsided[265], very much in keeping with the results reported in the study above.

Other Sensors

The promise of being able potentially to "see" an illness a day or two before symptom onset means we're likely to continue to see innovation in the capabilities and form factors of wearable devices. Building on the increased interest in personal well-being, arising from the pandemic, consumer electronic companies will redouble their efforts to market these non-invasive "indicators" to consumers looking for signs they may need a diagnostic test. Though vendors will be cautious about over-claiming their usefulness in disease detection so as not to attract regulatory scrutiny, I would expect suppliers to continue emphasizing potential health benefits of sensors-equipped wearables given that public awareness of asymptomatic and presymptomatic conditions remains high. A growing number of clinical-grade wearables will be deployed in hospital settings too, an example being Empatica EmbracePlus, which received CE certification for COVID-19 detection.

To continue to reach wider audiences, device makers will have to address the challenges that have blunted demand for wearables, such as poor battery life (especially in the case of smartwatches: many offer several other functions but may require daily charging, which makes night-time monitoring difficult). A relevant interesting report[266] from 2021 summarises promising developments in ferroelectric polymer transducers and organic diodes for use in imperceptible sensing applications and energy harvesting systems, which would enable self-powering devices, thereby removing the need for regular recharging which limits the convenience of current solutions.

As well as smartwatches and fitness trackers, a few other sensor approaches offer some additional ways to watch for potential infections:

Passive Exposure Sensor

Researchers at Yale School of Public Health have proposed a passive air sampler device that clips onto your shirt collar. The device assesses levels of exposure to SARS-CoV-2 (although it could equally be applied to other pathogens). It captures aerosols that deposit on a silicon polymer (polydimethylsiloxane or PDMS) surface, which is then tested using RT-qPCR to determine the level of Sars-CoV-2 (or another analyte). Project leader Dr. Godri Pollitt noted that the clip can detect low levels of virus - well below the estimated SARS-CoV-2 infectious dose - but could serve to identify exposure events early, alerting people to get tested or quarantine[267].

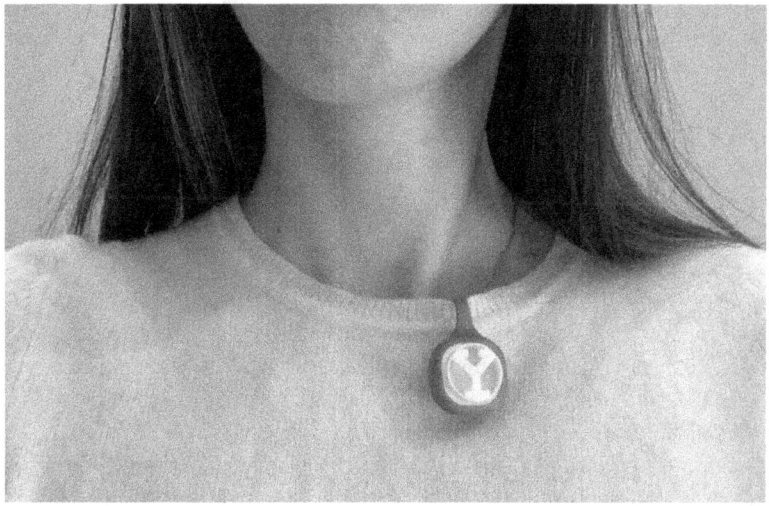

Figure 67: The Yale Fresh Air Clip. Source: Yale[268].

Acoustic Epidemiology and Diagnostics

For respiratory complaints, coughing is frequently a key symptom. Although there are obvious privacy-related concerns for continuous sound monitoring to assess coughing, it is conceivably a useful route of inquiry.

Artificial Intelligence, or more specifically Machine Learning, can be applied to analysing cough sounds and patterns to diagnose respiratory conditions. An interesting 2022 report[269] describes the role of technology in detecting biomarkers in cough sounds, specifically in the field of TB (which kills over 1m people annually). The paper also references other research on cough analysis for COVID-19[270], in which a classification algorithm was reported to detect COVID-19 infections, with 98% sensitivity and 94% specificity, among people with a cough, based on a sample of 5320 individuals. This area of study may eventually lead to a smartphone-based algorithm that could triage cough symptoms and identify cases requiring more urgent medical intervention.

Coughing Sensors

Just as the COVID-19 pandemic was beginning in March 2020, a group of researchers published a paper describing a system called *FluSense* that could monitor hospital waiting rooms for signs of ILI[271] by capturing crowd-level bio-clinical signals in an unobtrusive and privacy-sensitive manner - trained on more than 350,000 waiting room thermal images and 21 million non-speech audio samples from the hospital waiting areas.

An MIT report[272] described how an AI could be trained to detect indications of a COVID-19 infection in the cough of an asymptomatic person with sensitivity of 100% and a specificity of 83.2%. The authors conclude that *"AI techniques can produce a free, non-invasive, real-time, any-time, instantly distributable, large-scale COVID-19 asymptomatic screening tool"*.

In the consumer space, Amazon's Halo fitness band already includes microphones that can be enabled to assess the wearer's sentiment by analysing their voice, while a fascinating research project showed the value of Alexa smart speakers for passive detection of Agonal breathing, which can be an indicator of cardiac arrest[273]. But from a purely diagnostic point of view coughing is, of course, a very obvious symptom (compared to, say, temperature) so "detection" of coughing isn't a major focus. However, changes in the *nature* of a cough may be clinically useful if detected.

Dedicated devices such as this small chest-worn patch from VitalConnect (San Jose, CA), which partnered with the U.S. Department of Health and Human Service's Biomedical Advanced Research and Development (BARDA) to deploy the company's single-use, chest-mounted patch, in nursing homes to track vulnerable elderly patients[274], could be a useful early warning system for the vulnerable or those in shared living spaces. The patch adds cough monitoring in addition to use of devices using the more common metrics discussed above.

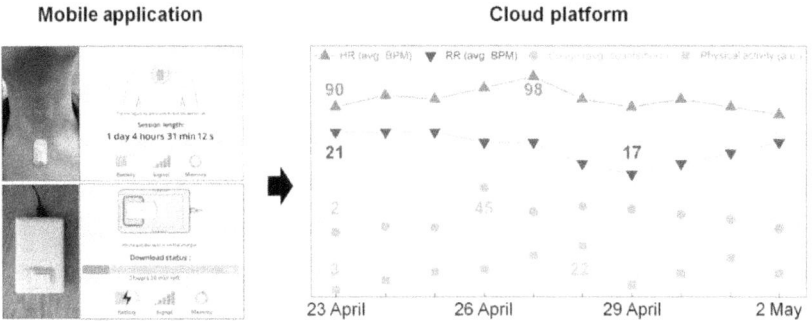

Figure 68: An example of the VitalConnect platform

Deviating for a moment from the viral focus of this book, I want to mention briefly some promising adjacent diagnostics work, looking at the potential of AI-powered tools to assist in tracking Parkinson's Disease (PD). It is a reminder of how new technologies in diagnostics can be applied to an almost endless array of diseases. In this study[275], data from 7,671 individuals was used to create an AI model to detect PD and estimate severity and progression. The system works in a touchless manner, by extracting breathing patterns from radio waves that bounce off a person's body during sleep.

Patient Friendly

Whether you regard promotion of the role of consumer devices in well-being as the medicalisation of consumers or the consumerisation of medicine, the broader use of such tracking devices simply to measure vital signs may, in fact, help with illness detection way beyond COVID-19. In an era of increasing telehealth, diagnosis can be more difficult, so the added datapoints provided by tracker devices may be especially useful. But, to avoid a flurry of false positives, there will need to be a concerted effort by regulators, together with comprehensive public education regarding the appropriate use and interpretation of these devices.

I would expect the cost of functional tracking devices to fall within reach of many consumers in the coming years, even in RLS, although certified devices may command a premium. Data suggest that vulnerable patient populations typically underreport their symptoms, so remote detection of disease through objective measures is a possible way to improve timely escalation of care[276].

Glucometers and Antibody Testing

We mentioned Continuous Glucose Monitoring (CGM) devices earlier. For many diabetic patients, they have significantly improved the management of the condition but there may be further uses for this technology. Although diagnostics tests typically rely on dedicated instruments and assays, examples are emerging of other healthcare-related devices being repurposed to assist in virus hunting, with huge attendant benefits for availability and cost reductions, compared to dedicated testing devices.

One interesting instance was reported in the Journal of the American Chemistry Society in Summer 2022[277], detailing how existing, widely available glucometers could be used for the quantitative detection of SARS-CoV-2 antibodies, with potential for detecting other targets too. This study showed that the glucose meter-based assay, containing the enzyme *invertase*, could reliably detect IgG antibodies for SARS-CoV-2 and its performance was comparable with commercially available laboratory or POC ELISA tests.

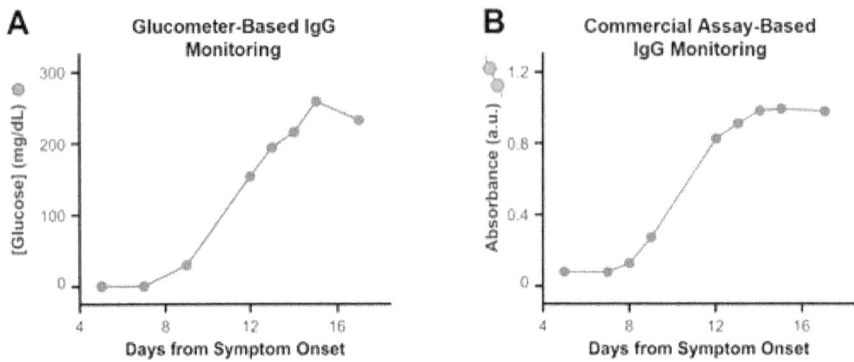

Figure 69: Comparing adapted Glucometer Antibody testing results vs lab test

The testing was carried out using a standard glucose meter from Nova Biomedical[278].

Chemistry vs Devices

2020 saw the phrase "Non Pharmaceutical Intervention" enter the common lexicon. The emergence of more accurate sensors, that can non-invasively feed algorithms continuous data for analysis, will see Non-Chemical Diagnostics grow in popularity. A bit like an automotive check engine light for humans, they may not tell you what's wrong but offer a non-specific indicator that further checks are advised.

Chapter 11: Emerging Diagnostic Innovations

Although PCR and Antigen tests were new names to most people before the COVID-19 pandemic, they are relatively mature diagnostic technologies. And while the extension of NAAT technologies to POC and domestic settings is already underway, there are many new diagnostic technologies at varying stages of development that will usher in a new era in our relationship with viruses and other pathogens. For future pandemics, a key question is what next generation diagnostic technologies might be available and what improvements will they offer?

As the pressure to increase laboratory testing capacity to cope with PCR ingredient shortages and COVID-19 surges, some scientists have revisited slightly older diagnostics methods such as Immunodiffusion[279] and Time-Resolved Förster Resonance Energy Transfer (TR-FRET)[280], as well as newer versions of staple technologies such as ELISA and Flow Cytometry, that could expand laboratory testing capacity. Refining existing proven methods can offer quick wins but, ultimately, the race is on to have more advanced technologies to bolster our fight against viral threats. In this chapter I'll mention recent advances in Flow Cytometry but then I'll focus on a few of the most promising new developments, not yet widely available, but offering exciting potential.

Flow Cytometry

Flow cytometry, a laser-based technique that analyses, counts and sorts cells, has been a dependable laboratory tool for decades. However, improvements in technology resolution have enabled flow virometry - the application of the same approach to smaller entities, viruses down to just 40nm in size[281].

While previous generation Flow Cytometry only worked with particles no smaller than 300nm, more recent versions of flow virometry have been used in the detection of HIV, HSV and Dengue Fever viruses:

Virus	Virion Particle Sizes
HIV[282]	120-150nm
HSV[283]	120-150nm
Dengue Fever[284]	45-60nm
SARS-CoV-2	70-90nm

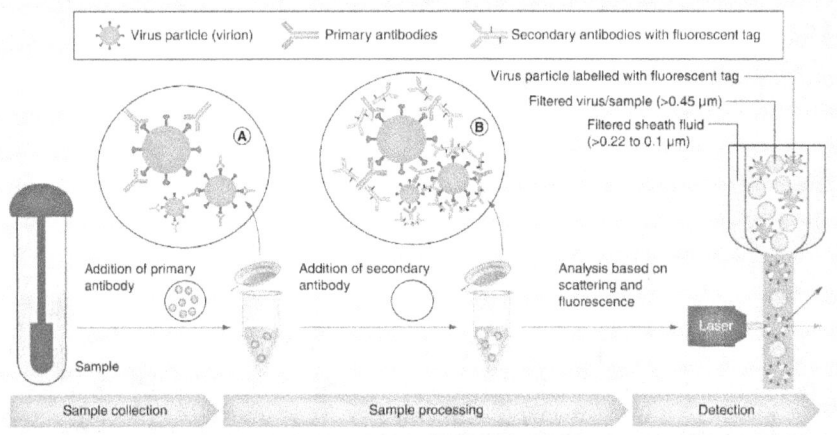

Figure 70: An illustration of Flow Virometry workflow

Although it offers potential to supplement PCR-based lab capacity (e.g., in the event of a shortage of PCR reagents), flow virometry as a method does still require biosafety labs certified to level 3 (BSL3) which are relatively rare.

Future Diagnostics

Although the refinement of existing technologies is a relatively low risk, low cost and reliable method to advance the field of diagnostics, the promise of breakthroughs is based largely on the development of novel technologies.

Each of these future diagnostic technologies would require at least an entire book to cover it in detail, so here I just want to provide a brief summary of some promising areas that researchers are excited about for the years ahead and which should support improvements in healthcare as well as assisting preparedness for any future epidemics/pandemics. Some of these technologies are new; others involve re-purposing technologies originally applied in adjacent testing or therapeutic areas.

In this Chapter, we'll explore:

- CRISPR-Cas
- Next Generation Sequencing (NGS)
- Microfluidics
- Others

CRISPR

CRISPR (pronounced "crisper") is most commonly considered as a means of editing genes, though it relates to a natural immune response process found in bacteria as a result of infection with phages (viruses). It stands for *Clustered Regularly Interspaced Short Palindromic Repeats* and refers to special sequences of DNA and associated proteins or enzymes that can identify and cut strands of DNA very precisely. For genetic editing, its power lies in the ability to find a specific piece of DNA in a cell, which can then be edited. CRISPR's use in diagnostics is based on this ability to *find* a sequence rather than the next step of editing it which is the domain of most research for potential genetic treatments.

Without going too far into the mechanics of CRISPR here, there are a number of types of CRISPR associated (Cas) nucleases (these are enzymes that can cut sequences) of particular interest. Six major types and more than 22 subtypes of Cas proteins have been identified but Cas12a and Cas13a are the ones most commonly used to date in SARS-CoV-2 related research, as some of these can be programmed to target viral RNA sequences. While Cas12a is DNA-specific, Cas13a works with RNA.

Interest in CRISPR-based diagnostic protocols has risen dramatically due to COVID-19, but work had already been underway on using CRISPR for detecting other infectious viruses. Two examples include Specific High-sensitivity Enzymatic Reporter unLOCKing (SHERLOCK)[285] and DNA Endonuclease-Targeted CRISPR Trans Reporter (DETECTR)[286], which were previously proven with Zika virus, cytomegalovirus and BK virus. These use isothermal amplification to amplify the target sequences in a sample where RNA-guided Cas12a or 13a nucleases recognise and bind target sequences of the amplified sample, resulting in cleavage of nucleic acid reporters for detection via fluorescence or LFT. These tests are low-cost and can be performed in as little as 60 minutes with POC-sized equipment.

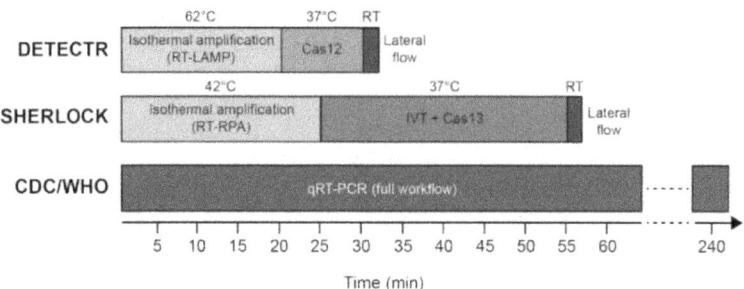

Figure 71: Image from Mammoth Biosciences' white paper comparing the diagnostic workflow times with DETECTR, SHERLOCK, and typical CDC/WHO gold standard RT-qPCR method

Sherlock Biosciences received EUA approval for its lab-run 1 hour SARS-CoV-2 CRISPR test kit in 2020 and has announced its intention to create a hand-held device (INSPECTR[287]) with similar technology[288]. In another development likely to boost CRISPR-based diagnostics, researchers have reported promising results from the use of Machine Learning to design more effective assays extremely rapidly[289].

CRISPR Multiplex and Microfluidics

CRISPR as a technique can also be extended to detect multiple targets. One research project[290] published in January 2021 describes Cas13-based assays capable of detecting SARS-CoV-2, MERS, and SARS, as well as influenza viruses such as, H1N1, H7N9, and H9N2 with a limit of detection (LOD) of 82 copies/μL. That compares with best-in-class PCR assays which typically have an LOD around 100 copies/μL[291], making this approach very promising (lower LOD is better).

CRISPR may be combined with other technologies to further improve diagnostic performance while reducing costs. A team of researchers, led by Dr. Cheri Ackerman from MIT, has described a CRISPR-Cas13 approach that uses microfluidics (see next section) to create a test capable of detecting a large number of pathogens across a large number of samples. Named CARMEN (Combinatorial Arrayed Reactions for Multiplexed Evaluation of Nucleic acids), it's a multiplexed assay that simultaneously differentiates over 169 human-associated viruses, including comprehensive subtyping of influenza A strains and multiplexed identification of dozens of HIV drug-resistance mutations. The miniaturisation enabled by microfluidics decreases reagent cost per test by more than 300-fold[292].

Low Cost CRISPR for RLS

In another interesting proof of concept, researchers at Harvard's Wyss Institute for Biologically Inspired Engineering recently developed a low-cost, easy to use POC-suitable solution that detects SARS-CoV-2 in saliva samples using SHERLOCK techniques. The battery powered reader unit (known as miSHERLOCK - minimally instrumented SHERLOCK) could cost as little as $15 and uses a smartphone as a display, making it potentially suitable for RLS. The authors discuss further potential applications beyond SARS-COV-2 as well as methods to reduce the cost per test further. They also note that the miSHERLOCK device demonstrated 96% sensitivity and 95% specificity compared to qPCR[293].

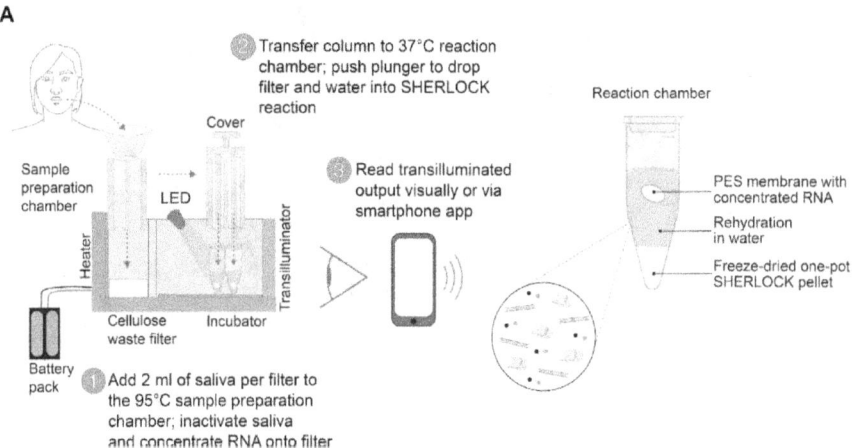

Figure 72: Low cost CRISPR - $15 battery-powered device

In a final example for this section, Fozouni et al[294] described the development of an amplification-free CRISPR-Cas13a assay, for direct detection of SARS-CoV-2 from nasal swab RNA, that can be read with a mobile phone-based microscope. The assay achieved ~100 copies/μL sensitivity in under 30 min of measurement time.

Since discovery, CRISPR diagnostic approaches have been difficult to deploy in RLS, but recent advances, where CRISPR is combined with microfluidics, show significant promise. Researchers[295] have described results using an electrokinetic microfluidic technique called isotachophoresis (ITP) to achieve results with reagent volumes more than 100 times lower than existing CRISPR assays, offering significant cost benefits.

CRISPR Therapeutics

Although we're focused on diagnostics here, researchers are also considering the potential for CRISPR-derived antiviral therapeutics[296] with early research underway on its efficacy against SARS-CoV-2. In a review of literature relating to the use of CRISPR during the COVID-19 pandemic, researchers[297] have noted greater focus on its application in the field of diagnostics, with less emphasis to date on treatments (therapeutics) than might be expected:

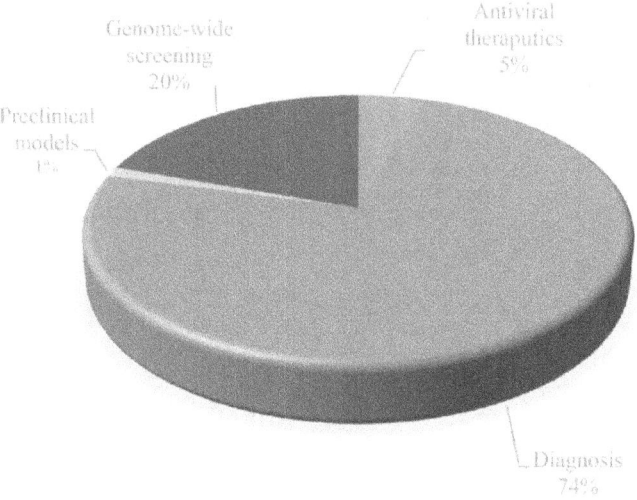

Figure 73: Categories of research using CRISPR for SARS-CoV-2

Abbott et al.[298], though, has expanded the application of CRISPR/Cas13 from its diagnostic function to therapeutic goals by its (memorably-named!) Prophylactic Antiviral CRISPR in the huMAN cells (PAC-MAN) approach. Contrary to traditional therapies, which have concentrated on triggering the human immune system to distinguish viral proteins and diminish viral entry into cells, this CRISPR/Cas13 system has focused on cleaving the viral RNA genome inside the infected cells or preventing the expression of protein-coding genes of the virus. This study showed it can *effectively degrade RNA from SARS-CoV-2 sequences and live influenza A virus (IAV) in human lung epithelial cells*. Delivery mechanisms remain a challenge but, according to the study's report: *with the development of a safe and effective system for respiratory tract delivery, PAC-MAN has the potential to become an important pan-coronavirus inhibition strategy.*

CRISPR-Cas is an extremely complex and exciting area that will play a huge role in biotechnology in the coming decades. If what you've read here is of particular interest to you, consider the following articles for more detail on CRISPR-Cas and its use in diagnostics[299],[300].

Next Generation Sequencing (NGS)

Unlike most testing methods that look for a specific target and then signal finding it, next-generation sequencing is an untargeted diagnostic method. It provides a readout of all genetic sequences in a patient sample and so can detect any pathogen, or pathogens, present. It is also key to tracking variants, discussed in Chapter 12.

NGS refers to a family of techniques including massively parallel signature sequencing, polony sequencing, 454 sequencing, Illumina technology, ion torrent technology, SOLiD DNA sequencing technology and DNA nanoball sequencing.[301] Beyond NGS, other emerging technologies include SMRT (Single Molecule Real Time) sequencing and Nanopore sequencing[302].

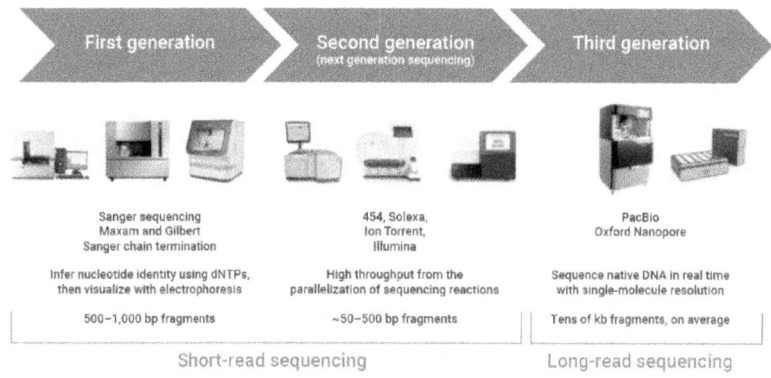

Figure 74: Rapid progress in genetic sequencing techniques

Sequencing identifies the precise order of the four nucleotide bases – Adenine (A), Guanine (G), Cytosine (C) and Thymine (T)/Uracil (U) - that make up a strand of DNA or RNA and determine its function. Work on sequencing dates back to the 1970s but recent advances have dramatically reduced the cost of sequencing and increased its speed. Compared to earlier sequencing techniques such as *Sanger* (also known as *Capillary Electrophoresis Sequencing - CES*) which ran a single DNA fragment at a time, NGS typically sequences millions of fragments simultaneously per run.

The ability to sequence samples quickly has been crucial during the COVID-19 pandemic, to track variants but also to provide the genomic sequence that has allowed the design of molecular tests. As mentioned in Chapter 6 on NAAT, the ability to design the primers quickly for SARS-CoV-2 RT-PCR tests relied on sequencing of the original strain of the virus. And, just as advances between the outbreak of SARS-CoV-1 and SARS-CoV-2 led to much quicker responses in 2020 than in 2003, the progress of NGS techniques will be similarly important and influential in speeding health system responses in future pandemics.

Sharing Sequences

Even since 2019/2020, the increased sequencing capacity provided by new techniques has enabled better surveillance of the pandemic that would have been possible earlier. Researchers all over the world who use NGS upload their findings into the GISAID EpiCoV Database at https://www.gisaid.org/hcov19-variants/. As at Feb 19, 2022, scientists in 154 countries had shared 1,459,312 Omicron genome sequences to the database. This sharing of nucleotide-level data allows for the tracking of mutations and the spread of the virus in great detail.

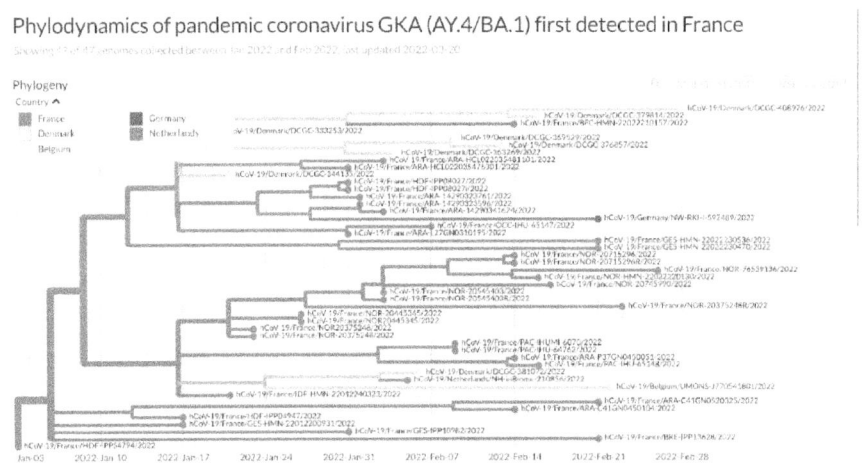

Figure 75: A screenshot of GISAID analysis of sequences uploaded from researchers

Note: Viral phylodynamics is defined as the study of how epidemiological, immunological, and evolutionary processes act and potentially interact to shape viral phylogenies. A phylogenetic tree is a branching diagram showing the evolutionary relationships based upon similarities and differences in physical or genetic characteristics[303].

NGS Devices

Although currently favoured only in research settings or public epidemiological/survey studies, due to its cost and relatively slow speed, advances in NGS technologies will likely see further clinical applications and even POC devices.

NGS devices can generate large amounts of sequence data at dramatically higher speed and lower cost than previous sequencing technologies. But, while it's very promising for the future of diagnostics to be able not only to identify the presence of a pathogen but to fully sequence it, the challenges of analysing the NGS output remain a limiting factor to wider use of the technology outside research facilities. For example, a $20,000 benchtop device from manufacturer Illumina[304] takes between 4.5 and 19 hours to run, and can produce up to 1.2gb of data per run. At the other end of the operational scale, Illuminia's largest sequencer (c$985,000) can produce 6000 gb during a c.40 hour run. The cost and quantity of data produced mean this technology is only really applicable in well-funded research settings.

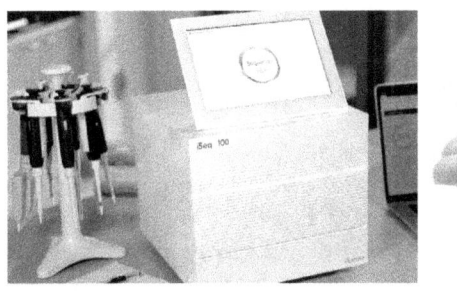
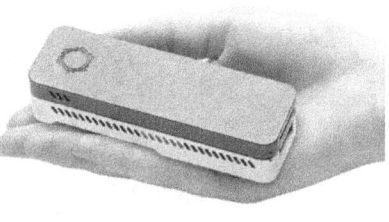

Figure 76: (L) An Illumina iSeq 100 benchtop device and (R) an Oxford Nanopore MinIon device

Nanopore Sequencing

Nanopore sequencing is a further type of sequencing technology that enables a single molecule of DNA or RNA to be sequenced without the need for amplification - and offers results in real-time. It works by monitoring changes to an electrical current as nucleic acids are passed through an array of tiny holes — nanopores — embedded in an electro-resistant membrane. Each nanopore corresponds to its own electrode connected to a channel and sensor chip, which measures the electric current that flows through the nanopore. When a molecule passes through a nanopore, the current is disrupted producing a signal that is then decoded, using algorithms to determine the DNA or RNA sequence in real time[305]. Approximately a quarter of all SARS-CoV-2 sequences completed so far have been carried out using Nanopore technology[306].

As illustrated above, Oxford Nanopore has created a portable (87gram) and affordable device called the MinION that costs just $1000 and is powered by a laptop[307], but can still output 50 Gb of data from a single flow cell during a

72-hour run at 420 bases per second. In 2015 the MinION was used in the field in Guinea to sequence Ebola virus samples during an outbreak.

Though initially focused on sequencing, Oxford Nanopore has established a division to explore the application of the technology for diagnostic use. An initial study, looking at bacterial identification to guide antibiotic treatment, identified the causative pathogen in 32/33 (97%) samples and contributed to antimicrobial treatment changes for 30 patients (67%)[308].

NGS Applications

For diagnostic uses, NGS can also be combined with an NAAT such as PCR to amplify DNA prior to sequencing, to focus on instances where a target pathogen is known or suspected to be present.

Among the applications of NGS in virology are[309]:

1. Discovering new pathogens in undiagnosed illness or outbreaks (e.g., the coronavirus which caused Middle East respiratory syndrome [MERS] first reported in Saudi Arabia in 2012), the novel highly divergent rhabdovirus Bas-Congo virus (BASV) and the novel polyoma viruses HPYV9 and Merkel cell polyomavirus (MCPyV);

2. Retrospective diagnosis of undiagnosed illness, for example, encephalitis, using stored autopsy samples;

3. Screening vaccines for contaminants;

4. Analysis of the quasi-species sequence composition of the viruses in a clinical sample, including detection of minor variants with new pathogenic implications, for example, drug resistance;

5. Investigation of the diversity and evolution of particular viral genomes;

6. Studies of the human virome in health and disease.

In an interesting piece of research looking at the potential application of rapid sequencing in a critical care setting, scientists described how they leveraged nanopore technology to reduce the time from arrival of the blood sample in the laboratory to the initial diagnosis to just over 7 hours[310]. Although still high, the appendix to their report noted that costs were justifiable in the context[311]:

We estimated the costs of our approach including DNA extraction, library preparation, sequencing, and computation and found those costs to range from $4971 - $7318. This is broadly comparable with similar rapid approaches previously reported using short read sequencing. Given the daily cost of critical care is more than $10,000, rapid genome sequencing diagnostics well below this figure have been shown to be significantly cost saving and, as a result, are reimbursed by several payers.

Many other fields may also benefit where improved understanding of viruses offers promise. Researchers previously involved in sequencing SARS-CoV-2 applied the same sequencing techniques to look at a potentially fatal condition called necrotizing enterocolitis (NEC). It afflicts premature infants, with a case fatality rate (CFR) approaching 1 in 3. Their research will help understand if it's possible to predict this rapid-onset disease by diagnosing viral components in at-risk infants' gut virome[312].

It seems likely that, in the coming years, further cost reductions and speed improvements will see the application of NGS increasing, especially in cases where conventional diagnostics fail to identify a cause.

Combinatorial Barcoding

Increasing testing capacity is of huge interest at a time of public health emergencies, remembering that constraints have been widely reported during the COVID-19 pandemic. Pooling is a technique in diagnostics where samples from multiple individuals are combined and tested in a single run. This increases testing capacity and can be quite effective in situations of low prevalence where it's expected most samples will be negative. However, if even a single sample included in the pooled specimen is positive, each sample has to be retested individually to trace the positive sample.

NGS offers significant promise to help improve pooling. Combinatorial barcoding is an emerging solution to pooling that combines the benefits of increased capacity but maintains the ability to pinpoint the owner of the positive sample(s). Salis et al from Penn State University have described[313] a massively parallel diagnostic assay (MPDA) that combines RT-PCR and Next-generation Sequencing (NGS) for diagnostic COVID-19 testing on up to 19,200 patient samples per workflow (compared to <500 with a conventional approach). Such capacity increases however pose their own logistical challenges for handling that number of swabs!

The technique uses 57,600 unique primers with barcodes to link patient samples to 3 amplicons (2 'N' proteins and a control). Next-generation sequencing of patient-specific barcodes and viral amplicon sequences are then mapped and counted, yielding verified read counts indicative of viral RNA levels. A NGS machine such as the Illumina NextSeq 550 takes about 14 hours to process a run and, while its price tag of $275,000 limits it to larger laboratories, the cost spread over the capacity gain is efficient. As another example, a study in Austria demonstrated a PCR and NGS combined protocol that showed excellent performance using pooled samples for SARS-CoV-2 detection, with the ability to expand to multiplex detection of Influenza and Rhinovirus[314]. Others working on similar solutions include the Broad Institute[315] and Octant[316].

Microfluidics

Microfluidics is another very fast-growing area of medical research - US regulator, the FDA, has seen substantial growth in the number of medical device submissions that use microfluidics, with an increase of more than 400% from 2013 to 2018, based on a three-year moving average[317].

Microfluidic technology is not a test per se but describes techniques to manipulate fluids (samples and reagents) in tiny channels. These miniature devices exploit the physical and chemical properties of liquids at a microscale. Compared to conventionally sized systems, microfluidics offers benefits including the ability to use smaller samples, reduce the quantities of reagents required and offer potentially faster reaction time and easier temperature control, as well as the more obvious benefit of portability.

Microfluidic devices employ channels as small as tens of micrometers. (As discussed in Chapter 2, a micrometer is just 0.001 mm and is also called a micron or symbolised as μm). Although not instantly familiar to most people as an example of microfluidics, many people already have a microfluidic device in their home - an inkjet printer. These printers manipulate ink droplets that are between 10 to 100 μm in diameter. In diagnostic applications, microfluidics allows for the creation of tiny devices that are essentially a lab-on-a-chip. While microfluidic devices can be made from a variety of materials including plastic, glass, polymers and silicon, in some cases they can be made from paper, which offers low cost and ease of production.

The Broad Promise of Microfluidics

Prior to the emergence of COVID-19, numerous studies have been looking to develop and deploy cost effective and portable microfluidic devices, including ones that use isothermal amplification at a micro scale. The use of microfluidic devices combined with smartphones, that offer portable display, camera and processing functions, may yield highly effective field/POC applications in RLS. For example, researchers[318] have created a microfluidic platform for the detection of Zika, Dengue (types 1 and 3) and Chikungunya virus in whole blood samples. Another project[319] describes a 10 minute assay for African Swine Fever Virus with 92.73% sensitivity, and 100% specificity. A 2017 study found that a microfluidics paper-based chip had 90% concordance with PCR tests for Ebola[320]. A 2019 study[321] proposed a system using CRISPR-Cas13a to generate results within 5 min. Likewise, investigators have shown promising results in creating microfluidics devices for POC HIV tests in RLS[322]. A comprehensive review by Zhuang et al[323] includes further microfluidics examples for Influenza, HBV, HCV, Zika and Dengue.

Aside from identifying viral pathogens, in 2017, Wu et al explored microfluidics as a potential way to improve timely chronic diseases (CD) diagnosis, prognosis/risk prediction and frequent disease monitoring combined, to improve the management of CD and even prevent their progression. The attractive concept of early CD diagnosis is often technically challenged by the lengthy and expensive diagnostic procedures in current clinical practice. Furthermore, the delay in obtaining CD diagnosis results is a major limiting factor in optimising healthcare resource allocation and coordination, which leads to significantly increased economic burden. In this context, rapid point-of-care (PoC) diagnosis is the key for improving the management of chronic health problems[324]. Jiang et al in 2021 described how the promising field of microfluidic diagnosis of cancer via liquid biopsy could be adapted to SARS-CoV-2[325] detection, offering improved performance over lateral flow assays. Indeed, in their 2020 paper, Hemming et al[326] described the use of microfluidics in the detection of cardiac marker Troponin I as *paving the way for the next generation of POC immunodiagnostics.*

More recently, Lin et al[327] have created a combined antibody/antigen microfluidic approach for SARS-CoV-2. Ziyue et al[328], combining Microfluidics with the CRISPR technologies discussed above, in March 2022 described their work to develop an instrument-free, CRISPR-based diagnostics of SARS-CoV-2, using a self-contained microfluidic system. The microfluidic chip integrates isothermal amplification, CRISPR cleavage and lateral flow detection in a single, closed microfluidic platform, enabling visual detection. In testing, the device achieved sensitivity of 94.1% and specificity of 100%.

Other Tech: Biosensors, Aptamers and More

Numerous other diagnostics technologies and techniques are at varying stages of development and will likely emerge as contenders for commercialisation in the coming years, at a faster pace than ever before. Among the most impactful will be those that promise POC breakthroughs, especially for RLS.

Biosensors & EIS

While microfluidics can use any number of detection technologies, most use miniaturised enzyme-linked immunosorbent assays (ELISAs), or NAAT. Biosensing mechanisms based on electrochemical impedance spectroscopy (EIS) have shown great promise because of their label-free operation and high sensitivity.[329] There are several other biosensing technologies but in the interests of brevity, I'll discuss just EIS here but I'm including some references for alternatives such as Surface-Enhanced Raman Scattering (SERS)[330], differential pulse voltammetry (DPV)[331] and square-wave voltammetry (SWV)[332]. Technologies such as Field Effect Transistors (FET) is another popular biosensor field evolving rapidly.

Li et al[333] have investigated the potential to use EIS sensors with microfluidics at POC to detect COVID-19. EIS is a highly sensitive electrochemical technique, capable of creating measurable signals resulting from small changes in chemical reactions or biomarker concentration. Often found in applications such as measuring corrosion of metals, in human diagnostic terms the first EIS-based immunosensor was proposed by Taylor et al (1991)[334]. In EIS-immunosensors, a difference in the electrical signal is caused by the binding of antibodies and its antigens on the sensor surface.

For a more detailed explanation of the workings of EIS, I'd recommend starting with Magar et al (2021)[335] but below I want to describe one promising project, led by Professor Cesar de la Fuente-Nunez at the University of Pennsylvania[336], as an example of a technology that was pivoted to COVID-19 detection but can be adapted to a diverse range of pathogens in future. The low cost and robust nature of this assay example are of particular interest.

Dubbed RAPID 1.0 (real-time accurate portable impedimetric detection prototype 1.0), this device is a simple, miniature (handheld) biosensor that uses EIS to capture the reaction between SARS-CoV-2 spike (S) protein and biosensor-mounted Angiotensin-Converting Enzyme-2 (ACE2), which is the receptor protein where SARS-CoV-2 attaches to human cells. Said to give results in just 4 minutes, the sensitivity and specificity of RAPID for nasopharyngeal/ oropharyngeal swab (85.3% and 100%) and saliva samples (100% and 86.5%) compare favourably to other POC tests. In testing for cross-reactivity potential, the test was shown to be accurate at detecting SARS-CoV-2 specifically and not delivering false positives in the presence of other viruses including three coronaviruses (MHV, murine hepatitis virus; HCoV-OC43, human coronavirus OC43; and human coronavirus 229E) and four non-coronavirus viral strains (H1N1; H3N2; influenza B; HSV2).

According to the project team, the test doesn't require sample preparation - saliva can be used directly. The authors estimate the cost of producing the test at $4.67, with easy production using standard commercially available screen printers. One laboratory-sized unit can produce 35,000 electrodes daily.

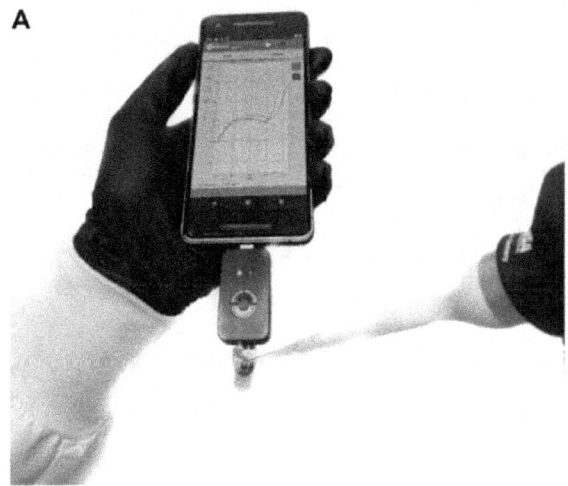

Figure 77: RAPID 1.0 with handheld device

Elsewhere, Ekrami et al. provides a summary of research[337] into EIS/Voltammetric tests for Influenza, Hepatitis, Dengue, Avian Flu and Chikungunya virus which will hopefully all receive additional focus after COVID-19.

Among further research work to create the next generation of biosensors - beyond the current standard field-effect transistors (FET) - using graphene, perhaps capable of detecting single molecules of pathogens, is that undertaken by a team at Toyohashi University of Technology in Japan. They have demonstrated a novel Fabry–Pérot interferometric (FPI) surface-stress sensor that could detect for prostate-specific antigen as small as 100 ag/mL (attograms per millilitre - attograms - are a quintillionth of a gram or 10^{-18})[338]. This technology remains years away from commercialisation but offers hope for future breakthrough devices.

Aptamers

As a key part of our immune response to infection, antibodies are core components of many diagnostics. Aptamers can be thought of as artificially created antibodies. They are single-stranded nucleotide sequences that bind very selectively to a specific target. They are a class of *ligand* - the biochemistry term for a molecule that binds to a receiving protein molecule or receptor. Compared to natural antibodies, aptamers are much easier and quicker to synthesize for a particular target, such as a virus. A process known as Systematic Evolution of Ligands by Exponential Enrichment (SELEX) is used to create an aptamer for a particular target. Aptamers for diagnostic applications can be used in lateral-flow devices or in biosensors.

Although they were first created a little over 30 years ago, interest in Aptamers has been growing dramatically in recent years and is accelerating further, with the promise of next generation *optimer ligands* technologies. Thanks to their ability to attach to targets ranging from small ligands such as heavy metal ions and small molecules, up to larger ligands such as proteins and cells and viruses, aptamers are likely to be further used in diagnostics.

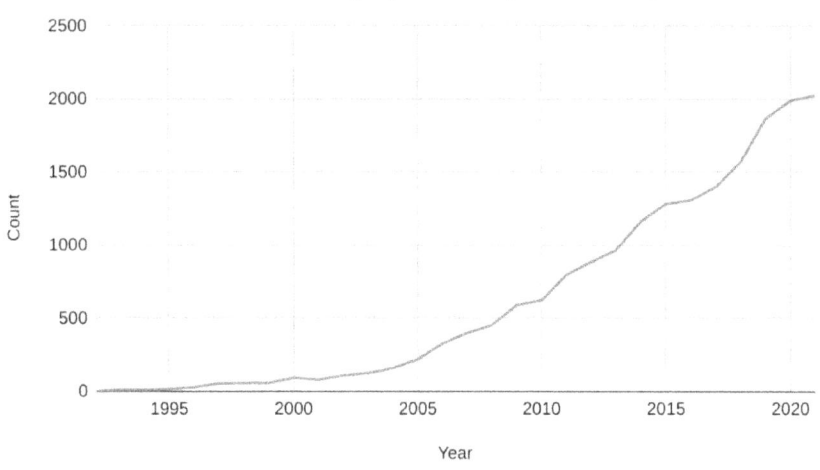

Figure 78: Growing interest in the role and use of Aptamers in the last 20 years

In the COVID-19 testing space, Swiss-based diagnostics firm Achiko received CE approval in May 2022 for its COVID-19 saliva rapid test, which uses an aptamer in place of an antibody to detect SARS-CoV-2 and runs on a spectrophotometer desktop device[339].

Zou, Xinran et al. provide an excellent and detailed overview[340] of the applications of Aptamers in Virus Detection and Antiviral Therapy for anyone looking to understand more than we have space for here on this topic.

Aptamer Biosensors

Biosensors are analytical devices that combine a bioreceptor and a transducer to measure a chemical reaction - a biological component that acts as the sensor and an electronic component that detects and transmits a signal. The biological element can be a nucleic acid, antibody, enzyme or an aptamer. When a sample is added, the bioreceptor recognizes and binds the target with high sensitivity and selectivity, and the transducer identifies the interaction between the analyte and the bioreceptor. Biosensors using aptamers are known as an aptasensors, which are further divided into types based on the transducer technology used, electrical or optical. There are at least six different types of optical aptasensor[341] alone, so we will likely see a wide variety of aptasensors of varying complexity evolve, to meet differing diagnostic requirements.

Other Biosensors

Although easier than traditional antibody approaches, Aptamers remain relatively complex to create. Looking at examples with low complexity and cost, in 2017, Nidzworski et al[342] described the use of a boron-doped diamond (BDD) biosensor to detect Influenza in throat or nasal wash specimens in 5 minutes. In another promising development, Turbé et al.[343] developed a biosensor that could analyse an untreated biological sample in one step and detect a target analyte using surface acoustic waves (SAW). The analysis is performed on a disposable biochip and is controlled by a pocket-sized reader that is expected to cost $30. The proof of concept was used to detect HIV antibodies (the technique could be extended across a range of pathogens) and delivered results in just 10 seconds, far below the Foundation for Innovative Diagnostic (FIND)'s target product profile of 5-minute result assays.

Blood: Beyond Theranos

Although I've focused on viral diagnostics, I do want to mention, very briefly, the continued interest in novel blood testing methods, a branch of diagnostic testing that is familiar to most people as part of routine medical investigations.

The collapse of Theranos, the start-up which promised lots of blood tests on just a few drops of blood instead of vials, has shaken consumer and investor confidence in claims of testing breakthroughs and toughened regulatory oversight. However, due to the benefits from any improvements in the ease and speed of blood testing, researchers are continuing to investigate this space, albeit with less hyperbolic claims and increased transparency than in the case of Theranos. For example, Israeli start-up, Sight Diagnostics, is developing a POC diagnostic device, shown below, that offers one of the most commonly-ordered blood tests - a Complete Blood Count (CBC) - in just 10 minutes, using two drops of blood from a finger prick. Sight's system uses digital fluorescent microscopy and computer vision algorithms that visually scan (each test generates about 6gb of data) and analyse the blood.

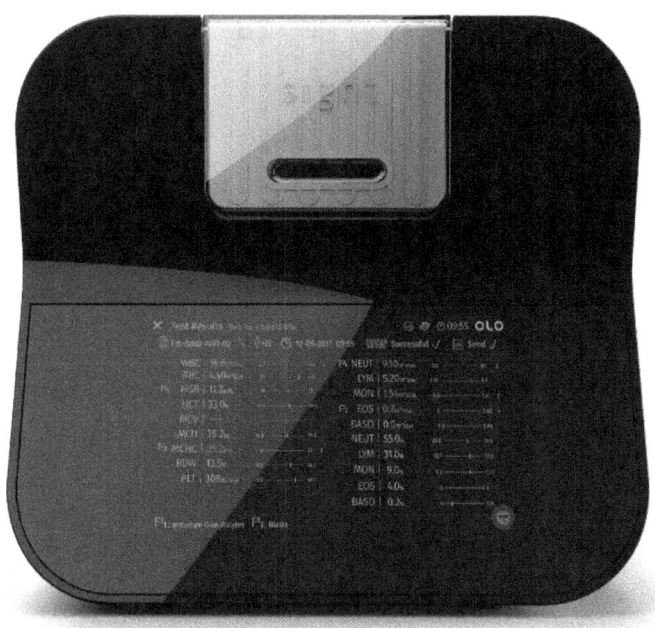

Figure 79: The Sight OLO® is a point-of-care blood analyser that performs a 5 part Complete Blood Count (CBC)

One other interesting advance in rapid blood testing is related to concussion injury. In early 2021, Abbott received FDA 510(k) clearance for the first rapid handheld traumatic brain injury (TBI) blood test. Although the current iteration requires plasma from a venous blood sample, a whole blood version would allow point of care tests. A negative test can be used to rule out the need for a head CT scan. This breakthrough promises to improve the standard of care for suspected brain injuries, while also potentially reducing unnecessary and costly CT scans.

From Diagnostics to Prognostics

Although the typical patient flow moves from presentation to diagnosis to treatment, there is the question of prognosis to consider in some situations, where the purpose of the diagnostic test is not necessarily to identify the pathogen but to better understand the prognosis, which may influence the therapeutic choice. In many instances, healthcare professionals may already be fairly sure of the etiological agent; what is of more concern is how the disease may evolve. For example, test developers are looking beyond simple binary positive/negative diagnostics for predictive biomarkers of COVID-19 severity that might be detectable early in disease onset and offer improved understanding of its pathogenesis.

In a pretty straightforward example, some research shows that even a person's blood type can be an indicator of severity for COVID-19: Zhao et al[344] found that blood type A patients were at significantly increased risk of infection compared with non-type A patients, while another report from Young et al summarises multiple similar studies[345].

In extreme cases, the pressure for a rapid diagnostic answer (what condition does a patient have?) may be accompanied by a desire to know what the prognosis is for that patient (how bad does this patient have it?). This may be driven by the requirement to prioritize or optimize the allocation of scarce treatments or resources. While there are established clinical assessment frameworks in ICUs, such as acute physiology and chronic health evaluation II (APACHE II) and sequential organ failure assessment (SOFA)[346], once again COVID-19 has seen development of new approaches that will contribute to the overall knowledge of the field.

cfDNA and Proteomics are two areas of interest in the search for tests that indicate not just the presence of a pathogen but the potential course of the disease:

cfDNA

Cell-free DNA (cfDNA) refers to extracellular DNA present in body fluids - small fragments of circulating DNA that are the "debris" of dead cells from across the body that may come from both normal and diseased cells. Analysing these fragments may yield vital clues to what's going on around the body - analysis can be done using PCR or Sequencing technologies described earlier. Primarily used as a screening test for non-invasive prenatal testing, oncology[347] and in organ transplantation as an indicator of rejection[348], the technology is being extended in further applications that may help with prognostics. For example, Researchers at Cornell University[349] have developed a blood test to quantify specific cell, tissue or organ injury due to COVID-19. Their trials confirm the utility of cfDNA profiling as a prognostic tool for the early detection and monitoring of cell and tissue injury due to COVID-19, as the concentration of cell-free DNA was significantly increased in patients later requiring intubation and correlated with the World Health Organization (WHO) ordinal scale for disease progression.

Though somewhat controversial and not currently FDA-approved, some firms are offering direct-to-consumer blood test kits using cfDNA to screen for cancers, at around $900 per test[350].

Proteomics

A proteome is the complete set of proteins expressed by an organism. Unlike our genome which is relatively stable, our proteome changes rapidly and significantly. Most diseases are manifested at the level of protein activity, and proteomics studies how specific proteins and changes relate to a given disease state. If we again take the publication of research papers as a proxy for interest in a topic, you can see that proteomics is gaining significant research attention.

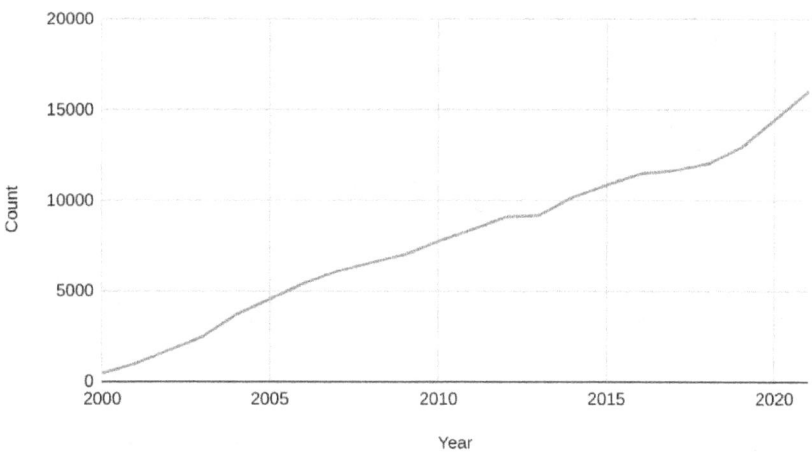

Figure 80: Proteomics on PubMed

The prognostic value of several biomarkers (e.g., CRP, IL-6, ferritin) and clinical scores for predicting disease progression in COVID-19 at early disease stages, e.g., at hospital admission, is now well established by two meta-analyses[351,352]. This research offers hope that patients at greater risk can be identified earlier.

Demichev et al[353] described a proteomic survival predictor for COVID-19 patients in intensive care based on two cohorts of patients with severe COVID-19. The study, which looked at 321 plasma protein groups across 50 critically ill patients at 349 timepoints, identified 14 proteins that showed trajectories different between survivors and non-survivors, and concluded: *"plasma proteomics can give rise to prognostic predictors substantially outperforming current prognostic markers in intensive care. Using a machine learning model which combines the measurements of multiple proteins, we were able to accurately predict survival in critically ill patients with COVID-19 from single blood samples"*.

The model correctly predicted the outcome for 18 out of 19 patients who survived and for 5 out of 5 patients who died.

Another area of interest for Proteomics is TB. Approximately one quarter of the world's population is infected with TB bacteria, but do not exhibit disease symptoms. Even though these people do not feel ill, they are at risk of developing active TB disease in the future and spreading it to others—more than 80% of TB cases in the US are due to untreated latent infection. To help to identify individuals at high risk of progressing to active disease, a team of scientists measured the levels of over 3,000 proteins (using a Somalogic[354] assay) in plasma collected from healthy TB-infected adolescents. They identified 135 proteins that were significantly different in those who developed active TB, compared to those who remained healthy, and they successfully validated two different combinations of three or five proteins that could predict the subset who developed the disease within a year. These were the first validated protein biomarkers with prognostic value for TB[355].

Genome Wide Association Studies

Genome Wide Associate Studies (GWAS) look to detect associations between genetic variants and disease progression. For researchers trying to better understand the pathogenesis of SARS-CoV-2 and why it leads to critical illness in less than 10% of infections[356], several studies are looking for genetic markers that may be indicative of protective effects or elevated levels of vulnerability[357],[358]. To date, these studies show that it may be possible to use genetic tests for more reliable risk stratification which in turn may guide therapeutic interventions. Combined with the viral load quantitative testing we described earlier, an HCP may be able to triage cases rapidly where the patient is at greater risk of severe illness.

Other Diagnostic Technologies

There are, thankfully, too many other diagnostic technologies being proposed and tested to cover here. Almost daily, there are new papers being submitted for peer review describing novel methods promising faster, smaller, cheaper or more accurate testing.

For anyone wishing to explore more technologies, among the ones I've recently read about are:

- Virolens® - a screening device, based on a nano-cellular microscope uses holographic imaging and artificial intelligence (AI) software technology to analyse saliva swab tests to detect (within just 20 seconds) the presence of the SARS-CoV-2 virus. Demonstrating an exciting proof of concept[359], 99.8% sensitivity and 96.7% specificity are claimed, based on the results of an internal in-vitro validation study, designed by the University of Bristol.

- In March 2022, a group of Korean researchers proposed a novel biosensing technique for an antigen test to detect and quantify viral particles, based on an optical phenomenon known as *slow light*, with an approach called a Gires–Tournois immunoassay platform (GTIP)[360]. The colorimetric nature of this technique allows for quantitative tests, not just binary positives/negatives and works with a standard optical microscope without the need for sample amplification.

- Among future alternatives to Lateral Flow tests, perhaps providing additional reach to diagnostics in conditions where existing rapid tests can struggle (e.g., short shelf-life of tests or unreliability in high temperature situations), is *molecularly imprinted polymer nanoparticles* (nanoMIPs) as outlined by McClements et al.[361] These are synthetic replacements for the antibodies required for existing antigen immunoassays.

It's worth emphasising again here that this book is intended to provide an introductory overview of the importance of viral diagnostics, together with some of the major relevant technologies, both in use and emerging. Other areas of medical diagnostics, e.g., imaging, are also, of course, seeing rapid evolution driven by technological advances, such as AI, and promise real potential. So, just as molecular diagnostic tools such as NAAT have proven invaluable for analysing nasal or saliva samples, diagnostics are emerging to look at tissue samples at molecular level. Examples include the slightly intimidatingly-named *matrix-assisted laser desorption/ionization (MALDI) trapped ion-mobility spectrometry (TIMS) time of flight (TOF)* imaging platform[362]. Careful collaboration will be vital, looking to combine these advances across all branches of diagnostics for overall patient benefit.

Chapter 12: Variants, Surveillance & Timing

As we conclude our review of technologies that may help us more effectively find and track viruses, it's important to highlight that viruses are a moving target. As they replicate, they change in ways that not only modify their impact on their hosts (e.g., causing more or less severe disease), but in ways that can make them harder to find - both for tests and sometimes for our body's natural defence mechanisms, such as antibodies.

Mutations may enable viruses to jump across species and then start spreading in humans. We need to be vigilant for novel viruses, as well as the return of old foes that were considered to pose little on-going threat. And, as we saw in previous Chapters, most tests are designed to look for a very specific target, to ensure accurate detection of a particular virus and not a cross-reaction with another virus. Despite the benefits of specific targeting, if the targeted area of the virus mutates, the test may fail and return a false negative.

Now that we've discussed the testing types, it's also important to understand how the timing of the test matters, as well as the tools available to public health authorities to monitor viruses at population scale rather than in individual tests.

Moving Targets

In another pandemic-induced addition to the public vocabulary, *variants* (with the Greek letters naming them) became frequent topics of conversation as SARS-CoV-2 became the first virus to be globally tracked at scale, with the latest genetic sequencing technology available to describe mutations in near real time.

Although many people worry more about variants that might evade vaccines or treatments, the ability to evade even detection, using current tests, is a major scientific concern. Therefore, ever-better understanding of the evolutionary dynamics of viruses is important, to ensure the tools used to manage public health responses remain effective. And while it may seem prudent to mass produce tests and have them ready in case of future waves, we must be cognisant that tests may struggle or even fail to identify variants at some point in the future.

Mutations, Variants and Strains

The terms mutations, variants and strains are often used interchangeably in popular coverage of viruses, but there are significant technical distinctions between them:

- A *mutation* refers to an *individual* change in a genetic sequence. So technically, scientists may identify a SARS-CoV-2 mutation, such as one called D614G. This refers to an aspartic acid-to-glycine substitution at position 614 of the spike glycoprotein[363]; a copying fault that altered a single nucleotide in the virus's 29,903-letter RNA code.

- A *variant* refers to a genetic sequence that has *one or more mutations*. It's important to note that a variant may differ by just one mutation or by many. A variant may or may not behave differently to the ancestral virus or others in the same lineage.

- A *strain* is a variant that has a demonstrably different phenotype (e.g., a difference in antigenicity, transmissibility, or virulence) as a result of the mutation(s).

Mutations are perfectly normal for viruses and, though different viruses mutate at different rates and in different ways, virologists fully expect viruses to evolve and change over time. Viruses reproduce at a very fast rate, so mutate and evolve at a much faster rate than large entities such as humans. Compared to viral DNA or RNA polymerases, the error rate in replicating the human genome is 6,000 times lower[364].

Mutation Mechanisms

Every time a virus replicates, there's a chance of a mutation, or an error in the copying/reproduction process. Most mutations can be thought of as being like typos in the string of letters that make up a strand of DNA or RNA code. Any mutation may be helpful, harmful or neutral to the virus in terms of infectiousness, ability to replicate or ability to evade immunity. Many mutations are tiny, inconsequential changes that quickly die out as they don't impact the transmissibility, host tropism (ability to infect different hosts), antigenicity or pathogenicity of the virus - i.e., most mutations are inconsequential glitches that do not significantly affect how the virus works[365].

However, some mutations may change symptoms[366], enable a virus to evade treatments, transmit or infect more rapidly, or even jump between species.

RNA Replication Errors

RNA is made up of building blocks known as nucleotides. These can be any one of four different types: A, G, C, or U. Every time the viral replication factory copies the genome, random genetic change can occur. For example, an A nucleotide at a particular position on the genome could change to a U nucleotide. This is known as a single nucleotide polymorphism, or SNP. The intrinsic error rate of coronavirus genome replication is in the order of 1×10^{-6} to 1×10^{-7} mutations per nucleotide per genome replication (1 mutation in 1-10 million nucleotides replicated). As the virus genome is almost 30,000 nucleotides long, then 1 mutation is introduced about every 33-330 replications. In an infected person, the peak number of virus genomes exceeds 100 million; therefore, the virus has the potential to mutate every nucleotide of its genome hundreds of times per infected person and so it follows that variant generation is common[367].

You may recall that, in Chapter 2, we discussed the distinction between RNA and DNA viruses. Here, the point of interest is that RNA viruses mutate more than DNA ones as they lack the inherent enzymes, called DNA polymerases, that copy DNA viruses, which can 'proofread' and fix errors quite effectively. Among RNA viruses, Coronaviruses like SARS-CoV-2 are less prone to mutations due to their having some limited ability to proofread during copying, errors do still occur, though not as fast as in other RNA viruses. As we'll see below, RNA viruses with more complex structures than SARS-CoV-2, such as Influenza, change more rapidly and not just via copying errors.

Drift and Shift

When discussing viral variants, it's worth noting that non-Coronaviruses also evolve using different mechanisms, alongside the polymerase copying described above. Looking to the future, as the world's attention moves away from the COVID-19 pandemic and SARS-CoV-2 variants, the resultant increased awareness of mutations and the potential impact on diagnostics should help us better understand how other pathogens mutate.

Influenza

Influenza, a highly prevalent virus that has been studied intensely for years and is the source of much of our prior knowledge about viral mutations, lacks even the limited proof-reading capabilities of SARS-CoV-2, and thus mutates more rapidly as it copies. Influenza mutations are most common in the genes that relate to the viral surface proteins *H*emagglutinin and *N*euraminidase (these proteins lend their first initials to flu subtypes. For example, the 2009 influenza pandemic was caused by Influenza A H1N1 virus.)

Small changes in a virus are referred to as *antigenic drift* when the number of mutations accumulates to cause a change that is substantial enough to evade our antibody response (whether natural or vaccine-induced). Antigenic drift is why the Influenza vaccine is updated annually and why we can get the flu more than once - this is usually caused when the drift is significant enough that our existing antibodies no longer recognise the mutated (drifted) antigen(s).

Larger changes in a virus are known as *antigenic shift,* where a virus is radically different from its ancestor strains. This occurs less frequently than drift and usually happens through a process known as *reassortment.* If you recall the section earlier, describing the structure of the Influenza virus, I noted the importance of the fact that internally, the RNA of Influenza is in 8 separate strands, unlike SARS-CoV-2's single strand. In cases where two different, but related, influenza strains infect a host cell at the same time, segments from the two influenza viruses' genome can combine to make a new strain of influenza virus. As coronaviruses do not have segmented genomes, they cannot *reassort.* They can, however, *recombine,* when two different coronaviruses infect the same cell, and at time of writing, this process is becoming more prevalent among SARS-CoV-2 strains[368], [369].

SARS-CoV-2 Mutations

Researchers have shown that, when a coronavirus replicates, around 3 percent of its copies contain a new random error or mutation[370]. The SARS-CoV-2 variant named *omicron* (B.1.1.529) has 50 mutations overall, with 32 mutations on the spike(S) protein alone. For comparison, the *delta* variant had nine mutations[371]. The SARS-CoV-2 error rate is relatively slow - Two SARS-CoV-2 viruses collected from anywhere in the world differ by an average of just 10 RNA letters out of 29,903 - a rate of change about half that of influenza and one-quarter that of HIV. [372]

A CATALOGUE OF CORONAVIRUS MUTATIONS

Various mutations have been detected in SARS-CoV-2 genomes, including the most prevalent one, D614G. The virus's genetic code has just under 30,000 nucleotides of RNA, or letters, that spell out at least 29 genes. The most common mutations are single-nucleotide changes.

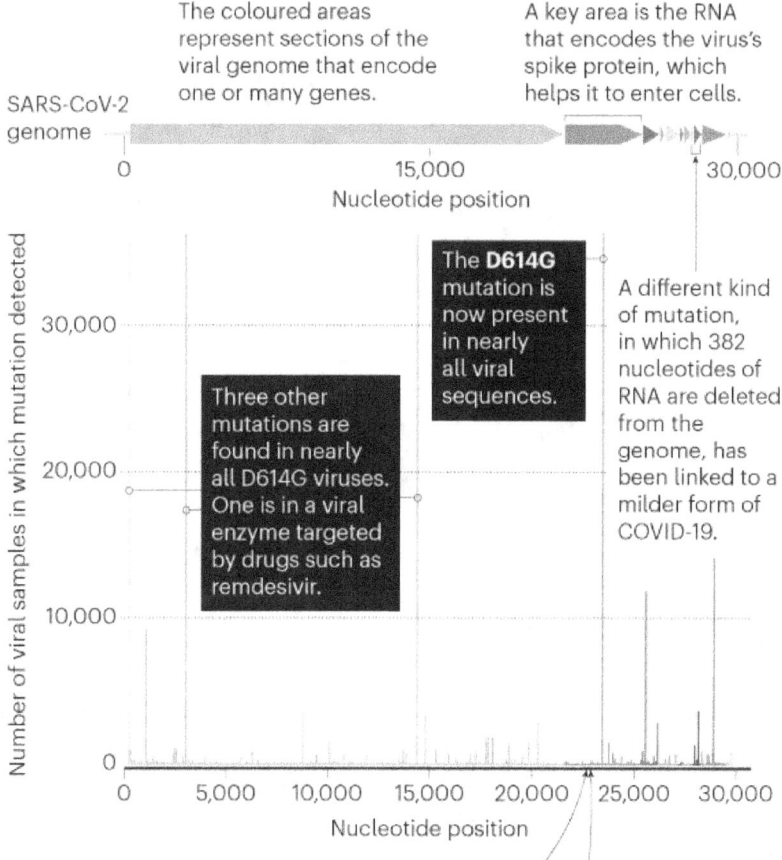

Figure 81: SARS-CoV-2 mutations. Source: ibid

The mutations of SARS-CoV-2 that have been tracked around the world can be represented visually to show the lineages that have developed as different mutations proliferate.

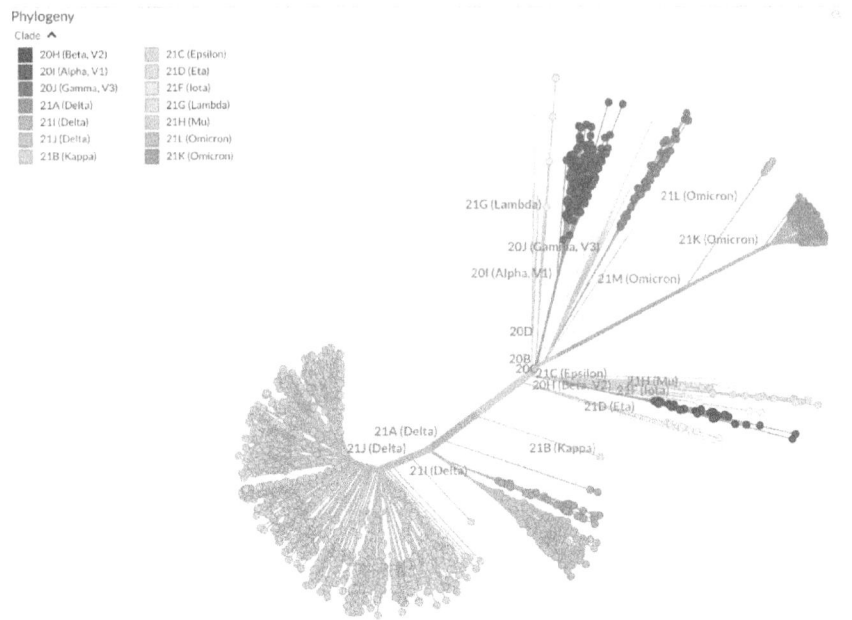

Figure 82: SARS-CoV-2 Phylogeny tree from GISAID data, generated April 9th, 2022 by the Author (see web for hi-res colour version) [373]

Diagnostics & Variants

On-going mutations are a major challenge for diagnostic tools targeting viruses. As mentioned earlier, the narrow focus of some tests can lead to false negatives when the targeted property mutates beyond the detectable range of the test. For example, when the Omicron variant of SARS-CoV-2 was identified, it emerged that several previously-used tests were less accurate against this variant. The typical mitigation for this is to use tests that look for a number of very specific elements of a virus, it being unlikely that all of the targeted areas would mutate at the same time.

As can be seen clearly in the Figure above, SARS-CoV-2 has diversified into multiple lineages which may each have different consequences for the performance of diagnostic tests approved for prior variants. So, to help better understanding of the impact of variants on in vitro diagnostic tests, the US National Institutes of Health's Rapid Acceleration of Diagnostics (RADx) initiative created a Variant Task Force[374].

PCR Tests and Variants

Continuing with the Omicron variant example, the emergence of that variant did lead to some tests having to be updated after the FDA warned they were no longer effective[375]:

- Applied DNA Sciences' Linea COVID-19 Assay Kit, has two viral targets on the SARS-CoV-2 genome and both cover the portions of the S-gene where these mutations occur and are not able to detect omicron.

- Meridian Bioscience single-target test can't detect omicron due to a nine-nucleotide deletion in the N-gene, which is the genetic target of their diagnostic.

SGTF

Other assays that detected multiple targets found an "advantage" with the variant. Dubbed S-Gene Target Failure (SGTF) - the failure of a test to detect the S gene, but still return a positive test based on the presence of two other targets (ORF1ab and N), implies the presence of SARS-CoV-2 omicron variant, as delta variant samples are positive on all 3 targets[376]. Given that a diagnostic RT-PCR test is faster and cheaper than sequencing positive samples to determine which variant is present, SGTF was, briefly, a useful indicator of the spread of omicron in some jurisdictions.

Although the alpha variant of SARS-CoV-2 had a similar mutation in the S gene, given the low prevalence of alpha by the time omicron was circulating widely, the SGTF was seen as a potential proxy for omicron infection vs delta. However, the second sub lineage of omicron, BA.2, lacks the test-evading S-gene mutation[377]. This highlights the ever-changing challenge and the importance of full genetic sequencing to track variants, rather than hoping diagnostic tests can discern variants reliably.

In mid 2022, the maker of the personal NAAT device, Cue, has submitted variant-specific assays to the FDA for EUA. These are intended to facilitate diagnosis of which variant a patient is infected with, in order to guide in the treatment of Omicron variants, which have been shown to evade some therapeutics while still responding to others.

Antigen Tests and Variants

In addition to the fact that RT-PCR tests which rely on the detection of genetic material may be fooled by mutations in the target genes, the emergence of omicron also raised concerns about the continued validity of some rapid antigen tests. As most antigen tests target the N(ucleocapsid) protein which is not significantly mutated in omicron, they were expected to remain effective.

In late December 2021, the FDA announced that early data from the National Institutes of Health's Rapid Acceleration of Diagnostics (RADx) initiative suggested that some antigen tests, while still capable of detecting omicron, would do so at reduced sensitivity[378], but remained useful and should continue to be used by the public. A December 2021 UK report[379] on the performance of selected antigen tests found no change in their ability to detect Omicron but did not assess any changes in the timing of sample collection. In a preprint report from January 2022, findings of a small study suggested that nasal-sample antigen tests may produce false negatives in cases of omicron infections, compared to saliva-based PCR tests[380]. If these findings are validated on a larger scale, it indicates the importance of adapting testing sampling and timing to ensure accuracy when facing variants.

Variants and Sample Collection

Returning to the topic of sample collection, with the added factor of variants, it's important to consider that a change in the pathogenesis of a virus may influence the optimal sampling approach. During the COVID-19 pandemic, the evidence on efficacy allowed for a switch from NP swabs to Nasal swabs, once the associated changes in sensitivity and specificity were found to be acceptable. Similarly, the emergence of the omicron variant led to reassessment of the appropriateness of salvia and oropharyngeal swabs, compared to the previously recommended and approved nasal tests. Although it may sound like a minor change, regulators were immediately concerned about ill-informed consumers repurposing nasal swabs to collect oropharyngeal samples. Short nasal swabs may not provide sufficient reach for a high-quality sample from the oropharynx located at the back of a person's throat. A well-intentioned user could miss the area and produce a false negative result because an insufficient sample was collected. In contrast, where advised and tested by regulators, collection of oral swabs or saliva samples would usually be accompanied with guidance regarding recommended intervals after eating, drinking or use of mouthwash or toothpaste, before testing.

The FDA has not authorized any at-home self tests with throat swabs and has warned of the potential dangers of sticking a swab near the throat. "When it comes to at-home rapid antigen COVID-19 tests, those swabs are for your nose and not your throat," the agency recently posted on Twitter. The warning came as some people started swabbing their throats with their at-home kits, having read about other countries where throat swabs are more common, and about extrapolating from some studies suggesting saliva samples tested using PCR can provide as reliable, or even more accurate results, than deep nasal samples used for PCR[381].

U.S. FDA acting commissioner Dr. Janet Woodcock told a Senate hearing[382] that the FDA could "act very rapidly" to approve the new method if research confirms its effectiveness but cautioned that test manufacturers would need to "change the test configuration to accommodate the larger swab."

Monitoring Variants

There's no way to stop viruses from mutating as long as they are circulating. However, any measures to reduce transmission, infection and severity serve to reduce the scope for viral replication and thus reduce the chances of a significant mutation, as explained by Andrew Pekosz, Virologist, Johns Hopkins[383]:

"Say, for example, it's a one in a million chance that a mutation will be advantageous to the virus. If you let the virus replicate itself 900,000 times, odds are that the advantageous mutation will occur. But if you limit the overall replication of the virus to 1,000 times, then it's much less likely that the random advantageous mutation is going to occur. And that's where public health interventions really help us a lot during this pandemic—by reducing the total amount of virus replication and therefore reducing the chances that the virus can improve or adapt."

Public health agencies that monitor mutations may give special labels to groups of variants that share a characteristic or attribute. These groups may contain variants that come from a single lineage, like an inherited trait in a family tree, or those that arise independently but behave similarly. Readers will recall that, In the case of SARS-CoV-2, variants are classified and labelled using letters of the Greek alphabet, e.g., the Delta and Omicron variants.

Variants are classified into different categories by the World Health Organization (WHO)[384] and the Centers for Disease Control and Prevention (CDC)[385]:

- A *variant of interest* is a SARS-CoV-2 variant that, compared to earlier forms of the virus, has mutations that are predicted to lead to greater transmissibility, evasion of the immune system or diagnostic testing, or to more severe disease.
- A *variant of concern* has been observed to be more infectious and more likely to cause breakthrough infections.
- A *variant of high consequence* is one for which current vaccines do not offer protection.

In the case of SARS-CoV-2, we've seen the emergence of variants that have increased transmissibility significantly and led to substantial reinfections but, as yet, we haven't seen dramatic negative changes in the severity of disease caused. Efforts are underway to adapt vaccines to better cope with new strains, while surveillance efforts have been bolstered by wider availability of low-cost sequencing technologies.

As mentioned, variants are a common and expected phenomenon within viral evolution. However, the ability of SARS-CoV-2 to mutate and reinfect people, soon after infection with a previous variant, together with the challenge of ensuring that variants don't evade detection as well as they can overcome our immune response, has pushed variant-testing to the top of the diagnostic agenda. The historical reliance on sequencing to identify a variant definitively is both time consuming and costly. Emerging tools are now promising the ability to differentiate accurately between variants without reliance on sequencing, but still offering the accuracy of single nucleotide mutation detection.

For example, a team of Chinese researchers has described the development of a cheap (less than USD 50 cent) paper-based test for SARS-CoV-2 variants[386] supported by a smartphone app. The test takes about 30 minutes and has successfully identified Alpha, Beta and Gamma, with 100% concordance with real-time quantitative polymerase chain reaction (RT-qPCR) and RNA sequencing, in throat swab samples. Another approach detailed by a team at UC, Irvine, can also identify specific variants of SARS-CoV-2[387] at a lower cost than CRISPR-based solutions.

Wastewater Surveillance

All the types of testing discussed elsewhere in this book rely on the collection and analysis of a sample from an individual person. But a useful method to assess infection levels at a community level is the analysis of sewage - many pathogens can be detected in sewage. Samples from sewage treatment plants can be analysed to gain a macro view of viral prevalence in a population. Such wastewater surveillance offers a uniquely broad view - including asymptomatic people, it can be analysed regardless of inequalities that may limit access to healthcare or clinical testing, though its reliability may be affected in areas with transient populations.

It's somewhat akin to pooled sample testing, but without the ability to go back and recheck an individual sample. As a technique, it's obviously useful only where there are sewage systems - not always the case in LMICs - but, compared to random individual sampling, it is a cost-effective way to "poll" an area for pathogen pervasiveness.

So, while it's of no use to detect individual cases, wastewater surveillance can tell if a virus is increasing or decreasing in intensity in a particular area, A study from New York wastewater, published in February 2022, used sequencing to identify cryptic variant lineages that weren't detected by other means[388]. In the US, the Centers for Disease Control and Prevention (CDC) established a National Wastewater Surveillance System (NWSS) in the fall of 2020. In the Netherlands, a publicly available online dashboard summarising the national wastewater surveillance system data is updated daily.

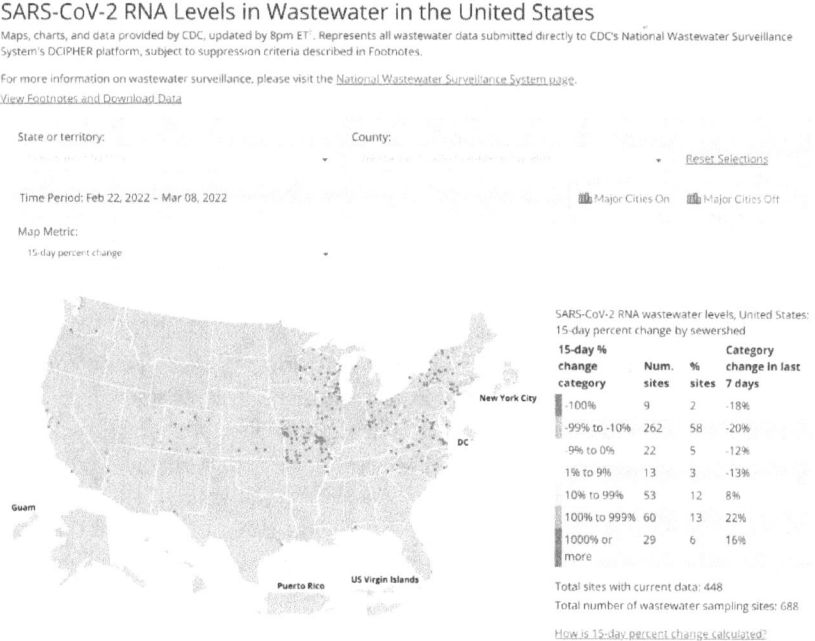

Figure 83: An example of the NWSS reporting available via the CDC[389].

In terms of the analysis technologies used for wastewater, RT-PCR is typically used, with NGS applied where variant tracking is required. A development of PCR technology, known as ddPCR (droplet digital PCR), has been shown in a wastewater study[390] to be very effective to quantify norovirus and adenovirus prevalence.

I want just briefly to highlight the potential public health use of wastewater surveillance or Wastewater-based epidemiology (WBE) beyond SARS-CoV-2 tracking. For example, in a paper[391] published in 2022, researchers noted its potential for real-time tracking of progress in attaining United Nations Sustainable Development Goals (SDGs): WBE currently is practiced in at least 55 countries, reaching about 300 million people. Expansion of WBE to 109,000 + treatment plants in 129 countries would increase global coverage 9-fold to 34.7%, or 2.7 billion, still excluding 5 billion people not served by centralized sewerage systems; lack of sanitation infrastructure means doubly disadvantaged populations, at risk of poor hygiene and cut off from the early-warning benefits of WBE.

The benefits of sewage monitoring were recognised as early as the 1920s, when it was used in monitoring typhoid and in the 1930s monitoring poliomyelitic viruses in the US. Its use in recent times has been broadened to include insights into pharmaceutical use, illicit drug levels and even hormonal indicators of hunger and stress such as ghrelin and cortisol. For public health researchers, WBE offers a large, anonymised sample set that may remove many of the collection biases in other approaches.

Surveillance

Surveillance has the potential to become a loaded word in public health terms, but in epidemiology, it pertains to the systematic collection of data regarding the occurrence of specific diseases, usually for public health planning for the prevention and control of disease. In most countries, there is some form of national disease surveillance system tied to diagnostic centres with mandatory reporting. For example, the US National Notifiable Disease Surveillance System[392] (NNDSS) has about 120 diseases under surveillance, including infectious diseases, bioterrorism agents, sexually transmitted diseases and some non-infectious conditions. Nearly 2.7 million disease cases are reported through NNDSS each year, from about 3,000 public health departments across the US. As of March 2022, there were 34 notifiable viruses listed on the NNDSS website (https://www.cdc.gov/nndss/), including SARS-CoV-2 (COVID-19) and SARS-CoV-1 (SARS).

Self-reporting

Surveillance of endemic diseases is difficult, as many cases will never come to the attention of health authorities. Where generic over the counter remedies are effective, or where most cases resolve without pharmaceutical treatment, it's very difficult to know the full extent of infections. For example, the true number of influenza cases each year is not known - typically only those cases severe enough to seek treatment are counted - more on this below. Approaches like antibody screening on blood donations or wastewater surveillance offer some level of insights.

During the earlier phases of the COVID-19 pandemic, authorities had centralised testing laboratories confirming cases via RT-PCR tests but, once rapid home testing became widely used, the statistical information became significantly less reliable, despite the setting up of self-reporting portals in many countries. In some instances, less than 10% of citizens who requested Government-supplied rapid tests uploaded any subsequent results, though UK Government figures suggest about two-thirds of LF test users did register their results.

The rise of at home testing poses something of a dilemma for public health officials and epidemiologists. While they support the use of tests to identify and isolate infectious people, the reporting certainty associated with laboratory-assessed samples provides statistical data to help track and manage epidemics/pandemics. A compromise may be the strong encouragement for users to upload their positive results anonymously. This is already the case via app-augmented testing products, but there is no guarantee that users will upload their results.

Organisational Testing

Most of the testing described in this book refers to testing of individuals, carried out at a public health level as some sort of national response to COVID-19, or by individuals at home. Another level of testing becoming more common is organisation-level testing, where an employer or other agency has taken responsibility for testing their workforce. This may place a significant burden on organisations, not only financially to implement the measures, but also in terms of expertise in designing such screening programmes.

For those interested in understanding more about the variables in testing at this level, the Center for Improving Medicine with Innovation and

Technology[393] (CIMIT) has made a free tool available at https://whentotest.org/.

Early Warning Systems

Several pharmaceutical firms are exploring the use of AI technologies to help identify variants or threats earlier than has been possible to date. For example, BioNTech, the German firm known as one of the pioneers of mRNA technology used in some COVID-19 vaccines, has developed a system it claims (in a preprint report[394]) is capable of identifying >90% of WHO designated variants, on average, two months in advance of traditional techniques. This system can analyse the c.10,000 SARS-CoV-2 variants identified each week and evaluate the potential threat of the mutations.

Other technologies, such as AlphaFold from Alphabet-owned DeepMind, that forecast protein structures from DNA samples have also been applied to SARS-CoV-2 variant analysis[395]. In late 2020, Microsoft announced a project, Premonition[396], which combines robotic sensing platforms, artificial intelligence, predictive analytics and cloud-scale metagenomics to autonomously monitor disease-carrying animals such as mosquitoes, robotically collect environmental samples, and then genomically scan them for biological threats, with the stated aim *to change the paradigm from reacting to known pathogens to continuously looking for them as they evolve in order to spot potential threats earlier, respond faster and develop new interventions before outbreaks occur.*

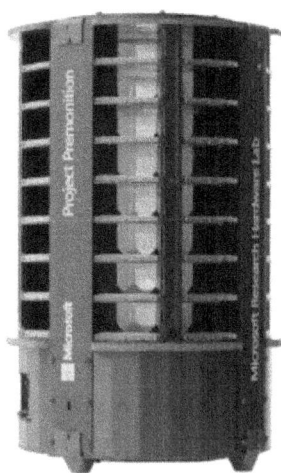

Figure 84: A Microsoft "Premonition" device to capture mosquitoes for automated analysis

CDC and Forecasting

In April 2022, the US CDC's Center for Forecasting and Outbreak Analytics (CFA) was officially launched to improve the nation's ability to prepare for and respond to infectious disease threats using data, modelling, and analytics[397].

The CFA has three core functions:

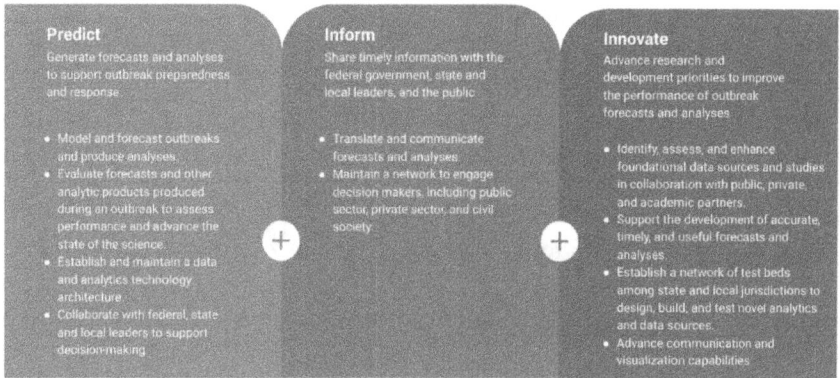

Figure 85: CDC's Center for Forecasting and Outbreak Analytics (CFA)

Machine Learning and Predicting Viruses

Although diagnostics will remain at the forefront of virus hunting, scientists are increasingly looking to new technologies from outside the realm of biotech to increase understanding of viruses and to guide the application of diagnostics.

As the scientific concern about zoonotic spill over grows, the branch of Artificial Intelligence (AI) known as Machine Learning (ML) is being harnessed to try to predict which animal virus reservoirs are most likely to evolve in ways that could see a virus jump to human populations. Where viruses of concern are identified, this may be a useful guide to prioritising diagnostic capacity.

A New York Times article in April 2022[398] describes a project in Georgetown University that has highlighted mousepox as a concern for potential spillover, while a 2015 paper[399] described the application of ML "to datasets describing the biological, ecological, and life history traits of rodents, which collectively carry a disproportionate number of zoonotic pathogens".

Influenza and Global Cooperation

There is plenty of precedent for extensive global cooperation on tracking viral outbreaks, under the auspices of the World Health Organisation. For example, although little-known outside Public Health circles, Global Influenza Surveillance and Response System - GISRS - is a vital global network dating back to 1952[400].

It has been estimated that, globally, c.300,000 to 645,000 seasonal influenza-associated respiratory deaths (4·0–8·8 per 100 000 individuals) occur annually[401], with an estimated 1 billion cases and 3 to 5 million severe cases.

GISRS operates as a global network of over 150 laboratories in 127 countries, areas or territories, continuously monitoring influenza viruses and other infectious diseases. Between 2014 and 2019, GISRS tested an average of 3.4 million specimens each year. This grew to 6.7 million tests annually for influenza and 44.2 million tests for SARS-CoV-2 in 2020 and 2021.

GISRS is the entity that makes biannual recommendations for seasonal influenza vaccine compositions for the northern and southern hemispheres, based on anticipated mutations. Although established to address influenza, GISRS serves as a scientific exchange across other diseases and played an important role in global investigations into SARS-CoV-2.

If little else comes from the pandemic but increased willingness to fund such initiatives, many lives will be saved. As Bill Gates put it in a recent TED talk, we need to spend billions to save millions of lives and trillions of dollars[402].

Timing

"COVID has turned out to be so difficult to control because so much of its transmission happens from people who don't know they're infected. The faster, easier and cheaper we can make it to find out if you're infectious, the better."

> Mark McClellan, M.D., Director of the Center for Health Policy at Duke University[403]

We talked, in Chapter 5, about the importance of sample collection, but I purposely left the topic of timing of tests until after we'd discussed the types of tests as different ones respond differently and are appropriate at different stages of the disease. Now it's time to explore that other critical aspect of testing - when the test is carried out. The pathogenesis of SARS-CoV-2 has highlighted this issue with particular clarity - the utility of diagnostics depends hugely on the stage of the disease. Now that we've also talked about variants, we can examine the challenge of test timing, mindful that mutations may create strains that change effective timings.

Incubation, Infectiousness and the Asymptomatic Challenge

One of the major challenges of SARS-CoV-2 is the amount of asymptomatic and presymptomatic transmission. Pathogenesis is the process by which viral infection leads to disease and includes several stages, with varying degrees of visibility. A full exploration of pathogenesis is beyond the scope of this book, but Chapter 45 of Medical Microbiology[404] provides a good overview for those seeking more detail.

The pathogenic stages of interest here are incubation, latency and infectiousness. The incubation period refers to the period after exposure but before the presence of the virus causes signs or symptoms. This period can range from a few days to weeks. The second important phase is that of infectiousness (or shedding) - the period during which a person may transmit the virus to others. The final term here is latency - the period between exposure and infectiousness. Diseases that are communicable before becoming symptomatic (i.e., where the incubation period and latency period are not the same) are especially difficult to contain as without testing of asymptomatic/presymptomatic people, there's no way to be aware of spread.

For comparison, here are some typical incubation ranges for common viruses:

Viral Agent	Clinical Manifestation	Incubation Period in Days (Days from Exposure to Symptoms)	
		Range	Most Typical
SARS-CoV-1	SARS	3-7	4-6
SARS-CoV-2	COVID-19	2-10	3-6
Varicella-zoster virus	Chickenpox	10-21	14-16
Treponema pallidum	Syphilis	10-90	21

HAV	Hepatitis-A	14-50	28
HBV	Hepatitis-B	50-90	60-90
HIV	AIDS	<1 year to 15 years	

When comparing SARS-CoV-1 to SARS-CoV-2, a critical difference is that there has been no reported instance of SARS transmission by a carrier before symptom onset[405]. In other words, the incubation period and latency period were the same for SARS-CoV-1. This means that symptom onset is a reliable indicator to take steps to stop the spread of SARS. However, with SARS-CoV-2, it is desirable to identify infection earlier, as waiting for symptom onset may miss presymptomatic infectiousness as shown below.

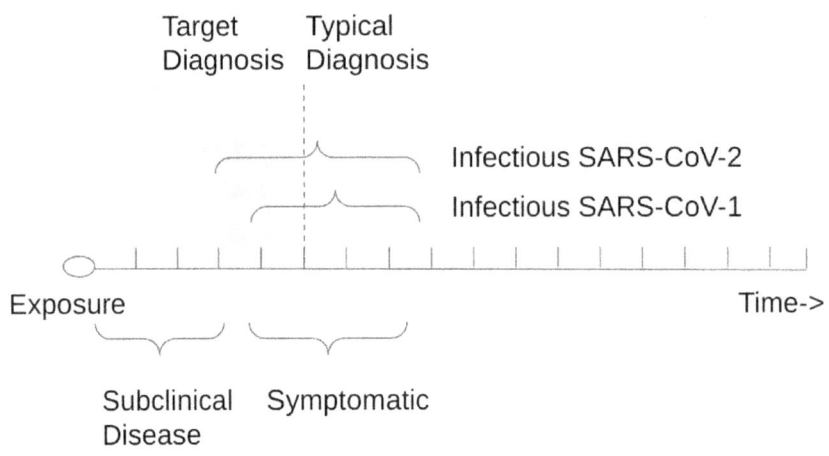

Figure 86: Earlier Diagnosis than typical is desirable (target shaded area)

Timing and Types of Test

Some tests will not work at all until a certain elapsed time in the progression of the infection - testing too early or too late, or with the wrong type of test for the point in time, will yield misleading or useless results.

- NAATs are most likely to return a positive result earliest after exposure to a pathogen. Their reliance on amplified samples enables them to detect low viral loads, but conversely, their sensitivity also means they may return a positive result long after a person has ceased to be infectious.

- Antigen tests are more reliable at detecting infection at higher viral loads associated with peak infectiousness but can struggle to detect the early phases of infection. The improved performance of antigen tests as viral load increases is why serial testing with them is often recommended to increase the chances of testing at the optimal time.

- Antibody tests are unlikely to work until after the peak of infection and, depending on the antibody class they are targeting, will not turn positive until seroconversion takes place, potentially days or weeks after initial infection.

The following diagram shows typical timing effectiveness for different types of test after exposure:

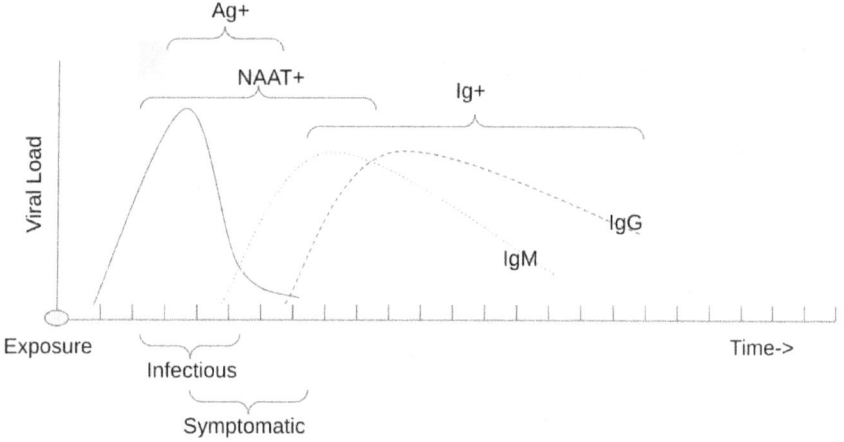

Figure 87: Viral Load vs When Types of Test are Positive (+)

As you can see in the diagram, as the viral load increases during incubation after exposure, NAATs are likely to be first able to detect a positive case, while Antigen (Ag) tests are usually most effective slightly later, but still in time to detect infectious levels. NAATs are also likely to show positive when viral load levels are below the detection threshold for Antigen tests. During the latter part of the COVID-19 pandemic, there has been much focus on the use of serial Antigen testing to offset deficiencies in their sensitivity - repeating a rapid antigen test at intervals may offset the false negative window (shaded in the diagram above). Antibody tests (Ig) are only likely to return a positive result much later in the course of the disease, signalling a past infection.

Individual Variations

While understanding patterns in viral behaviour, then adapting testing strategies to fit the most common pattern is crucial, the large variation in individual responses should not be overlooked. A 2022 report into the infectiousness of SARS-CoV-2 patients found the response to the virus varies widely between people - so, while there are clear typical timelines, different individuals, for poorly understood reasons, display substantial heterogeneity in dynamics of SARS-CoV-2 replication and shedding, making it very difficult to define an infectiousness threshold[406].

Researchers looking at other viruses have noted similar challenges: transmission heterogeneity has also been implicated in the epidemic spread of several other important viral pathogens, including measles and smallpox[407].

Other Testing & Surveillance Examples

Beyond SARS-CoV-2, I want to emphasize again the opportunities to apply the learnings of 2020/22 to other viral threats and to public health generally into the future. For reasons of equity, wellbeing of populations and health systems costs it is imperative to do so.

As useful as viral surveillance can be, there is a crucial need both to improve means to detect novel viruses and to extend the reach of testing for known pathogens. Public Health officials hope that increased familiarity with self-testing, thanks to COVID-19 rapid tests, may help in campaigns to control other diseases. Despite concern that self-testing means people may receive worrying results without any professional counselling and that results may not be reported, the availability of self-tests for more conditions may increase reach in cases of stigmatised infections or lack of access to (affordable) testing facilities.

It's encouraging that the diagnostics industry is creating more effective tests for more pathogens than ever before. From home self-tests, using lateral flow technology, for syphilis (a bacterial rather than viral infection) to 70-minute desktop PCR tests for viruses that cause viral meningitis, encephalitis and herpes[408], to novel methods for rapid detection of Ebola[409] virus (EBV), our viral testing toolkits are expanding at an unprecedented rate.

Even detection of age-old diseases is now within the grasp of new and affordable testing technologies. The mosquito is the deadliest animal in the world in terms of the number of deaths in which it is directly involved[410], spreading diseases and viruses such as malaria, dengue, West Nile, yellow fever, Zika, chikungunya and lymphatic filariasis. These often have similar symptoms and require tests to determine which is the cause, to enable early, appropriate treatment and level of response. For example, Zika virus (primarily transmitted by Aedes aegypti mosquitoes) is largely asymptomatic, or results in mild symptoms in adults, but results in developmental disorders in new-born babies if the mothers are infected during early pregnancy.

Until recently, Zika detection relied on lab-based PCR tests, but researchers at the University of Illinois Urbana-Champaign have developed a LAMP-based instrument that can be clipped onto a smartphone to test rapidly (25 minutes) for Zika virus in a single droplet of blood[411].

Langya

Finally, on this topic of surveillance, let's remain acutely conscious of the need, not alone to expand our thinking to better cope with known threats, but to accompany that with constant vigilance. Virologists and epidemiologists the world over were warning, before the COVID-19 pandemic, that such an event was highly likely. They caution that another pandemic is almost a certainty, if we don't maintain a very high degree of alertness and readiness to respond, even to what may prove to be false alarms, rather than assume a pandemic will only happen once in a generation.

In a further topical example of the importance of virus hunters in a world of increasing zoonotic threats, Summer 2022 saw the publication of a paper[412] identifying a new virus that, thankfully, so far at least, does not show evidence of easy human to human transmission.

The virus, named Langya henipavirus (LayV), can cause respiratory symptoms such as fever, cough and fatigue; it is genetically closely related to two other henipaviruses known to infect humans — Hendra virus and Nipah virus, which can cause serious problems. Henipaviruses belong to the Paramyxoviridae family of viruses, which also includes measles and mumps. The paper notes that only 35 people have been infected since 2018, with no connection between the cases, with shrews believed to be the host animals.

Hopefully by the time you read this, Langya won't have become a commonly known virus, and will join the long list of viruses under surveillance that pose a minimal risk to humans but, as we learn more about viruses, we need to invest in global surveillance to ensure we're aware of emerging threats and ready to respond effectively to them. Alongside that, concerted efforts will remain necessary to reduce the impact of known threats, especially in lower and middle income countries where many diagnostic and viral surveillance technologies available elsewhere have been beyond reach.

Chapter 13: Reducing the Disease Burden

As a final topic before wrapping up this discussion of diagnostic advances, I want to highlight the importance of ensuring that whatever improvements in diagnostic capabilities we see, post pandemic, are distributed equitably around the world and that every effort is made to adapt our new-found knowledge and capabilities to address previously intractable health challenges.

Healthcare Inequality

Global healthcare inequalities have been highlighted to a degree during the COVID-19 pandemic, with various global efforts to improve the distribution of vaccines to LMIC. But the pandemic has also seen much talk of eagerness to "return to normal". That's not something we should aspire to - "normal" for millions around the world means lack of access to vital diagnostic tests that can help save lives. Admittedly, much more needs to be done than just providing diagnostics. But it is a vital and achievable step towards greater healthcare equality and, thanks to the COVID-19 pandemic, it's more achievable than it was just a couple of years ago.

Regular access to medical facilities and well-equipped laboratories offering an array of diagnostic services has ensured that less than 5% of deaths in developed nations are due to infectious diseases. In the world's poorest nations, however, more than 50% of deaths are from infectious diseases[413]. Overlooked before and amidst the global focus on COVID-19, myriad other health challenges remain in poorer parts of the world. Diseases such as tuberculosis (TB), malaria and HIV continue to take a heavy toll, causing millions of deaths annually, especially in LMICs across parts of Africa, Asia, and Latin America.

While moving from lab-based tests to POC and domestic testing may see quicker times to test results in well-off nations, the availability of lab-free testing in RLS/LMICs can make the difference between access to a test and no diagnostics at all.

A 2007 Rand report[414] highlighted the potential benefits of new diagnostics in stark terms:

- A quick, easy-to-use test for bacterial pneumonia could save at least 405,000 children's lives each year
- A widely accessible, easy-to-use diagnostic for antenatal syphilis would save at least 138,000 lives and avert more than 148,000 stillbirths annually
- A rapid, easy-to-use test for TB could save approximately 400,000 lives per year
- A test for malaria that requires no laboratory infrastructure could save nearly 300,000 lives and avoid almost 450 million unnecessary treatments (resulting in more than 1 million additional lives saved) annually

Note: Lives saved include those saved through treatment of the disease and those saved indirectly through reduction of overtreatment with antibiotics. Estimates assume that treatment is available if required following testing.

The Disease Burden

It's important to spend some time discussing non-COVID-19 challenges which, while not top-of-mind, remain significant in certain locations and/or demographics. A number of diseases have seen some improvements in test availability in recent years but could benefit from a move to next generation tests. Although we've focused on viruses in this book, we'll also refer in this section to some other pathogens such as Malaria (parasite) and TB (bacteria) to highlight the scope, beyond just viruses, of the technologies discussed in this book.

Malaria

Despite advances in treatments over the years, Malaria remains a leading cause of death and illness worldwide. Globally, the World Health Organization estimates that, in 2020, 241 million clinical cases of malaria occurred, and 627,000 deaths resulted, mostly of children in Africa[415].

Malaria is caused by a parasite known as Plasmodium, so it is neither bacterial nor viral like the other diseases discussed. There is a vaccine now, *RTS S*, (trade name Mosquirix) but diagnostics for malaria remain important in the quest to reduce the death rate. The gold standard test for malaria is microscopy of a blood smear, using a Giemsa stain. However, this test requires a laboratory and trained reviewer, so rapid antigen tests may be more practical in LMIC where malaria is prevalent.

Malaria symptoms tend to be quite non-specific with fever, headache and body pains making diagnosis without a test quite difficult. Once diagnosed, the provision of an antimalarial drug is usually highly effective. But Malaria can progress quite rapidly, so fast POC testing is preferable to lab-based PCR or microscopy options. In 1999, the WHO put in place a testing and education plan to support the use of rapid testing and as of 2020, there are more than 200 malaria rapid tests on the market - with 2.7 billion sold between 2010 and 2019[416]. Malaria antigen tests target proteins produced by malaria parasites in infected blood[417]. Some assays detect a single parasite species, while others can distinguish between different species.

Testing the Malaria Tests

A 2019 review[418] of the performance of rapid malaria tests concluded that a WHO co-ordinated programme to comparatively assess different rapid tests, *"combined with policy changes has been influential in the acceptance of malaria RDTs as a case-management tool, enabling a policy of parasite-based diagnosis prior to treatment. Publication of product testing results has produced a transparent market allowing users and procurers to clearly identify appropriate products for their situation, and could form a model for introduction of other, broad-scale diagnostics".*

Assay manufacturers who improved and resubmitted their products after initial WHO testing saw a doubling of acceptable performance: *Fifteen products met the procurement criteria on initial evaluation, compared with 31 on repeat evaluation. The RDT evaluation programme also served as a model for establishing and ensuring performance standards for RDTs detecting other diseases. To date, a leishmaniasis and Ebola RDT evaluation programme have been established using protocols adapted from malaria product testing.*

It seems clear there may be lessons learned from this process that could also be applied to the regulation of rapid tests for SARS-CoV-2 and other pathogens.

In a potential complication for patients with a specific hereditary condition - a deficiency of the enzyme glucose-6-phosphate dehydrogenase (G6PD) - who receive a positive test for malaria, one recommended treatment (primaquine) can trigger a severe blood disorder known as acute haemolytic anaemia. G6PD deficiency affects more than 400 million people worldwide and there is considerable geographical overlap between the prevalence of G6PD deficiency and the prevalence of malaria. Diagnostic advances are addressing this challenge, with the emergence of a rapid test for G6PD to replace the laboratory-based spectrophotometric/fluorescent spot testing (FST) methods formerly used. In testing[419], an LFT rapid assay showed as 90% sensitive in determining individuals with severe deficiency and 84.8% sensitive in determining individuals with moderate or severe deficiency. In another promising development, researchers in Thailand have reported 90% sensitivity and 97% specificity using LAMP isothermal NAAT[420].

Tuberculosis (TB)

According to the CDC[421], TB is the leading infectious disease killer in the world, claiming 1.5 million lives each year. Of the estimated 10 million individuals who became ill with TB in 2018, approximately three million how is this known were "missed" by health systems and do not get the care they need, allowing the disease to continue to be transmitted.

TB poses a particular diagnostic challenge - only about 5% of those infected will develop the disease within a short period of time. The vast majority will instead see the bacteria remain dormant in what's known as latent tuberculosis infection (LTBI). It is estimated that one-third of the world's population is latently infected with tuberculosis. Overall, an estimated 5% of people infected with LTBI will reactivate in their lifetime.[422]

Further complicating pursuit of availability of rapid POC TB testing is the requirement for any test to be able to identify rifampicin-resistant variants, as that's an important factor in treatment choice.

The traditional approach to TB diagnosis is laboratory-based smear microscopy, which suffers from relatively low sensitivity of only 60% and doesn't differentiate resistant variants. More recently, RT-PCR has been used to detect the RNA of the Mycobacterium tuberculosis bacterium with studies showing sensitivity of up to 90%[423].

In very encouraging news, given that 95% of TB cases are in RLS/LMIC, a POC PCR test from Cephid called Xpert® MTB/RIF was endorsed by the WHO in 2010 and has been used to conduct millions of tests, with a 2-hour turnaround per test. A systematic review in 2014[424] found the benchtop machine delivered a pooled sensitivity of 88% and specificity of 98% compared with culture, despite being operated by non-specialist staff.

Acceptably sensitive LFTs for TB have yet to be developed but several efforts are underway and in 2016 the WHO published an update regarding the use of isothermal LAMP testing for TB[425], which will likely lead to miniaturised NAAT capabilities in the coming years. For those looking for a deeper overview of the TB diagnostics market, UNITAID's comprehensive *Diagnostics Technology Landscape 5th Edition, 2017* report is freely available[426].

HIV

Although it is by definition difficult to quantify, researchers believe that up to 60% of people worldwide who have HIV are undiagnosed[427]. This is despite the widespread availability of rapid tests, and the emergence of highly effective treatments for those diagnosed. The research indicates that many people in at-risk groups cannot afford self-tests, although there is hope of competition driving prices down as new and improved tests come to market. Current HIV self-tests tend to be antibody tests that aren't effective until about 3 months after infection; molecular tests that could detect infection earlier could offer increased chances of identifying an infection before someone spreads it unknowingly, but these are not available as a domestic test.

Children suffer tremendously from infectious diseases. It's their leading killer worldwide; over 58 percent of deaths in children under five are due to infections, with a list of horrors that includes tetanus, malaria, measles, HIV, pertussis as well as countless pathogens causing fatal pneumonia and diarrhoea[428]. In the case of HIV, let's look at an example of the importance of improved diagnostics in infant cases.

The WHO notes[429] that in cases of HIV, the mortality of untreated, perinatally infected infants reaches 52% by 24 months of age. A preprint systematic review of laboratory-based, standard-of-care infant testing found that the mean turnaround time from sample collection to the results received at the clinic was 44.5 days[430]. POC NAAT tests for HIV are WHO-approved and can provide results in less than an hour. A systematic review of the clinical impact of using same-day point-of-care infant diagnosis, compared to laboratory-based technologies, found the overall proportion of infants living with HIV initiating treatment within 60 days was 90% when tested at the point of care compared to 54% when testing using the standard of care.

Enteric Viruses

Though recent popular focus and most of this book have been on the threat posed by respiratory viruses, it's important to note that enteric viruses which cause acute gastroenteritis are a significant source of mortality, especially in children, in some parts of the world. Several types of enteric viruses affect humans, including Norovirus, Rotavirus and Astrovirus; RT-PCR tests are typically used to identify these pathogens.

For those interested in a comprehensive summary of how diagnostic technologies are being applied to enteric viruses, the article *"Advances in Diagnostic Approaches for Viral Etiologies of Diarrhea: From the Lab to the Field"*[431] offers an accessible overview and, as you can see from the figure below, it covers many of the technologies described in this book but with an enteric, rather than respiratory, focus.

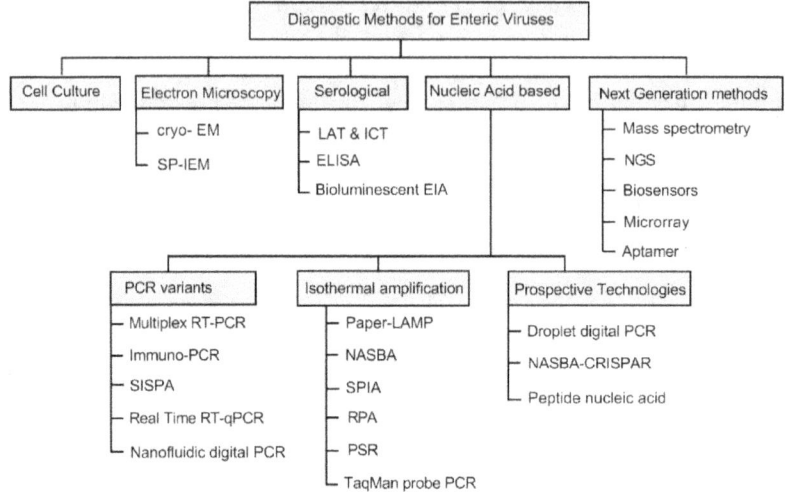

Figure 88: Diagnostics for Enteric Viruses

Polio

Polio has been in the news at the time of writing too. Though largely eradicated, continuing vigilance is essential to avoid significant recurrences.

As noted in a letter from Dr. Mary Bassett, the health commissioner of New York State, to the New York Times in August 2022[432], Polio made a shock return to the US, with the first case in New York State since 1990 leading to paralysis. She reminded the public that *about 70 percent of people who contract polio have no symptoms. About 25 percent of people infected experience symptoms that are mild or flu-like — headache, fatigue, fever, stiffness, muscle pain, nausea, a sore throat — all of which could be mistaken for many other illnesses. Fewer than 1 percent of infected individuals develop paralysis. Of those paralyzed, 2 to 10 percent die when their breathing muscles become immobilized.* Dr Bassett continued: *"This is where we are. The emergence of new pathogens like Covid-19 or unusual presentations of more recently identified viruses in the U.S., like monkeypox, will be only the beginning. Polio, an ancient scourge, can come back. The good news is that we can change this grim scenario."*

In a promising example of how new techniques can offer faster results, the Poliovirus Sequencing Consortium, an international collaboration between academic and public health researchers focused on detecting polio, has developed a method that combines PCR and nanopore sequencing, to detect and sequence poliovirus from stool and environmental samples, improving time to result by 3-7 days over current culture-based methodologies[433]. The use of nanopore sequencing offers significantly reduced costs over traditional Sanger sequencing.

Healthcare Equity

As we saw earlier, the pandemic threw into sharp relief the inequalities in access to healthcare, even within richer countries, let alone LMICs. In many countries, State funded RT-PCR testing programmes meant most groups were able to access testing, but not without having to travel to a testing centre. As at-home tests became available, many countries offered subsidies or even free test kits. It may be optimistic to think that public health policy makers will focus on ensuring that marginalised groups will continue to have access to diagnostics in the future, but the imperative to continue to hunt COVID-19, as it becomes endemic, may offer an opportunity to broaden access to other tests.

In the US, the CDC is using its Social Vulnerability Index to determine the location of over 1,000 free testing sites, as part of a program known as Increasing Community Access to Testing (ICATT), targeting individuals who are under/un-insured and at higher risk for severe COVID-19. Many of these testing sites are unattended - providing free testing kits for people to carry out sampling themselves and drop off to be sent for PCR testing at a lab. This initiative is delivered using a CDC/private testing firm partnership. In other countries, where the health infrastructure is less developed, alternative approaches to improving access to testing are taking shape.

In 2020, the WHO established its COVID-19 Technology Access Pool (C-TAP) initiative to facilitate timely, equitable and affordable access to COVID-19-related products. This framework allows for the licensing of tests to be produced in local facilities. For example, in 2022[434], a South African pharmaceutical company, Biotech Africa, was able to manufacture Spain's National Research Council (CSIC) COVID-19 serological test.

"The most effective way to get – and keep – ahead of COVID-19 is to keep testing," said Dr Tedros Adhanom Ghebreyesus, WHO Director-General. "This new agreement means we can take advantage of untapped manufacturing capacity so more people in more countries can have easier access to affordable diagnostics."

Diagnostics in Resource Limited Settings

By some estimates, deploying rapid, laboratory-independent diagnostic tests for just four infections (bacterial pneumonia, syphilis, malaria, and tuberculosis) could prevent more than 1.2 million deaths each year in developing countries

Drain et Al, 2013[435]

It may be naive, but I'm optimistic that a long-term dividend of the investment in COVID-19 diagnostic technologies will be improved healthcare in resource limited settings (RLS) and in low/middle income countries (LMIC). For communities that lack access to laboratory facilities for testing, any improvement in access to diagnostics is potentially a massive breakthrough. Extending availability of next generation isothermal and LFIA tests around the globe is vital to tackling health inequalities while also aiding defence against future pandemics. Of course, any improvements in diagnostics must be matched by concomitant improvements in access to treatments but, as a first step, availability of affordable, accurate diagnostics, without the need for laboratories, is now more attainable than ever.

I find it hugely disappointing that there's an official list of World Health Organisation "neglected diseases"[436]; surely the 2020 pandemic proved that tests for novel diseases can be created quickly, given enough scientific focus. Recreating even a fraction of the effort mobilised for SARS-CoV-2 could dramatically improve disease outcomes for millions of people.

Prior investigations into the efficacy of improved POC diagnostics reinforce the potential - and the imperative - to harness the progress of the 2020 pandemic for meaningful improvements: according to a 2015 study[437] of multidrug-resistant TB (MDR-TB), the deployment of NAAT POC Cephid Xpert MTB/RIF[438] test was an important contributor to improved case detection and rapid treatment initiation, with resultant interruption of transmission and reduced mortality. The median time to treatment (TTT) reduced from 28 days in 2011 to 8 days in 2013. TB, though, still kills some 4,000 people *per day* globally (2020 figures), with delayed diagnosis a major contributor to the high mortality and ongoing transmission challenges in RLS.

The last decade has seen great strides in making diagnostics more widely available in LMICs, through the efforts of organisations such as the Bill & Melinda Gates Foundation and Grand Challenges Canada. Now, the pandemic has created new opportunities to repurpose diagnostic developments beyond domestic testing in high income countries. While they may not be equipment free, a device such as the Cue or Detect, with cartridges for pathogens other than SARS-CoV-2, could be used to supplement improved LFT solutions, given their relatively low cost and low power requirements.

Many researchers have been motivated to assess novel approaches to COVID-19 diagnostics in RLS. One interesting example is a $300 PCR machine[439], made using standard Sous-Vide cooking devices, that can process a relatively high throughput of 96 samples per run. And, in an interesting proof of concept, published in Jan 2022[440], scientists from Queen Mary University of London demonstrated a "lab-in-a-backpack" device that is as effective as commercially available COVID-19 tests at detecting SARS-CoV-2. The compact kit uses a Saliva-based LAMP test and is relatively inexpensive to make, costing $51 per unit.

Other potential avenues may involve the use of smartphone cameras combined with low-cost saliva testing kits such as one from the University of Santa Barbara[441] trialled with SARS-CoV-2 and Influenza. As far back as 2017[442], researchers combined a Thermos and a smartphone to demonstrate an isothermal POC diagnostic concept for Herpes (HSV-2). As smartphone cameras continue to improve and drop in price, they will offer additional promise as reading devices.

WHO POC Guidelines for SARS-CoV-2

In September 2020, the WHO announced target product profiles (TPP), describing the desired parameters for point of care tests, with an emphasis on achieving broad distribution[443]:

In an effort to guide research and development efforts and assist donors, technical agencies and ministries of health to select products that best respond to public health needs, WHO (with input from clinicians, public health experts and laboratory scientists) has developed prioritized target product profiles (TTPs) outlining 'acceptable' and 'desirable' characteristics. Due to the urgency of the current situation, the proposed target product profiles are focused on priority use case scenarios to address the greatest needs and are tailored to emerging or existing technologies. This should not discourage SARS-CoV-2 biomarker research or the drive towards superior performance targets or more innovative or more simplified testing formats. Furthermore, as the need for COVID-19 tests crosscuts all cultures, climates and economies, test characteristics that often lead to reduced access to testing such as elevated price, high complexity and requirements for cool or cold chain have been carefully considered. The proposed 'desirable' requirements reflect the specifications that would allow for the broadest uptake and in turn public health impact and should be the target for developers who are starting out or developing new tests and for the next generation of emerging assays.

The TPP aims for POC tests offering:

- Sensitivity of at least 70%
- Specificity of at least 97%
- Results delivered in under 40 min
- Individual test cost of less than $20
- Equipment/diagnostic machines cost of under $3,000
- Minimal training requirements of no more than a few hours

The WHO acknowledges that any given system may not meet all of these criteria but believes it offers useful guidance to manufacturers. Those systems that meet some of the criteria may still offer valuable diagnostic capacity in some situations.

Among the devices in this category are Mesa Biotech's handheld "Accula" RT-PCR system that offers a SARS-CoV-2 assay via an LF readout, capable of a result in about 30 minute and Talis Biomedical's Talis One which uses loop-mediated isothermal amplification (LAMP) for results in under 30 min.

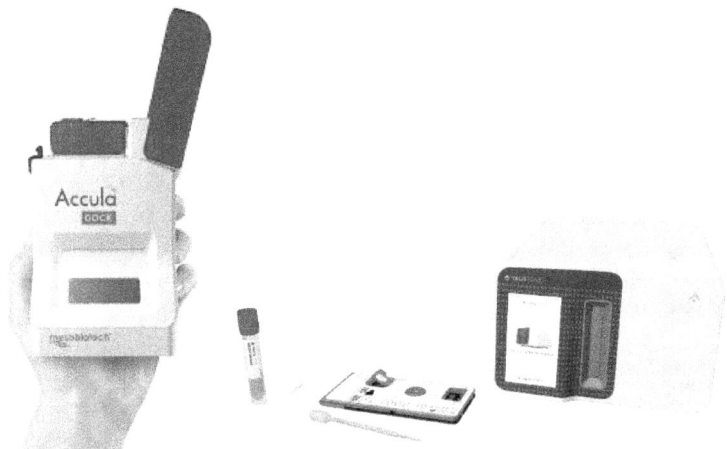

Figure 89: (L) Mesa Biotech Accula and (R) Talis One

Encouragingly, while the Abbott and Cephid POC systems have received the earliest approvals, a number of solutions are emerging from other companies, showing the accelerated progress generated by the COVID-19 pandemic. There are too many other vendors to list here, so I've included links to

FinddX and FDA sources in the Appendix providing up to date lists of all known vendors.

Before we move on from innovative devices aiming to improve access to diagnostics, I'd like to bring together a few themes of this book. Let's take a look at an example of how isothermal NAAT (in this case LAMP) is being applied to creating POC testing for Zika virus, the last major outbreak of which was in 2015 in Latin America. The standard test for Zika is a lab-based RT-PCR assay, thus limiting its use in RLS. However, the research shown below reports accuracy results for LAMP-based tests of up to 95.24%.

The following diagram shows the variety of approaches to deployment of isothermal NAAT in POC solutions, including many of the technologies mentioned earlier for reading the results of the amplified sample:

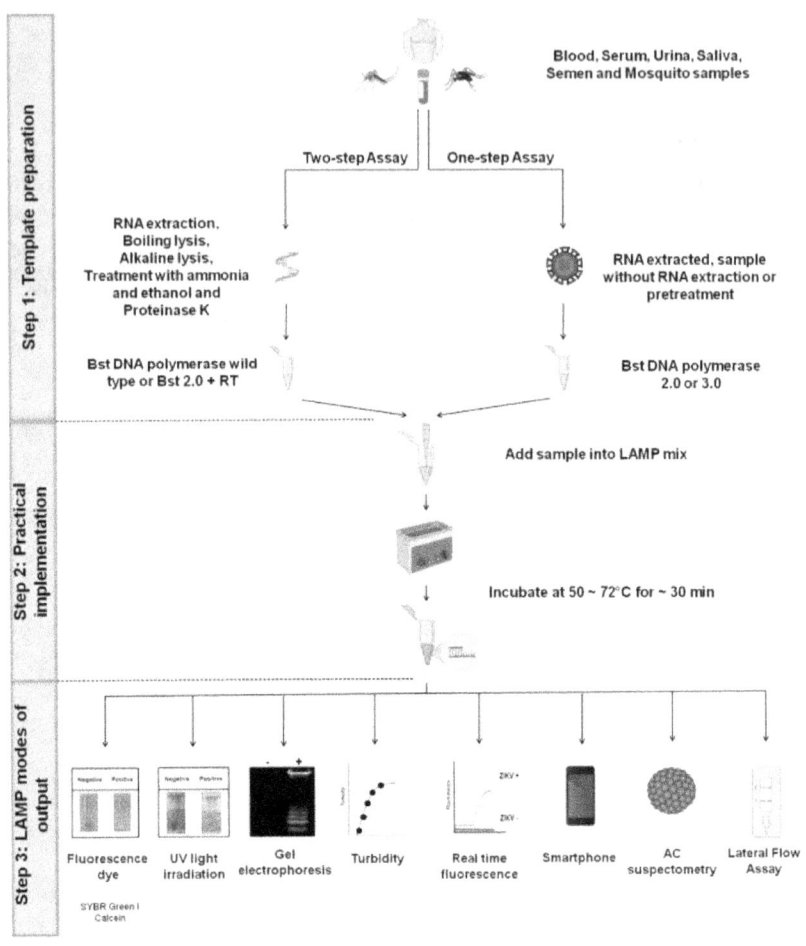

Figure 90: LAMP for Diagnosis of Zika Virus: A Review[444]

Affordable LFTs

As well as the device-based developments which may bring greater testing capabilities to remote locations, even more widespread benefits could result from ensuring that instrument-free testing methods reach under-served populations. We saw in Chapter 7 that the production cost for an LFT can be less than a couple of dollars. However, this may not be low enough to enable widespread use in LMICs.

Each year, approximately 1.3 million women living with HIV become pregnant and just under 1 million pregnant women are infected with syphilis. In late 2021, the WHO announced an initiative to make a dual HIV/syphilis rapid diagnostic test available for under $1, via a partnership between the Clinton Health Access Initiative (CHAI), MedAccess and SD Biosensor, to help in the fight to eliminate mother-to-child transmission (EMTCT) of HIV and syphilis[445].

In a promising step towards improving access, the Foundation for Innovative New Diagnostics (FIND) and Unitaid launched a scheme in July 2020, to drive equitable access to high quality rapid antigen tests (Ag RDTs) for SARS-CoV-2[446]. The plan includes access to tests for less than $2.50 each, as well as technology transfer and investment funds for local production capacity, which could be repurposed after demand for COVID-related tests is met. At the time of the announcement, FinddX estimated that, while high-income countries were conducting 252 tests per 100,000 people each day, in LMICs the rate is 10 times lower, at just 24 tests per 100,000 people[447].

When Neglected Diseases Aren't

Public Health experts around the world are used to outbreaks. But while these tended to go unnoticed outside of the dedicated teams involved, there is now broader interest. High Income countries' recent reports of Monkeypox and Polio cases give some insight into the scale of the ever-present challenge of viral threats to humanity - but remind us that it still takes occurrence of cases outside LMIC populations to mobilise substantial international response and resources.

MonkeyPox Testing

On July 23rd 2022, the WHO declared Monkeypox (MPX) a Public Health Emergency of International Concern (PHEIC), the highest level of alarm that the WHO can declare. Although not as readily transmissible as SARS-CoV-2, epidemiologists were worried about the disease spreading outside countries it had historically been present in, primarily tropical rainforest areas of central and west Africa.

Researchers have for decades highlighted the potential for a serious monkeypox outbreak, with warnings in papers such as this one in 1998[448] and another in 2008[449]. Despite its endemic presence in Africa for over 50 years, the lack of large outbreaks elsewhere has left it as a neglected tropical disease[450].

"This virus has been spreading in marginalized and vulnerable populations [in Africa] for decades, and we've done nothing about it. We have known that monkeypox is a potential problem for decades."

Dr. Anne Rimoin, UCLA epidemiology professor[451]

Monkeypox virus is a zoonotic disease, primarily of rodents, but was first identified in monkeys. The first human case was reported in 1970 in Africa, with the first Western case in 2003. Unlike SARS-CoV-2 which is an RNA virus, MPX is a DNA virus, a member of the Orthopoxvirus genus in the family Poxviridae. Unlike SARS-CoV-2 or Influenza, it typically presents with visible skin lesions, but does also manifest non-specific fever, headache and asthenia (fatigue) symptoms.

PCR tests on skin lesion swabs are the standard means of detecting MPX; as of Summer 2022, no tests that use saliva swabs or at-home tests are available or approved. In the US, the CDC has an orthopoxvirus PCR test that detects most non-smallpox related orthopoxviruses, including MPX. Note that, as a DNA virus, the RT process is not required, so a PCR test is used rather than the RT-PCR required for SARS-CoV-2. An available antibody test is CorDx's Monkeypox Virus IgM/IgG Ab Test, an LFT for MPX antibodies.

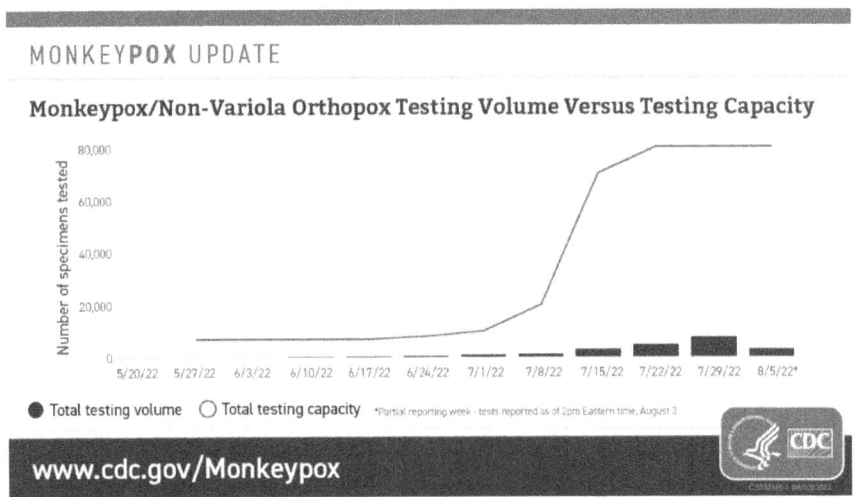

Figure 91: US National Monkeypox weekly laboratory testing capacity in mid-2022 grew from 8k to 80k. Source: CDC[452]

Perhaps coming too soon after SARS-CoV-2 for the full diagnostic dividend to be available to fight it, the importance of the availability of testing for MPX is nonetheless clear already in the early phase of the outbreak. According to the diagnostics tracking service, FIND; as of August 2022, the Monkeypox test directory[453] lists 111 tests, the vast majority of which are PCR assays, and are lab-based - with just 9 rapid antigen tests, 3 of which are for research use only.

In late August 2022, CorDX[454] announced it had received CE marks for three monkeypox diagnostics - in forms that will be familiar to readers from Chapter 6, 7 and 8.

- The Monkeypox Virus Fluorescence PCR Kit, used for the qualitative detection of monkeypox virus nucleic acid in human rash exudates/whole blood/plasma samples.
- The Monkeypox Virus Ag Test, a lateral flow chromatographic immunoassay for the qualitative detection of monkeypox virus antigen in human rash exudates and blood samples.
- The Monkeypox Virus IgM/IgG Ab Test, a lateral flow chromatographic immunoassay used for the qualitative detection of monkeypox virus IgM and IgG antibodies in human whole blood/serum/plasma samples.

For those wondering about the mutations discussed in Chapter 12, the 2022 monkeypox outbreak already shows 47 mutations from a 2017 outbreak in Nigeria, reminding us that viruses are a moving target.

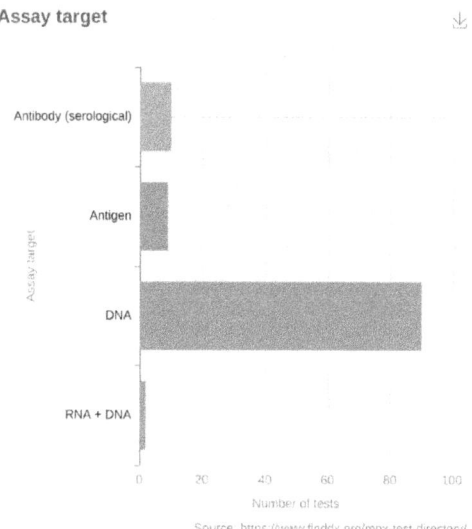

Figure 92: August 2022 Available Monkeypox tests

Drug Resistance

The COVID-19 pandemic has served as a sharp reminder of the difficulty of containing disease geographically and should serve as a warning of the importance of preparation for tackling predicted health challenges. Prior to the pandemic, a growing concern amongst science and medical professionals was the emergence of drug resistance among pathogens. As a final example of the potential benefits of harnessing improved diagnostics across the globe, let's talk briefly about drug resistance.

In a major systematic analysis of bacterial antimicrobial resistance published in the Lancet in 2022[455], researchers highlighted that Antimicrobial resistance (AMR) poses a major threat to human health around the world: they estimated 4·95 million (3·62–6·57) deaths were associated with bacterial AMR in 2019, including 1·27 million (95% UI 0·911–1·71) deaths attributable to bacterial AMR and concluded that bacterial AMR is a health problem whose magnitude is at least as large as major diseases such as HIV and malaria - and potentially much larger. The UK Health Security Agency referred to the threat of AMR as a "hidden pandemic"[456].

Improved diagnostics offer an important route to reducing the unnecessary or inappropriate use of antibiotics, which will assist in mitigating the growing problem of AMR. A 2006 report on the contribution of new diagnostics to reducing the global burden of acute lower respiratory infections (ALRI) in children highlighted[457]:

"Multiple drug resistance is increasing; for example, 25.5% of S. pneumoniae strains in South Africa, 53.2% in the Far East and 21.1% in Mexico are resistant to any three classes of drugs, excluding penicillin….For H. influenzae type b, resistance rates to penicillin and amoxicillin of 30–50% have been reported in Indonesia, Singapore, Thailand, the Philippines and Vietnam, 25–30% in Argentina and Venezuela, and ≤50% in hospital isolates in Guatemala. The prevalence of antibiotic resistance probably reduces the possibility of treating ALRI effectively (that is, significantly altering the probability of death) and increases the risk of complications and mortality).

What Happens Next?

Many reports have demonstrated that COVID-19 disproportionately impacted people of colour and under-resourced regions. Limited access to testing in these communities exacerbated the impact of the pandemic. Use of POC devices could help significantly in bridging the social divide in COVID-19 and other pandemics in the future.

Valera et al, 2021[458]

In a promising initiative, The Lancet Commission on Diagnostics[459] offers a model for an international alliance to oversee the implementation of efforts to overcome barriers to the expansion of diagnostics to LMICs. It's now possible for any country to create a national diagnostics strategy with far less need for the prohibitively expensive laboratory infrastructures that were the only option in the past. With advances in POC and low-cost tests for conditions such as diabetes, hypertension, HIV, tuberculosis, syphilis, and hepatitis B, which collectively account for a large share of the global burden of disease, historically underserved populations can hope to gain access to testing capabilities that were previously impractical.

The Lancet Commission noted that "47% of the global population has little to no access to diagnostics, with only 19% of the people in low- and middle-income countries having access to simple diagnostics for conditions such as malaria".
Lowering the amount of people without access to diagnostics to 10% of the population could reduce the annual number of unnecessary deaths in LMICs by 1.1 million per year.

Given that the Commission 's work predated some of the pandemic-inspired breakthroughs, I would expect that many of the recommendations and aspirations outlined are now even closer to being attainable, thanks to the acceleration in diagnostics in the last two years. For anyone interested in more detail than we can cover here on the topic of improved policy for LMIC diagnostics, the Lancet Commission Report is essential reading[460].

If one good thing can come from the COVID-19 pandemic, my hope is that it would be the application of these diagnostic breakthroughs to under-served populations, not just the expansion of faster, convenient domestic testing only to those that can afford it.

Chapter 14: Conclusion

Diagnostics are essential weapons in our arsenal against emerging pathogenic threats. As the COVID-19 pandemic has shown us, rapid and widespread testing capabilities can determine the course of a pandemic. Technologies that enable us to develop novel tests quickly, that provide results accurately and efficiently, and to distribute these tests rapidly and cost-effectively, will all be needed to tackle this and future outbreaks.

Centers for Disease Control and Prevention (CDC), 2020[461]

The COVID-19 pandemic has cost millions of lives, inflicted trillions of dollars of economic losses and upended the assumptions of billions of people. But amongst the damage, the scientific progress it has spurred presents us with an opportunity to make decisions that can save more lives in the future than those the disease ended prematurely.

A Pandemic of Questions

How has COVID changed our relationship with well-being, both individually and at a societal level? What new tools can we apply to improve our health and reduce disease transmission - what "war-time" technological advances will continue in our daily lives? Acknowledging that delays in the Covax programme have once again emphasised inequity in the global distribution of healthcare, how do we ensure that advances in diagnostic technologies may be applicable to LMIC and RLS?

More than ever, the COVID-19 pandemic has forced us to address the why, who, how, when, and where of testing. These questions must be directed methodically now to other infectious diseases, to establish a hierarchy of conditions, the testing and treatment of which would benefit to the greatest extent from advances in diagnostic technologies and disease awareness.

As we focus on the current challenge of COVID and mutations, it is important to ask ourselves the right questions so that we can pick out enduring trends and opportunities. Ultimately, patients are unlikely to care about the category of the test being used, but will stand to benefit from improvements, in the cost, speed, ease and accuracy, that have accrued in the last two years. But increased testing is not without risks. False positives, false negatives and distracting proxy indicators can cause real harm. Like many tools, diagnostics must be deployed carefully and appropriately to derive maximum benefits.

Our Relationship with Viruses

Modern diagnostic technologies have changed our relationship with viruses, but much work remains to be done to understand them. For instance, we don't know why the same virus can kill one person but be totally asymptomatic in another. Until the advent of enhanced diagnostics, we assumed the absence of illness meant the absence of the pathogen; now, though, we can detect them even when they aren't wreaking havoc in our bodies but are latently present or fended off by our immune system without our knowledge, leaving only trace antibodies as evidence that tests can find now.

A study published in JAMA[462], covering over 200 adults in late 2021/early 2022, identified that more than half (56%) were unaware of having an Omicron-variant COVID-19 infection. The study relied on the detection of antibodies to determine prior infection in the absence of a positive PCR or Antigen test. Although it's positive that the disease was so mild that it went completely undetected or dismissed as inconsequential, it highlights the continuing risk of asymptomatic transmission, which runs the dual risk of infecting others who may have a severe case, as well as offering more scope for variants to emerge, due to uncontrolled spread. The study clearly highlights the need for improved diagnostic tools for early detection of asymptomatic cases.

We've seen in stark terms the impact a virus can have at a global level. Though little consolation to those who lost loved ones to COVID-19, it's not the worst viral threat we could face. There are other viruses with higher case fatality rates (CFR) that urgently require more attention, for example Nipah virus (NiV), which has a CFR of 40-70%[463]. Or a virus with the transmissibility of SARS-CoV-2 and the CFR of MERS would pose a massive challenge.

As our scientific understanding of viruses improves, researchers are studying their role in diseases not typically thought of as viral. Should these research paths prove to be significant, the role of viral diagnostics will expand far beyond the already vast importance they hold for public health. Although this book is focused on viral diagnostic advances of recent years and on emerging test technologies, it is important to emphasize the role viruses may play in triggering other diseases and to incorporate any new knowledge in the development of testing and surveillance advances.

Multiple Sclerosis

Multiple sclerosis (MS) is a chronic demyelinating disease of the central nervous system. The underlying cause of this disease is not known, but Epstein-Barr virus (EBV) is thought to be a possible culprit, despite the rarity of MS on the one hand but the fact that about 95% of humans are infected with EBV, on the other. Using data from millions of US military recruits monitored over a 20-year period, Bjornevik et al. determined that Epstein-Barr virus infection greatly increased the risk of subsequent multiple sclerosis (risk of MS increased 32-fold after infection with EBV but was not increased after infection with other viruses, including the similarly transmitted cytomegalovirus) and that it preceded the development of disease, supporting its potential role in the pathogenesis of multiple sclerosis[464]. If EBV is further implicated in the occurrence of MS, perhaps improved diagnostics and sequencing of EBV can contribute to efforts to combat MS.

Alzheimers

A 2022 study[465], published in the Journal of Alzheimer's Disease by researchers at the University of Oxford and Tufts University, suggests that the onset of Alzheimer's disease may be triggered by the activation of two common viruses, varicella zoster virus (VZV) and herpes simplex virus 1 (HSV-1). Non-viral diagnostics are beyond the scope of this book, but there are myriad interesting adjacent investments being made in the area of dementia diagnostics, with initiatives such as the Alzheimer's Drug Discovery Foundation (ADDF) Diagnostics Accelerator being funded by high profile philanthropists including Bill Gates and Jeff Bezos[466].

Current Testing Choices

There are plenty of immediate lessons to be taken from the COVID-19 pandemic about diagnostic tests. Though at times lacking in scientific grounding, high profile debates about the relative roles for lab-based testing vs domestic/rapid tests have raised awareness of the trade-offs involved in testing. Just what level of accuracy is acceptable for rapid tests compared to the lengthy turnaround times for lab-based testing?

NAAT and Antigen tests are likely to remain the most common diagnostic test technologies on the frontline of detecting the majority of new and existing pathogens. The advances in miniaturisation, simplification and cost reduction, particularly due to isothermal NAAT, offer great hope for POC and domestic use and, importantly, the extension of rapid testing to RLS. Possibly supplemented using continuous monitoring sensor technologies, at least in some high-risk cohorts, it's not unreasonable to forecast more targeted use of testing in the years ahead, with less reliance on centralised laboratories. Inpatient stays could be reduced with a concomitant decrease in iatrogenic and nosocomial events, which would reduce the strain on health services.

Epidemiologist Michael Mina, formerly of Harvard, has used an analogy of coffee when describing lab tests vs rapid home tests for SARS-CoV-2[467]. He likens lab tests to professionally made Espresso coffee from a coffee shop and compares rapid tests to instant coffee. Though the espresso is "better", the instant option may be quicker, easier and cheaper than going to a coffee shop, if you just want a cup of coffee. To his analogy, I'd add the new layer of "capsule coffee" to represent the home NAAT devices we talked about in Chapter 9. The capsule coffee proposition is a domestic machine that promises coffee as good as your barista in your home - but it requires the purchase of a dedicated device, special capsules and it's still more expensive than instant coffee.

Testing Futures

In recent years, the technological breakthroughs in the field of diagnostics have been nothing short of breath-taking. The promise of genetic sequencing (NGS) and manipulation techniques (CRISPR-Cas), along with microfluidics and biosensors are, astonishingly, only some of the emerging tools that will define the next few decades; other advances in, AI-powered imaging and the application of consumer healthcare devices to early warning, should give us great hope. As widening availability of tests via laboratories and point of care devices, using NGS and CRISPR technologies, becomes more common, digital devices such as wearables may offer a completely non-invasive way to signal when a test is advised.

Awareness and Preparedness

Detecting and containing infectious disease outbreaks has long been a key pillar of public health, alongside education on improving health-related behaviours. But it has long been a slightly invisible speciality, frequently overlooked by policy makers who prioritise threats that pose a greater "clear and present danger".

Addressing the threat posed by novel and potentially fatal pathogens requires not only the capacity to create better diagnostics, vaccines and treatments but also a commitment to surveillance and the development of expertise. The

COVID-19 pandemic has dramatically altered the landscape in diagnostic technology, creating renewed awareness and funding for new technologies to improve our defences against legacy pathogens and to better prepare for future epidemics or pandemics which, unfortunately, are highly likely. Governments around the globe need to invest billions in improving health services, investing in scientific expertise and health education.

For a more detail analysis of the pandemic from a policy point of view and for improving preparedness for future events, I'd recommend the following books:

- Preventable by Devi Sridhar[468]
- Preventable by Andy Slavitt[469]
- How to Prevent the Next Pandemic by Bill Gates[470]

Personal Health vs Public Health

On an individual level, COVID-19 has familiarised billions of people with the concept of at-home testing and, in particular, taking precautionary tests to detect presymptomatic infections. In the long term, the COVID-19 pandemic may come to be seen as a turning point in the at-home testing market; building the level of consumer awareness that might have taken years or even decades, happened in a year. If only a small percentage of people were to take steps to test for endemic viruses, such as influenza and reduce their contacts in the event of a positive test, millions of infections could be eliminated each year.

I anticipate that the NAAT home testing devices such as the Cue and Detect will be targeted at the well-being market already conquered by Fitbit, Apple Watch and Peloton. Consumers who take an interest in their health and fitness will undoubtedly be interested in understanding whether they have a common cold or something more serious.

Public Health Policy

The role of public health policy makers will continue to be scrutinised to learn what could have been done better. Already, the US CDC has announced reforms[471] aimed at improving its agility of response following criticism of its COVID-19 handling and initial posture on Monkeypox.

In an April 2022 letter to the Lancet[472], leading UK scientists working in Pathology and Laboratory Medicine (PALM) noted the imperative to harness the advances and focus of the pandemic to ensure better preparedness for future pandemics.

As early as August 2020, the Association of British HealthTech Industries published its recommendations[473]:

- Develop national oversight and leadership of a holistic approach to diagnostics, aimed at reducing fragmentation and aligning and co-ordinating outputs
- Place diagnostics at the centre of population health management by developing expertise and increasing investment in the sector
- Ensure systems and resource is in place to retain and build upon the existing partnership and collaboration
- Retain the infrastructure built to support COVID-19 testing to accelerate adoption of new diagnostic delivery models
- Put in place critical enablers so that patients have access to innovative and lifesaving diagnostics

A 2021 Roche report[474] advised that the government should consider how COVID-19 testing infrastructure could be repurposed for early disease screening, so as not to lose the long-term benefits that could accrue from the emergency infrastructure put in place.

The Diagnostic Dividend

The unprecedented investment in diagnostic technologies that we've seen since 2020 means we're better positioned than ever before to manage our relationship with viruses. As a result of the pandemic, we now have:

- A wider public awareness of testing
- Better understanding of the testing process
- Improved performance of tests
- More capable point of care tests
- Domestic Consumer NAAT
- Enhanced understanding of wearables' role in diagnosis
- Further investment in more technologies
- More prepared Regulatory Frameworks

The rapid progress made since 2020 in creating and scaling diagnostic testing capabilities and capacity has the potential to radically improve global health. Advances in miniaturising high quality testing devices may rank as one of the most important dividends of the Covid-19 pandemic. The learnings from increased awareness of testing procedures will help improve infection control, while the ability to quickly and correctly identify viral infections will play a part in tackling the very concerning problem of inappropriate antibiotic use: the European Health Action Plan on AMR and the O'Neill Report on "Tackling Drug-resistant infections globally" both point to rapid diagnostics as a key instrument in tackling AMR[475].

Harnessing the Pandemic

A striking feature of my research of this topic was the speed of change - articles that were the very latest just 6 months ago now seem to be massively out of date. This is a fast-moving area which brings both cause for optimism and concern. What troubles me most is the notion that we don't build on what we've learned at such great cost.

While most people focus on when the pandemic will end and life can return to "normal", inevitably there are things that won't return to normal, one of which will be our relationship with viruses and how we find them - the important challenge is to make that a change for the better for *all* humanity.

The COVID-19 pandemic has forced much reflection across the world, and fundamental reassessments of things that were taken for granted. For example, the common wisdom was that workers should assemble in an office daily and that vaccines took decades to create, approve and distribute. The resilience and adaptability of humans under pressure has seen us question the very future of work and deliver scientific breakthroughs in astonishing timelines. Problems we thought were beyond us came within our reach to solve thanks to global investment, focus and cooperation.

As the world moves out of emergency mode regarding COVID-19 (notwithstanding the very real possibility of recrudescence) we should challenge ourselves to redouble our efforts on problems we've ignored or tackled only ineffectively. The pandemic dividend should be a renewed belief in our capabilities to achieve the seemingly impossible when faced with an urgent crisis. What we've learned about infectious diseases, diagnostics and public health interventions can reduce the global disease burden, as long as we stop accepting the inevitability of health inequality.

Appendices

A1: DNA and RNA Viruses
A2: Sampling Options
A3: COVID-19 Tests
A4: SARS/MERS Immunology Dividend

Appendix 1: Common DNA & RNA Viruses

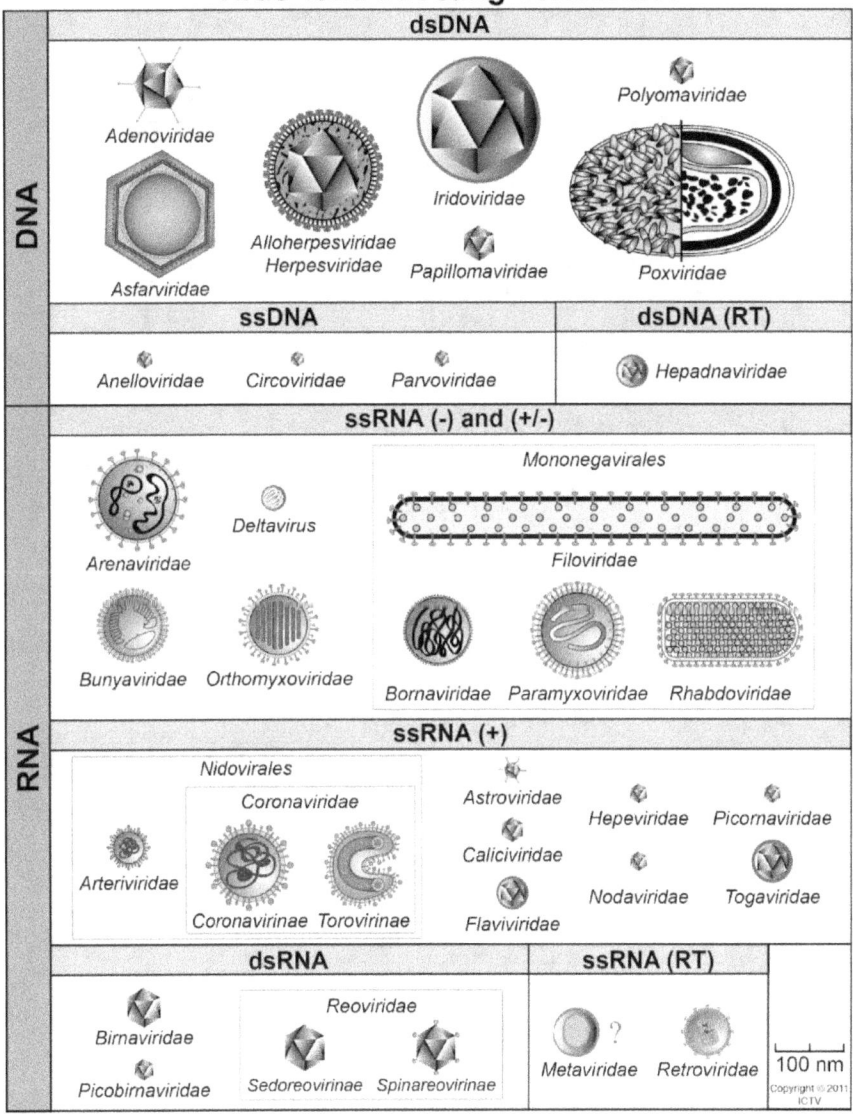

Figure 93: Virus Taxa from ICTV[476]

Table 1. DNA viruses.

Genome composition		Replication site	Envelope	Family	Genus	Common species example
Double stranded	Linear	Cytoplasm	Y	Poxviridae	Orthopoxvirus	Variola, Vaccinia, Monkeypox viruses
					Molluscipoxvirus	Molluscum contagiosum virus
					Parapoxvirus	Orf virus
		Nucleus	N	Adenoviridae	Mastadenovirus	Human adenovirus A - G
			Y	Herpesviridae	Simplexvirus	Herpes simplex virus 1 + 2
					Varicellovirus	Varicella-Zoster virus
					Cytomegalovirus	Cytomegalovirus
					Roseolovirus	Human herpesvirus 6 + 7
					Lymphocryptovirus	Epstein-Barr virus
					Rhadinovirus	Human herpesvirus 8
	Circular		N	Polyomaviridae	Polyomavirus	BK virus, JC virus
				Papillomaviridae	Alphapapillomavirus	Human papillomavirus 32, 10, 61, 2, 26, 53, 18, 7, 16, 6, 34, 54, 90
					Betapapillomavirus	Human papillomavirus 5, 9, 49, 92, 96
					Gammapapillomavirus	Human papillomavirus 4, 48, 50, 60, 88, 101, 109, 112, 116, 121
					Mupapillomavirus	Human papillomavirus 1, 63
					Nupapillomavirus	Human papillomavirus 41
	Circular; Rev. transcribing		Y	Hepadnaviridae	Orthohepadnavirus	Hepatitis B virus
Single stranded	Linear		N	Parvoviridae	Bocavirus	Human bocavirus
					Erythrovirus	Human parvovirus B19

Table 2. RNA viruses

Genome composition		Replication site	Envelope	Family	Genus	Common species
Double stranded	Linear	Cytoplasm	N	Reoviridae	Rotavirus	Rotavirus A, B, C
Single stranded	Linear; Neg. sense	Nucleus	Y	Orthomyxoviridae	Influenzavirus A-C	Influenza A, B & C viruses
				Filoviridae	Ebolavirus	Cote d'Ivoire, Sudan, Zaire ebolaviruses
					Marburgvirus	Lake Victoria marburgvirus
				Rhabdoviridae	Lyssavirus	Rabies & Australian bat lyssavirus
				Paramyxoviridae	Henipavirus	Hendra, Nipah viruses
					Morbillivirus	Measles virus
					Respirovirus	Human parainfluenza virus 1 + 3
					Rubulavirus	Human parainfluenza virus 2 + 4, Mumps virus
					Metapneumovirus	Human metapneumovirus
					Pneumovirus	Respiratory syncytial virus
	Linear; Ambisense			Arenaviridae	Arenavirus	Lymphocytic choriomeningitis virus
				Bunyaviridae	Hantavirus	Hantaan virus
					Nairovirus	Crimean-Congo haemorrhagic fever virus
	Circular; Neg. sense			Deltavirus	Deltavirus	Hepatitis delta virus
	Linear; Pos. sense	Cytoplasm	N	Coronaviridae	Alphacoronavirus	Human coronavirus 229E & NL63
					Betacoronavirus	Betacoronavirus 1, Human coronavirus HKU1, SARS & MERS-CoV
				Caliciviridae	Norovirus	Norwalk virus
					Sapovirus	Sapporo virus
				Hepeviridae	Hepevirus	Hepatitis E virus
				Picornaviridae	Aphthovirus	Foot-and-mouth disease virus
					Enterovirus	Enterovirus A-D (inc. coxsackie-, echo- & poliovirus), Rhinovirus A-C
					Hepatovirus	Hepatitis A virus
					Parechovirus	Human parechovirus
				Astroviridae	Mamastrovirus	Human astrovirus
			Y	Togaviridae	Alphavirus	Barmah Forest, Chikungunya, O'nyong-nyong, Ross River, Sindbis virus
					Rubivirus	Rubella virus
				Flaviviridae	Flavivirus	Dengue, Japanese encephalitis, Murray Valley encephalitis, Yellow fever, West Nile (Kunjin) viruses
					Hepacivirus	Hepatitis C virus
	Linear; Rev. transcribing			Retroviridae	Deltaretrovirus	Human T-lymphotropic virus 1 + 2
					Lentivirus	Human immunodeficiency virus 1 + 2

Source: https://www.ogmagazine.org.au/17/2-17/virology-guide-basics/

Appendix 2: Sampling Options in More Detail

This appendix provides more detail on some of the sampling options discussed in Chapter 5.

Nasal Options: Depth Matters

Perhaps as you might intuitively expect, nasal specimens are the most common starting point when seeking specimens to test to identify viral respiratory conditions. Although a nasal sample may sound simple, the CDC defines three different types, which require different collection swabs. The "nose" is a complex part of the human anatomy and has its own medical speciality - otolaryngology, often referred to as Ear, Nose and Throat or ENT.

Prior to the Covid-19 pandemic focus on testing, there wasn't a large body of research addressing the variance between nasal sites and, in fact, a recent study concluded that guidelines about the different types of nasal sampling sites were frequently inconsistent across jurisdictions and amongst individual HCP. It may seem overly pedantic to focus on where exactly in the nose a sample is collected, especially if studies show only a small impact on test accuracy resulting from how/by whom a sample is collected. But remember that, while a 1% difference may sound insignificant, at population scale it still involves a substantial number of people who may receive potentially incorrect results, with the associated consequences.

Nasal & Oral Options

The major types of samples in this category include:

Nasal:
- Anterior Nares/Nasal (AN) – takes a sample from just inside the nostrils
- Mid-turbinate (MT) – takes a sample from further inside the nose
- Nasopharyngeal (NP) – takes a sample from deep inside the nose, reaching the back of the throat

Oral:
- Oropharyngeal (OP) – takes a sample from the middle part of the throat (pharynx) just beyond the mouth
- Saliva samples are collected by spitting into a tube rather than using a nose or throat swab.

3 Noses

Although the 3 nasal sites listed above may sound reasonably well-defined, in practice the execution of testing may not be consistent; even when carried out by a trained healthcare professional, there is still room for interpretation or improper technique.

Numerous studies in the last two years, comparing the specimen sites, have greatly advanced the understanding of variations between sites, the specimens collected and the variations in analyte levels that impact testing.

A team of Danish researchers seeking to quantify the risk of false negative results from variations in collection techniques and to provide clearer guidelines for specimen collection found considerable disagreement and vagueness in existing literature describing sampling procedures[477]. Obviously, people's nasal passages vary in size, but the team defined the following average depths:

- NP - 9.4cm
- MT - 4.17cm
- AN - 1.95cm

The researchers highlighted instructions-for-use manuals that underestimated the required NP depth down to as little as 4 cm - vastly increasing the potential for false negatives. They also noted that the MT depth of 4cm was almost twice the depth recommended by the CDC.

Let's look in a little more detail at the 3 nasal sites and discuss the pros and cons of each one:

Nasopharyngeal (NP)

NP swabbing is the most established approach for collecting respiratory samples in healthcare settings. In addition to being the early standard testing method for the presence of SARS-CoV-2, the NPS is also frequently used for samples for the detection of other viruses including influenza, rhinovirus, adenovirus, respiratory syncytial virus (RSV), human metapneumovirus

(HMPV) and non-polio enterovirus (EV). A number of pathogenic bacteria, such as Streptococcus pneumoniae, that may be present on the nasopharynx can also be collected by NPS.

NPS is proven to result in high quality samples, when carried out with good technique by a trained healthcare professional. However, it is relatively uncomfortable for patients and can increase the risk of exposure for the HCP, especially if patients cough during the procedure. It also requires relatively expensive swabs, which may be in short supply. In the pandemic, the sudden spike in testing requirements led to a shortage of the NP swabs and so testing decisions became a trade-off of availability vs what might have been desired or required by policy.

Due to the outward appearance of the nose, there can be a tendency to assume the path to the nasopharynx is "up" the nose, but it is actually along the floor of the nose. The NP swab should be inserted horizontally to a depth of approx 9cm or approximately equal to the distance from nostrils to outer opening of the ear. This will be uncomfortable for the patient but should not be painful.

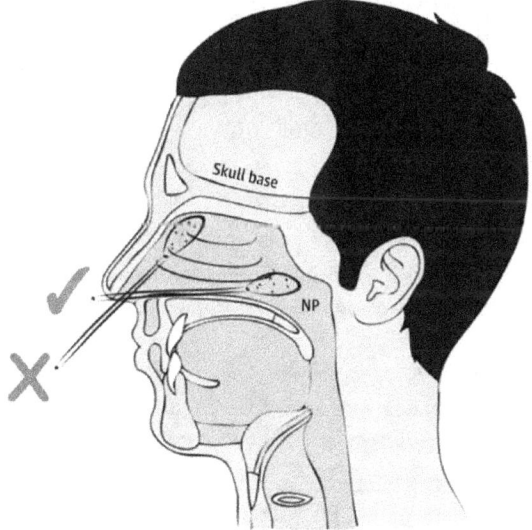

Figure 94 - NP Swabbing [478] *- Insert Horizontally, not Upwards*

Pros	Cons
Accuracy when done correctly	Requires HCP in PPE Can't be self-administered Requires long Swab Relative discomfort

Nasal Mid-Turbinate (MT)

Similar to the NPS, the Nasal Mid-Turbinate (MT) swab is inserted horizontally into the nasal passage, but only to about half the depth of a NPS.

Anterior Nares (AN)/Nasal

The final and least invasive style of nasal test is the Anterior Nares - AN swab (sometimes simply referred to as Nasal). This sampling is done by inserting a swab just about 2cm up the nose vertically. This type of swabbing is the most common method for at home tests, where samples are self-collected by users unlikely to have any training in sample collection. Users don't typically find this sampling at all uncomfortable.

Comparisons

The literature comparing the accuracy of various specimen types for respiratory virus testing is vast now and growing rapidly. The variety of approaches makes an objective comparison difficult, but in this section, I'll highlight some comprehensive studies. It appears that in many cases, MT provides a reasonably accurate sample with significantly lesser levels of discomfort. AN samples generally provide lower quality samples but, thanks to their suitability for self-collection, offer a far greater population reach than professionally-administered NPS, while still offering acceptable results.

Influenza Sampling

A study of 484 subjects across 4 hospital EDs, published in 2017[479], was designed to determine the optimal specimen type for influenza testing, comparing the 3 nasal collection sites. The researchers concluded that MT was the sampling method of choice: *Compared with the reference standard nasopharyngeal swab specimen, midturbinate swab specimens provided a significantly more comfortable sampling experience, with only a small sacrifice in sensitivity for influenza detection. Nasal swab specimens were significantly less sensitive than midturbinate swab.*

	NP	MT	AN
Sensitivity	100%	98%	84.4%
Specificity	100%	98.5%	99.1%
Discomfort level (0-5 where 5 is highest discomfort)	3	1	0

MT and AN

A 2021 study[480] comparing the results from MT and NP swabs for detection of SARS-CoV-2 introduces two additional parameters that we'll discuss in more detail later in this Appendix: the impact of who collects the specimens and when they are collected relative to the course of the disease. Highlighting that the samples were collected by trained personnel, the study found that 80% of NP tested positive compared to 64% of the MT samples. However, these results diverged later in the disease course, with retesting a week later showing 76% for NP vs just 45% on MT - indicating that MT is less sensitive for lower viral loads.

A meta-analysis of studies comparing the relative sensitivity of anterior nares and nasopharyngeal swabs for initial detection of SARS-CoV-2 published in 2021[481] found that AN are less sensitive (82% - 88%) than NP swabs (98%).

Swab Composition & Transport

In an interesting, in-depth review published as a preprint in 2020[482], researchers explored the impact of swab choice and use on sample collection. They noted that the *swab composition and structure have a significant impact on the main properties of the swab i.e., absorption, capture, extraction and recovery efficiency of collected sample*, with different swabs exhibiting potentially result-impacting variations: *Less than 25%, 30% and 55% SARS-CoV-2 RNA was recoverable from swab types 1, 2 and 3 respectively, indicating that most of the viral particles either were left in buffer or were entrapped by the swab material.*

When approving a test, regulators will look at the specimen collection as part of the testing process. For example, in their technical evaluation of the Abbott ID Now Covid test, UK regulators noted the importance of swabs[483]:

- For optimal test performance, use the swabs provided in the test kit. Alternatively, rayon, foam, HydraFlock® Flocked swab (standard tip), HydraFlock® Flocked swab (mini tip), Copan Mini Tip Flocked Swab, or Copan Standard Flocked swabs can be used to collect nasal swab samples.
- Puritan PurFlock Standard Tip Ultra Flocked Swabs, Puritan PurFlock Mini Tip Ultra Flocked Swabs and Copan Standard Rayon Tip Swabs are not suitable for use in this assay.

Among our pandemic preparedness learnings should be the need for further research on the suitability of alternative swab materials, so that any potential shortages of NP swabs can be offset by other compositions. For example, this study[484] found that despite the WHO recommending only synthetic fibres for SARS-CoV-2 testing sample collection, cotton-tipped swabs demonstrated equivalent performance at a lower price. From an economic point of view, even if small variations in the unit costs seem unimportant, scaling to population size or for use in LMIC can make small unit cost variations significant in total.

In an interesting piece of ingenuity, researchers at Boston University Medical Center demonstrated the viability of 3-D printed (and sterilised) swabs of their own design to mitigate supply chain shortages[485].

Swab Risks

All forms of nasal swab are considered minimally invasive and extremely unlikely to cause any harm. If there are concerns about the risk level of swabs, it should be noted that the levels of iatrogenic harm (that caused by a healthcare professional in the course of a patient interaction) relating to diagnostic collection are tiny. A study published in the Journal of Otolaryngology[486] found that the frequency of complications requiring treatment in the ED was 1.24 per 100,000 performed SARS-CoV-2 tests. Extremely rare broken swabs were removed via nasal endoscopy under local anaesthesia, whereas any nasal bleeds (epistaxis) required no specialist treatment.

Swabs and Transport

Where samples need to be sent to a laboratory for analysis they are usually transported, once collected, to the laboratory in a preservative buffer solution. This is usually a Viral Transport Medium (VTM) but researchers seeking to alleviate shortages during the Covid-19 pandemic have shown that Phosphate Buffered Saline (PBS) is also viable[487], as are Minimum Essential Medium (MEM) and Saline[488].

A VTM is suitable for the collection, transport, preservation and long-term freeze storage of viral samples that can maintain organism viability for 48 hours at room temperature. Although a viral transport medium is preferred, studies[489] have shown that dry swabs are capable of preserving RNA respiratory viruses without requiring a transport medium.

Appendix 3: COVID-19 Tests

For up-to-date details on available COVID-19 tests, you can refer to the following resources:

WHO:
https://extranet.who.int/pqweb/vitro-diagnostics/coronavirus-disease-covid-19-pandemic-%E2%80%94-emergency-use-listing-procedure-eul-open

US FDA Molecular Tests:
https://www.fda.gov/medical-devices/coronavirus-disease-2019-covid-19-emergency-use-authorizations-medical-devices/in-vitro-diagnostics-euas-molecular-diagnostic-tests-sars-cov-2

US FDA Antigen Tests:
https://www.fda.gov/medical-devices/coronavirus-disease-2019-covid-19-emergency-use-authorizations-medical-devices/in-vitro-diagnostics-euas-antigen-diagnostic-tests-sars-cov-2

US FDA Antibody Tests:
https://www.fda.gov/medical-devices/coronavirus-disease-2019-covid-19-emergency-use-authorizations-medical-devices/in-vitro-diagnostics-euas-serology-and-other-adaptive-immune-response-tests-sars-cov-2

For an up-to-date list of Covid-19 tests (NAAT, Antigen and Serology) with EUA check here:
https://www.fda.gov/medical-devices/coronavirus-disease-2019-covid-19-emergency-use-authorizations-medical-devices/in-vitro-diagnostics-euas

Tracker for commercially available and in development diagnostics

https://www.finddx.org/covid-19/pipeline/?section=show-all#diag_tab

The Johns Hopkins Bloomberg School of Public Health - offers a good summary and detail on testing types here:

https://www.centerforhealthsecurity.org/covid-19TestingToolkit/molecular-based-tests/current-molecular-and-antigen-tests.html https://www.centerforhealthsecurity.org/covid-19TestingToolkit/serology/Serology-based-tests-for-COVID-19.html

Appendix 4: The SARS/MERS Immunology Dividend

Readers interested in the scientific dividend of SARS and MERS Immunology research for tackling SARS-CoV-2 may find the following article interesting:

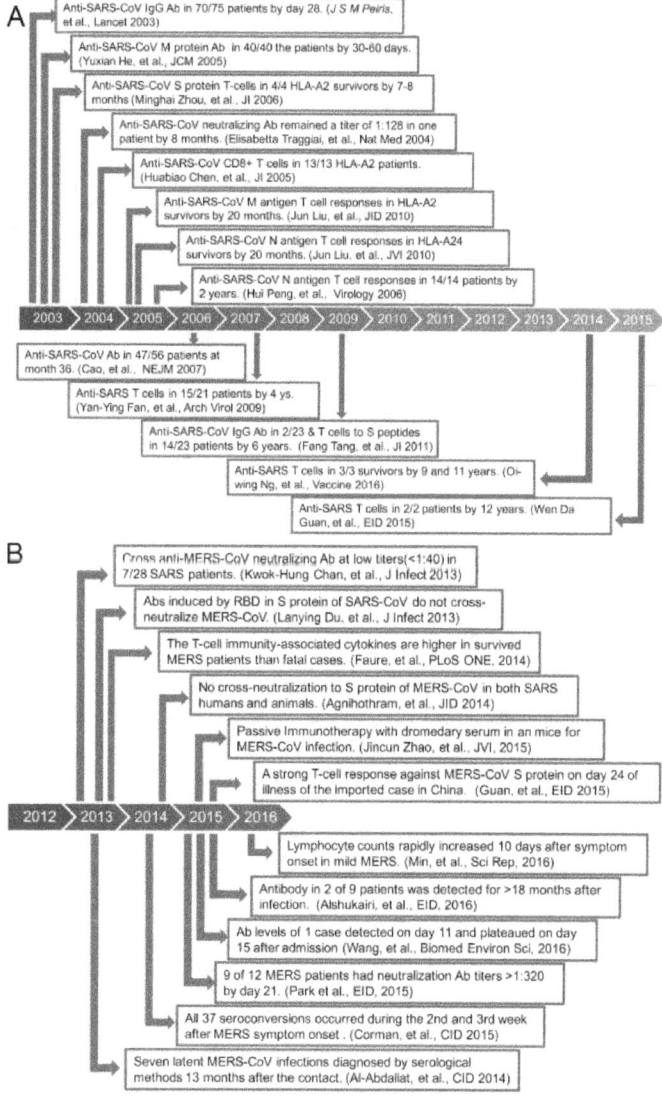

Figure 95: Immunology Learnings from SARS-CoV and MERS-CoV [490]

Abbreviations/Glossary

2019-nCoV	Original name for SARS-CoV-2
ACE2	Angiotensin Converting Enzyme
Ab	Antibodies
Ag	Antigen
AN	Anterior Nares
BAL	Bronchoalveolar Lavage
CDC	Centers for Disease Control & Prevention (USA)
cDNA	Complementary DNA
cfDNA	Cell-Free DNA
CFR	Case Fatality Rate
CGM	Continuous Glucose Monitor
CLIA	Chemoluminescent Immunoassay
CLIA	Clinical Laboratory Improvement Amendments
CRISPR	Clustered Regularly Interspaced Short Palindromic Repeats
CST	Consumer Self Test
CT	Cycle Threshold
DNA	Deoxyribonucleic acid
DPSO	Days Post symptom onset (sometimes written as POS, post onset of symptoms)
DRC	Direct To Consumer
EBV	Epstein-Barr Virus
ECDC	European Centre for Disease Prevention and Control

EIS	Electrochemical Impedance Spectroscopy
ELISA	Enzyme-linked immunosorbent assay
EUA	Emergency Use Authorization
FDA	Federal Drug Administration (USA)
GC-MS	Gas Chromatography Mass-Spectrometry
GISAID	Global Initiative on Sharing All Influenza Data
HCP	Healthcare Professional
HRV	Heart Rate Variability
Ig	Immunoglobulin
IL	Interleukin
kbp	kilobase pairs
LAMP	Loop-mediated isothermal amplification
LDT	Lab-Developed Test
LFA/LFT	Lateral Flow Assay/Test
LMIC	Low and Middle Income Countries
LOD	Limit of Detection
MERS	Middle East Respiratory Syndrome
MRSA	Methicillin-Resistant Staphylococcus Aureus
MT	Mid Turbinate
N	Nucleocapsid
NAAT	Nucleic Acid Amplification Technique
NGS	Next Generation Sequencing
nm	Nanometer
NP	Nucleocapsid Protein
NP(s)	Nasopharyngeal (Swab)
NPI	Non-Pharmaceutical Intervention

NSP	Non-Structural Protein	
nt	nucleotide	
OP	Oropharyngeal	
ORF	Open reading frame	
OTC	Over The Counter	
PPG	PhotoPlethysmography	
POC	Point-Of-Care	
RADx	Rapid Acceleration of Diagnostics	
RDT	Rapid Diagnostic Test	
RHR	Resting Heart Rate	
RLS	Resource Limited Settings	
RSV	Respiratory Syncytial Virus	
RT-PCR	Reverse Transcription-Polymerase Chain Reaction	
S	Spike	
SARS	Severe Acute Respiratory Syndrome	
SELEX	Systematic Evolution of Ligands by Exponential Enrichment	
SGTF	S-Gene Target Failure	
SP	Spike Protein	
ssRNA	single-strand Ribonucleic Acid	
STD/STI	Sexually Transmitted Disease/Infection	
TMV	Tobacco Mosaic Virus	
TTR	Time To Result	
VOC	Variants of Concern	
VOC	Volatile Organic Compounds	
VTM	Viral Transport Medium	
WBE	Wastewater-based Epidemiology	

| WHO | World Health Organization |

Further Reading & References

Viral diagnostics is a complex, fascinating and vital discipline.

Several of the books I have found useful are referenced below.

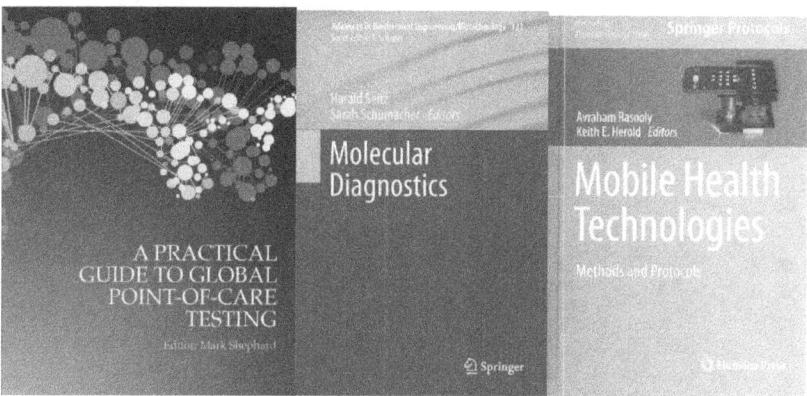

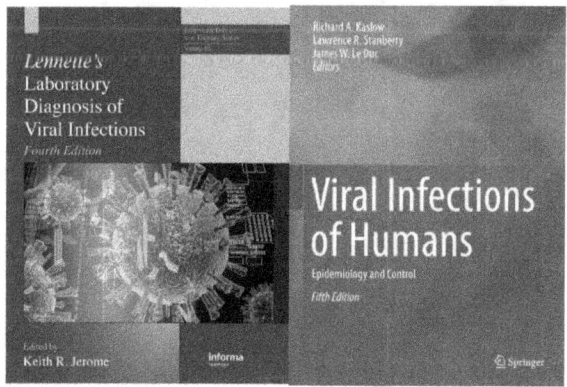

Fenner and White's Medical Virology (Fifth Edition)
Full book available for free download from:
https://www.sciencedirect.com/science/article/pii/B9780123751560000102#t0015

Acknowledgements

This book is dedicated to the scientists and others working to develop diagnostic innovations to keep humanity safe and improve global health.

My thanks as always to my family, and my friends, including Marie, Orlagh, Louise, Luke, Caroline, Lorraine, Susan, Sylvia, Henning, Matt, Aideen, David, Phelim, Sinead, Rob, Trish, Adam, Ian, Lar, Caroline P, Simon, Fergal, Lottie, Ken, Pat, Claire, Jeremy, Colin, Eric, Alice, Avril, Sudha and the Mastercard Team.

References

This section details the nearly 500 references to the amazing work of researchers and scientists and others contained in this book. Any errors or omissions will be updated on the website.

[1] Rosenfeld L. Clinical chemistry since 1800: growth and development. Clin Chem. 2002;48:186–97
[2] Dokouhaki P, Blondeau JM. Advances in laboratory diagnostic technologies in clinical microbiology and what this means for clinical practice. Clin Pract. 2012;9:347–52. doi: 10.2217/cpr.12.32
[3] https://www.finddx.org/
[4] Lecoq H. Découverte du premier virus, le virus de la mosaïque du tabac: 1892 ou 1898? [Discovery of the first virus, the tobacco mosaic virus: 1892 or 1898?]. C R Acad Sci III. 2001;324(10):929-933. doi:10.1016/s0764-4469(01)01368-3
[5] K.E. Jones et al., "Global Trends in Emerging Infectious Diseases," Nature 2008; 451: 990–993.
[6] Beyond coronavirus: the virus discoveries transforming biology
[7] ibid
[8] Petabase-scale sequence alignment catalyses viral discovery | Nature
[9] Woolhouse, Mark et al. "Human viruses: discovery and emergence." Philosophical transactions of the Royal Society of London. Series B, Biological sciences vol. 367,1604 (2012): 2864-71. doi:10.1098/rstb.2011.0354
[10] https://www.sciencedirect.com/science/article/pii/B9780123751560000023
[11] https://www.hsph.harvard.edu/news/press-releases/epstein-barr-virus-may-be-leading-cause-of-multiple-sclerosis/
[12] Micron equals one-millionth of a meter, whereas nanometer is equal to one-billionth of a meter. Micron is symbolized as 'μm' and nanometer is represented as 'nm'. Micron is also sometimes referred to as a micrometer.
[13] https://www.pbs.org/spillover-zika-ebola-beyond/about-viruses/virus-explorer/
[14] https://www.pnas.org/content/118/25/e2024815118
[15] Artasensi, Angelica & Mazzotta, Sarah & Fumagalli, Laura. (2021). Back to Basics: Choosing the Appropriate Surface Disinfectant. Antibiotics. 10. 613. 10.3390/antibiotics10060613. CCA4 License
[16] https://cen.acs.org/pharmaceuticals/drug-discovery/How-Pfizer-scientists-transformed-an-old-drug-lead-into-a-COVID-19-antiviral/100/i3

[17] https://talk.ictvonline.org/taxonomy/
[18] https://www.frontiersin.org/articles/10.3389/fimmu.2020.552909/full
[19] Etienne EE, Nunna BB, Talukder N, Wang Y, Lee ES. COVID-19 Biomarkers and Advanced Sensing Technologies for Point-of-Care (POC) Diagnosis. Bioengineering. 2021; 8(7):98. https://doi.org/10.3390/bioengineering8070098
[20] https://www.frontiersin.org/articles/10.3389/fimmu.2020.552909/full
[21] https://eu.usatoday.com/in-depth/graphics/2020/10/13/flu-covid-19-how-tell-difference-seasonal-influenza/5880649002/
[22] Joint United Nations Programme on HIV / AIDS UNAIDS. Intercountry Team for Eastern and Southern Africa. SAfAIDS News. 1998 Dec; 6(4):12-3.
[23] Wain-Hobson S, Sonigo P, Danos O, Cole S, Alizon M. Nucleotide sequence of the AIDS virus, LAV. Cell. 1985;40(1):9-17. doi:10.1016/0092-8674(85)90303-4
[24] https://www.webmd.com/hiv-aids/news/20220128/moderna-hiv-vaccine
[25] "Medical gallery of Mikael Häggström 2014". WikiJournal of Medicine 1 (2). DOI:10.15347/wjm/2014.008. ISSN 2002-4436. Public Domain.
[26] https://www.scientificamerican.com/article/viruses-can-help-us-as-well-as-harm-us/
[27] https://bmcbiol.biomedcentral.com/articles/10.1186/s12915-014-0071-7
[28] Viral Infections of Humans: Epidemiology and Control, 5th Edition, Richard A Kaslow et al, New York : Springer, cop. 2014.
[29] To Catch a Virus, John Booss, Marilyn J. August. ISBN: 978-1-555-81507-3 March 2013 ASM Press
[30] https://www.academia.dk/Blog/wp-content/uploads/KlinLab-Hist/LabHistory2.pdf
[31] Harrison, T. R, 4th Edition
[32] John Booss, Marilyn J. August, ISBN: 978-1-555-81507-3, Wiley, 2013
[33] Huebner 1959 Public Health Rep
[34] Hsiung GD. Progress in clinical virology--1960 to 1980: a recollection of twenty years. Yale J Biol Med. 1980;53(1):1-4.
[35] BMJ 2020;369:m1547
[36] Almeida, J. D., P. Atanasiu, D. W. Bradley, P. S. Gardner, J. E. Maynard, A. W. Shuurs, A. Voller, and R. H. Yolken. 1979. Manual for Rapid Laboratory Viral Diagnosis. World Health Organization, Geneva, Switzerland
[37] Christopher J. Burrell, Colin R. Howard, Frederick A. Murphy, Chapter 10 - Laboratory Diagnosis of Virus Diseases, Editor(s): Christopher J. Burrell, Colin R. Howard, Frederick A. Murphy, Fenner and White's Medical Virology (Fifth Edition), Academic Press, 2017, Pages 135-154, ISBN 9780123751560, https://doi.org/10.1016/B978-0-12-375156-0.00010-2.
[38] https://www.fda.gov/medical-devices/in-vitro-diagnostics/home-use-tests
[39] https://pubmed.ncbi.nlm.nih.gov/?term=sars-cov-2+test&sort=&filter=dates.2020%2F1%2F1-2021%2F12%2F31&filter=dates.2020%2F1%2F1-2021%2F12%2F31
[40] https://www.reuters.com/business/imf-sees-cost-covid-pandemic-rising-beyond-125-trillion-estimate-2022-01-20/
[41] Rose G., "Strategy of prevention: lessons from cardiovascular disease", Br Med J 1981; 282: 1847-51.
[42] https://ec.europa.eu/info/research-and-innovation/research-area/health-research-and-innovation/coronavirus-research-and-innovation/diagnostics_en

[43] https://www.nih.gov/news-events/news-releases/nih-launch-public-private-partnership-speed-COVID-19-vaccine-treatment-options
[44] https://www.poctrn.org/
[45] https://www.nih.gov/research-training/medical-research-initiatives/radx/radx-programs
[46] https://www.COVIDresponseadvisors.org/newsletter as at Feb 23 2022
[47] https://www.breakingnews.ie/ireland/supply-lines-for-antigen-tests-are-not-elastic-amid-massive-demand-says-paul-reid-1238928.html
[48] https://www.wsj.com/articles/how-the-COVID-19-test-was-won-11646456601
[49] https://www.theatlantic.com/health/archive/2022/03/ba2-variant-rapid-testing/627591/
[50] https://www.defense.gov/News/Releases/Release/Article/2488793/dod-awards-2318-million-contract-to-ellume-usa-llc-to-increase-domestic-product/
[51] Hasell, J., Mathieu, E., Beltekian, D. et al. A cross-country database of COVID-19 testing. Sci Data 7, 345 (2020). Our World in Data (https://ourworldindata.org/coronavirus).
[52] Apollo's Arrow, Nicholas A. Christakis, Little, Brown US, 2020
[53] Hasell, J., Mathieu, E., Beltekian, D. et al. A cross-country database of COVID-19 testing. Sci Data 7, 345 (2020)
[54] https://ourworldindata.org/coronavirus-testing
[55] https://www.bbc.com/news/health-59895258
[56] https://www.finddx.org/COVID-19/test-tracker/
[57] https://chs.asu.edu/diagnostics-commons/testing-commons
[58] John Booss, Marilyn J. August, ISBN: 978-1-555-81507-3, Wiley, 2013
[59] https://www.bccresearch.com/market-research/healthcare/point-of-care-diagnostics-report.html
[60] https://ir.quidel.com/news/news-release-details/2021/Quidel-Announces-Preliminary-Revenue-for-Fiscal-Third-Quarter-2021/default.aspx
[61] https://abbott.mediaroom.com/2021-10-20-Abbott-Reports-Third-Quarter-2021-Results-Achieves-Strong-Double-Digit-Earnings-Growth-and-Raises-Guidance
[62] Keith R Jerome (ed), ISBN 9780429142222, 2016 by CRC Press
[63] C J, Y P, Sf B, Rj B. "More men die with prostate cancer than because of it" - an old adage that still holds true in the 21st century. Cancer Treat Res Commun. 2021;26:100225. doi:10.1016/j.ctarc.2020.100225
[64] Asch DA, Patton JP, Hershey JC. Knowing for the sake of knowing: the value of prognostic information. Med Decis Making 1990;10:47–57.
[65] https://www.valueinhealthjournal.com/article/S1098-3015(10)60377-4/pdf
[66] Wilson JMG, Jungner G. Principles and practice of screening for disease. Geneva: World Health Organization; 1968.
[67] Dobrow MJ, Hagens V, Chafe R, Sullivan T, Rabeneck L. Consolidated principles for screening based on a systematic review and consensus process. CMAJ. 2018;190(14):E422-E429. doi:10.1503/cmaj.171154
[68] http://www.who.int/bulletin/volumes/86/4/07-050112/en/
[69] Kaier, Klaus et al. "Mechanical ventilation and the daily cost of ICU care." BMC health services research vol. 20,1 267. 31 Mar. 2020, doi:10.1186/s12913-020-05133-5
[70] https://www.fda.gov/news-events/press-announcements/coronavirus-covid-19-update-fda-authorizes-first-oral-antiviral-treatment-covid-19
[71] https://twitter.com/POTUS/status/1498852509745623045
[72] European Centre for Disease Prevention and Control. COVID-19 testing strategies

and objectives. 15 September 2020. ECDC: Stockholm; 2020

[73] https://www.fda.gov/emergency-preparedness-and-response/mcm-legal-regulatory-and-policy-framework/emergency-use-authorization

[74] https://eur-lex.europa.eu/legal-content/EN/TXT/HTML/?uri=CELEX:32017R0746&from=EN#d1e2117-176-1

[75] https://www.nejm.org/doi/full/10.1056/NEJMp2023830

[76] Clinical Laboratory Improvement Amendments - the US federal regulatory standards that apply to all clinical laboratory testing performed on humans.

[77] https://www.fda.gov/news-events/press-announcements/fda-roundup-january-4-2022

[78] Pinto, Ligia & Shawar, Ribhi & O'Leary, Brendan & Kemp, Troy & Cherry, James & Thornburg, Natalie & Miller, Cheryl & Gallagher, Pamela & Stenzel, Timothy & Schuck, Brittany & Owen, Michele & Kondratovich, Marina & Satheshkumar, Panayampalli & Schuh, Amy & Lester, Sandra & Cassetti, M. & Sharpless, Norman & Gitterman, Steven & Lowy, Douglas. (2022). A Trans-Governmental Collaboration to Independently Evaluate SARS-CoV-2 Serology Assays. Microbiology Spectrum. 10.1128/spectrum.01564-21.

[79] https://www.fda.gov/media/135659/download

[80] https://www.fda.gov/media/155039/download

[81] https://www.pewtrusts.org/-/media/assets/2021/10/understanding-the-role-of-lab-developed-tests-in-vitro-diagnostics.pdf

[82] https://www.cdc.gov/coronavirus/2019-ncov/lab/guidelines-clinical-specimens.html

[83] https://www.ogmagazine.org.au/17/2-17/virology-guide-basics/

[84] Natalie N Kinloch, Gordon Ritchie, Chanson J Brumme, Winnie Dong, Weiyan Dong, Tanya Lawson, R Brad Jones, Julio S G Montaner, Victor Leung, Marc G Romney, Aleksandra Stefanovic, Nancy Matic, Christopher F Lowe, Zabrina L Brumme, Suboptimal Biological Sampling as a Probable Cause of False-Negative COVID-19 Diagnostic Test Results, The Journal of Infectious Diseases, Volume 222, Issue 6, 15 September 2020, Pages 899–902, https://doi.org/10.1093/infdis/jiaa370

[85] Xia, Jianhua et al. "Evaluation of coronavirus in tears and conjunctival secretions of patients with SARS-CoV-2 infection." Journal of medical virology vol. 92,6 (2020): 589-594. doi:10.1002/jmv.25725

[86] https://www.thelancet.com/journals/ebiom/article/PIIS2352-3964(20)30278-4/fulltext

[87] https://jamanetwork.com/journals/jamainternalmedicine/fullarticle/2775397

[88] https://cen.acs.org/analytical-chemistry/diagnostics/Saliva-tests-show-promise-widespread/98/web/2020/08

[89] https://www.science.org/content/article/saliva-could-hold-clues-how-sick-you-will-get-covid-19

[90] https://www.thelancet.com/journals/laninf/article/PIIS1473-3099(11)70368-1/fulltext

[91] https://pubmed.ncbi.nlm.nih.gov/34718065/

[92] Gobeille Paré, S, Bestman-Smith, J, Fafard, J, et al. Natural spring water gargle samples as an alternative to nasopharyngeal swabs for SARS-CoV-2 detection using a laboratory-developed test. J Med Virol. 2022; 94: 985- 993. doi:10.1002/jmv.27407

[93] https://www.thelancet.com/journals/laninf/article/PIIS1473-3099(21)00146-8/fulltext

[94] https://www.sciencedirect.com/science/article/pii/S1386653220301840

[95] https://pubmed.ncbi.nlm.nih.gov/34431684/

[96] https://www.nejm.org/doi/full/10.1056/NEJMsr2022263

[97] Nikolai, Olga et al. "Anterior nasal versus nasal mid-turbinate sampling for a SARS-CoV-2 antigen-detecting rapid test: does localisation or professional collection matter?." Infectious diseases (London, England) vol. 53,12 (2021): 947-952. doi:10.1080/23744235.2021.1969426
[98] https://pubmed.ncbi.nlm.nih.gov/33326503/
[99] Dhiman N, Miller RM, Finley JL, et al. Effectiveness of patient-collected swabs for influenza testing. Mayo Clin Proc. 2012;87(6):548-554. doi:10.1016/j.mayocp.2012.02.011
[100] Murray MA, Schulz LA, Furst JW, et al. Equal performance of self-collected and health care worker-collected pharyngeal swabs for group a streptococcus testing by PCR. J Clin Microbiol. 2015;53(2):573-578. doi:10.1128/JCM.02500-14
[101] Todsen T, Bohr A, Hovgaard LH, Eið RC, Benfield T, Svendsen MBS, Kirkby N, Konge L, von Buchwald C, Melchiors J, Tolsgaard M. Valid and Reliable Assessment of Upper Respiratory Tract Specimen Collection Skills during the COVID-19 Pandemic. Diagnostics. 2021; 11(11):1987. https://doi.org/10.3390/diagnostics11111987
[102] https://www.fda.gov/medical-devices/letters-health-care-providers/recommendations-providing-clear-instructions-patients-who-self-collect-anterior-nares-nasal-sample
[103] Tonen-Wolyec S, Dupont R, Awaida N, Batina-Agasa S, Hayette MP, Bélec L. Evaluation of the Practicability of Biosynex Antigen Self-Test COVID-19 AG+ for the Detection of SARS-CoV-2 Nucleocapsid Protein from Self-Collected Nasal Mid-Turbinate Secretions in the General Public in France. Diagnostics (Basel). 2021;11(12):2217. Published 2021 Nov 27. doi:10.3390/diagnostics11122217
[104] https://www.azova.com/testing/ellume/
[105] Seo J, Shim S, Park H, Baek J, Cho JH, Kim N-H. Development of Robot-Assisted Untact Swab Sampling System for Upper Respiratory Disease. Applied Sciences. 2020; 10(21):7707. https://doi.org/10.3390/app10217707
[106] Discovering the Secret of Diseases by Incorporated Tear Exosomes Analysis via Rapid-Isolation System: iTEARS Liang Hu, Ting Zhang, et al. ACS Nano 2022, Publication Date:July 20, 2022 https://doi.org/10.1021/acsnano.2c02531
[107] https://www.kateto.net/covid19/COVID19%20CONSORTIUM%20REPORT%208%20TEST%20JULY%202020.pdf
[108] https://foodmarble.com/
[109] https://lumen.me/
[110] https://www.fda.gov/news-events/press-announcements/coronavirus-covid-19-update-fda-authorizes-first-covid-19-diagnostic-test-using-breath-samples
[111] https://healthcare-in-europe.com/en/news/spironose-the-electronic-nose-that-knows-about-covid-19.html
[112] GRANDJEAN D, ELIE C, GALLET C, JULIEN C, ROGER V, DESQUILBET L, et al. (2022) Diagnostic accuracy of non-invasive detection of SARS-CoV-2 infection by canine olfaction. PLoS ONE 17(6): e0268382. https://doi.org/10.1371/journal.pone.0268382
[113] For a detailed history of PCR, consider *Making PCR: A Story of Biotechnology* by Paul

Rabinow, University of Chicago Press, 1996. ISBN: 978-0226701462
[114] https://www.thelancet.com/journals/laninf/article/PIIS1473-3099(04)01044-8/fulltext
[115] https://www.thermofisher.com/ie/en/home/clinical/clinical-genomics/pathogen-detection-solutions/covid-19-sars-cov-2/multiplex.html?icid=WB45478
[116] https://discoverysedge.mayo.edu/2020/03/27/the-science-behind-the-test-for-the-covid-19-virus/
[117] Maitra, Pulak & Jamal, Mohammad Abu & Karim, Md. Rezaul & Islam, Md & Iqbal, Safia & Haque, Rashedul. (2014). A comparative study on microscopy, RDT and RT-PCR for detection of malaria parasites. International Journal of Biosciences (IJB). Vol. 5. p. 366-371. 10.12692/ijb/5.9.366-371.
[118] https://www.technologynetworks.com/diagnostics/articles/qpcr-analysis-how-a-qpcr-machine-works-and-qpcr-protocol-356835
[119] https://www.telegraph.co.uk/news/2022/02/04/shambolic-covid-pcr-testing-rules-meant-one-three-isolated-never/
[120] Oh, Hyunju et al. "A Closer Look into FDA-EUA Approved Diagnostic Techniques of COVID-19." ACS infectious diseases vol. 7,10 (2021): 2787-2800. doi:10.1021/acsinfecdis.1c00268
[121] https://www.ncbi.nlm.nih.gov/pmc/articles/PMC7128059/
[122] https://www.cdc.gov/coronavirus/2019-ncov/lab/multiplex.html
[123] https://www.thermofisher.com/ie/en/home/clinical/clinical-genomics/pathogen-detection-solutions/covid-19-sars-cov-2/influenza-a-b-rsv-multiplex.html#product-details
[124] http://www.genesystem.co.kr/sub/corona.php
[125] https://www.ncbi.nlm.nih.gov/pmc/articles/PMC8564276/
[126] https://www.ncbi.nlm.nih.gov/pmc/articles/PMC80298/
[127] https://pubmed.ncbi.nlm.nih.gov/32502334/
[128] https://www.labome.com/method/PCR-Machines.html
[129] https://www.frontiersin.org/articles/10.3389/fsens.2021.752600/full
[130] https://www.ncbi.nlm.nih.gov/pmc/articles/PMC7024801/
[131] https://www.ncbi.nlm.nih.gov/pmc/articles/PMC8802757/
[132] Oh, Hyunju et al. "A Closer Look into FDA-EUA Approved Diagnostic Techniques of Covid-19." ACS infectious diseases vol. 7,10 (2021): 2787-2800. doi:10.1021/acsinfecdis.1c00268
[133] Kyosei, Yuta et al. "Antigen tests for COVID-19." Biophysics and physicobiology vol. 18 28-39. 10 Feb. 2021, doi:10.2142/biophysico.bppb-v18.004
[134] https://www.researchandmarkets.com/reports/4805627/lateral-flow-assays-global-market-trajectory
[135] https://link.springer.com/article/10.1007/s00216-008-2287-2
[136] https://www.fujifilm.com/ie/en/news/hq/358e
[137] https://www.cytivalifesciences.com/en/us/solutions/lab-filtration/knowledge-center/lateral-flow-assays-what-can-we-expect-for-the-future
[138] https://www.sciencedirect.com/science/article/pii/S2667276621000470
[139] https://bdveritor.bd.com/en-us/main/bd-veritor-plus-system/how-it-works
[140] https://lumosdiagnostics.com/
[141] https://www.sciencedirect.com/science/article/pii/S0925400518306087
[142] https://www.jiac-j.com/article/S1341-321X(21)00297-X/fulltext

[143] Dinnes J, Deeks JJ, Berhane S, et al., Cochrane COVID-19 Diagnostic Test Accuracy Group. Rapid, point-of-care antigen and molecular-based tests for diagnosis of SARS-CoV-2 infection. Cochrane Database Syst Rev2021;3:CD013705. doi:10.1002/14651858.CD013705.pub2. pmid:33760236
[144] https://www.ecdc.europa.eu/en/publications-data/options-use-rapid-antigen-tests-covid-19-eueea-first-update
[145] https://pubs.acs.org/doi/10.1021/acs.analchem.0c03740
[146] https://www.fda.gov/medical-devices/safety-communications/home-covid-19-antigen-tests-take-steps-reduce-your-risk-false-negative-fda-safety-communication
[147] Caroline Chartrand et al, Diagnostic Accuracy of Rapid Antigen Detection Tests for Respiratory Syncytial Virus Infection: Systematic Review and Meta-analysis, 2015, Journal of Clinical Microbiology, P 3738-3749, V 53- N 12. https://journals.asm.org/doi/abs/10.1128/JCM.01816-15
[148] Chu et al. (2011) Performance of rapid influenza H1N1 diagnostic tests: a meta-analysis. Influenza and Other Respiratory Viruses DOI: 10.1111/j.1750-2659.2011.00284.x.
[149] https://pubmed.ncbi.nlm.nih.gov/27836481/
[150] https://www.cdc.gov/flu/professionals/diagnosis/clinician_guidance_ridt.htm (updated October 25, 2016)
[151] https://www.ncbi.nlm.nih.gov/pmc/articles/PMC6156320/
[152] https://www.prnewswire.com/news-releases/cordx-granted-ce-mark-for-worlds-first-combo-influenza-rsv-covid-19-self-test-301559170.html
[153] https://www.wsj.com/articles/at-home-covid-19-tests-might-cost-too-much-for-regular-use-11619602221
[154] https://www.intelligentfingerprinting.com/covid-19-lateral-flow-saliva-test/?lang=en-US
[155] https://www.med-technews.com/news/COVID-19-Medtech-News/birmingham-biotech-passes-phase-3a-for-lateral-flow-test/
[156] Celis, José E et al. "Plastic residues produced with confirmatory testing for COVID-19: Classification, quantification, fate, and impacts on human health." The Science of the total environment vol. 760 (2021): 144167. doi:10.1016/j.scitotenv.2020.144167
[157] https://microbeonline.com/epitope/
[158] Goh, Y.S.; Chavatte, J.M.; Jieling, A.L.; Lee, B.; Hor, P.X.; Amrun, S.N.; Lee, C.Y.; Chee, R.S.; Wang, B.; Lee, C.Y.; et al. Sensitive detection of total anti-Spike antibodies and isotype switching in asymptomatic and symptomatic individuals with COVID-19. Cell Rep. Med. 2021, 2, 100193.
[159] Liu, X.; Zheng, X.; Liu, B.; Wu, M.; Zhang, Z.; Zhang, G.; Su, X. Serum IgM against SARS-CoV-2 correlates with in-hospital mortality in severe/critical patients with COVID-19 in Wuhan, China. Aging 2020, 12, 12432–12440.
[160] https://www.idsociety.org/practice-guideline/covid-19-guideline-serology/
[161] https://www.frontiersin.org/articles/10.3389/fimmu.2014.00520/full
[162] https://www.ncbi.nlm.nih.gov/pmc/articles/PMC8491436/
[163] https://www.labcorp.com/coronavirus-disease-covid-19/providers/antibody-test
[164] Gorse GJ, Patel GB, Vitale JN, O'Connor TZ. Prevalence of antibodies to four human coronaviruses is lower in nasal secretions than in serum. Clin Vaccine Immunol. 2010;17(12):1875-1880. doi:10.1128/CVI.00278-10
[165] https://www.ncbi.nlm.nih.gov/pmc/articles/PMC7184472/

[166] https://extranet.who.int/pqweb/sites/default/files/documents/Status_COVID_VAX_02March2022.pdf
[167] https://www.technologynetworks.com/diagnostics/blog/covid-19-antibody-testing-s-vs-n-protein-340327
[168] https://www.cdc.gov/coronavirus/2019-ncov/lab/resources/antibody-tests-guidelines.html
[169] https://www.sciencedirect.com/science/article/pii/S1286457920300861
[170] Guo, Li et al. "Profiling Early Humoral Response to Diagnose Novel Coronavirus Disease (COVID-19)." Clinical infectious diseases : an official publication of the Infectious Diseases Society of America vol. 71,15 (2020): 778-785. doi:10.1093/cid/ciaa310
[171] https://www.technologynetworks.com/immunology/articles/antibody-vs-antigen-testing-for-covid-19-336486
[172] https://www.jimmunol.org/content/186/12/7264.long
[173] https://www.ncbi.nlm.nih.gov/pmc/articles/PMC7499300/
[174] https://www.ncbi.nlm.nih.gov/pmc/articles/PMC8491436
[175] https://www.ncbi.nlm.nih.gov/pmc/articles/PMC8491436/
[176] Wu M, Wu S, Wang G, Liu W, Chu LT, Jiang T, Kwong HK, Chow HL, Li IWS, Chen TH. Microfluidic particle dam for direct visualization of SARS-CoV-2 antibody levels in COVID-19 vaccinees. Sci Adv. 2022 Jun 3;8(22):eabn6064. doi: 10.1126/sciadv.abn6064. Epub 2022 Jun 3. PMID: 35658040; PMCID: PMC9166397.
[177] https://www.360dx.com/immunoassays/hong-kong-based-team-develops-rapid-microfluidic-sars-cov-2-antibody-test
[178] Ludolf, Fernanda et al. Detecting anti-SARS-CoV-2 antibodies in urine samples: A noninvasive and sensitive way to assay COVID-19 immune conversion. Science Advances, doi:10.1126/sciadv.abn7424. https://www.science.org/doi/abs/10.1126/sciadv.abn7424
[179] Butler D, Coyne D, Pomeroy L, et al. Confirmed circulation of SARS-CoV-2 in Irish blood donors prior to first national notification of infection. J Clin Virol. 2022;146:105045. doi:10.1016/j.jcv.2021.105045
[180] https://www.ncbi.nlm.nih.gov/pmc/articles/PMC7383527/
[181] https://www.fda.gov/medical-devices/coronavirus-disease-2019-covid-19-emergency-use-authorizations-medical-devices/in-vitro-diagnostics-euas-serology-and-other-adaptive-immune-response-tests-sars-cov-2
[182] https://www.ft.com/content/f28e26a0-bf64-4fac-acfb-b3a618ca659d
[183] https://www.medrxiv.org/content/10.1101/2020.06.02.20120345v1.full-text
[184] https://jamanetwork.com/journals/jama/fullarticle/2785530
[185] https://www.cebm.net/covid-19/what-is-the-role-of-t-cells-in-covid-19-infection-why-immunity-is-about-more-than-antibodies/
[186] https://www.ncbi.nlm.nih.gov/pmc/articles/PMC7837622/
[187] https://www.sciencedirect.com/science/article/pii/S0166354216304016?via%3Dihub
[188] https://www.nature.com/articles/s41586-020-2550-z
[189] Von Essen MR, Kongsbak M, Schjerling P, Olgaard K, Odum N, Geisler C. Vitamin D controls T cell antigen receptor signaling and activation of human T cells. Nat Immunol. 2010;11(4):344-349. doi:10.1038/ni.1851

[190] https://www.ncbi.nlm.nih.gov/pmc/articles/PMC8482551/
[191] https://www.med-technews.com/news/Covid-19-Medtech-News/t-cell-test-on-offer-to-detect-immune-responses-to-covid-19/
[192] https://www.360dx.com/covid-19/roche-readies-covid-19-t-cell-test-determine-patient-immune-response
[193] https://www.sciencedaily.com/releases/2021/09/210902124937.htm
[194] https://www.fda.gov/news-events/press-announcements/coronavirus-covid-19-update-fda-authorizes-adaptive-biotechnologies-t-detect-covid-test
[195] https://t-detect.com (reviewed by Author, April 30th, 2022)
[196] https://www.technologynetworks.com/diagnostics/blog/a-skin-test-to-measure-t-cell-immunity-to-sars-cov-2-347298
[197] https://www.centerforhealthsecurity.org/our-work/pubs_archive/pubs-pdfs/2020/200422-national-strategy-serology.pdf
[198] Jahn UR, Van Aken H. Near-patient testing--point-of-care or point of costs and convenience?. Br J Anaesth. 2003;90(4):425-427. doi:10.1093/bja/aeg082
[199] Kumar, Mukesh, and Suri S Iyer. "ASSURED-SQVM diagnostics for COVID-19: addressing the why, when, where, who, what and how of testing." Expert review of molecular diagnostics vol. 21,4 (2021): 349-362. doi:10.1080/14737159.2021.1902311
[200] https://www.frontiersin.org/articles/10.3389/fbioe.2020.602659/full#B21
[201] https://www.minipcr.com/
[202] https://info.biomeme.com/mobile-qpcr-thermocyclers
[203] https://www.abbott.com/IDNOW.html
[204] https://pubmed.ncbi.nlm.nih.gov/32434706/
[205] Assay Techniques and Test Development for COVID-19 Diagnosis, Linda J. Carter et al, ACS Central Science 2020 6 (5), 591-605 DOI: 10.1021/acscentsci.0c00501
[206] Renzoni, A.; Perez, F.; Ngo Nsoga, M.T.; Yerly, S.; Boehm, E.; Gayet-Ageron, A.; Kaiser, L.; Schibler,
M. Analytical Evaluation of Visby Medical RT-PCR Portable Device for Rapid Detection of SARS-CoV-2.
Diagnostics 2021, 11, 813. https:// doi.org/10.3390/diagnostics11050813
[207] https://www.numan.com/fear-nothing/fear-nothing-blood-test
[208] https://www.fda.gov/medical-devices/device-approvals-denials-and-clearances/510k-clearances
[209] https://www.advamed.org/sites/default/files/resource/30_10_11_10_2010_Study_CAgenda_makowerreportfinal.pdf
[210] https://www.fda.gov/news-events/press-announcements/coronavirus-covid-19-update-fda-issues-authorization-first-molecular-non-prescription-home-test
[211] https://www.cuehealth.com/about/press/cue-health%27s-connected-point-of-care-covid-19-test-demonstrates-97.8percent/
[212] https://www.cuehealth.com/about/press/cue-announces-$30-million-funding-contract-from-u.s.-department-of
[213] https://www.fda.gov/media/138826/download
[214] https://www.cnbc.com/2021/09/24/cue-health-googles-provider-of-covid-19-tests-just-held-its-ipo.html
[215] https://www.sec.gov/Archives/edgar/data/1628945/000114036121030058/nt10023122x6_s1

.htm
[216] https://circlepod.co/
[217] https://www.360dx.com/regulatory-news-fda-approvals/lucira-health-nabs-ce-mark-covid-19-covidflu-molecular-tests
[218] https://protondx.com/products/
[219] https://www.domusdx.com/
[220] https://www.genomeweb.com/molecular-diagnostics/domus-diagnostics-launch-point-care-infectious-disease-molecular-diagnostics
[221]
[222] https://roverdx.com/
[223] https://www.360dx.com/pcr/rover-diagnostics-developing-all-optical-rapid-point-care-qpcr-platform
[224] Blumenfeld, N.R., Bolene, M.A.E., Jaspan, M. et al. Multiplexed reverse-transcriptase quantitative polymerase chain reaction using plasmonic nanoparticles for point-of-care COVID-19 diagnosis. Nat. Nanotechnol. (2022). https://doi.org/10.1038/s41565-022-01175-4
[225] https://pubs.acs.org/doi/full/10.1021/acscentsci.8b00625
[226] https://www.pewresearch.org/fact-tank/2020/01/09/about-one-in-five-americans-use-a-smart-watch-or-fitness-tracker/
[227] https://www.philips.ie/c-dam/b2bhc/master/sites/west/pdfs/proceedings_electronics.pdf
[228] https://aktiia.com/uk/blood-pressure-monitor/
[229] Castaneda, Denisse et al. "A review on wearable photoplethysmography sensors and their potential future applications in health care." International journal of biosensors & bioelectronics vol. 4,4 (2018): 195-202. doi:10.15406/ijbsbe.2018.04.00125
[230] https://www.mayoclinic.org/healthy-lifestyle/fitness/expert-answers/heart-rate/faq-20057979
[231] Quer, G., Gouda, P., Galarnyk, M., Topol, E. J. & Steinhubl, S. R. Inter- and intraindividual variability in daily resting heart rate and its associations with age, sex, sleep, BMI and time of year: retrospective, longitudinal cohort study of 92,457 adults. PLoS ONE 15, e0227709 (2020).
[232] https://www.cdc.gov/nchs/data/nhsr/nhsr041.pdf
[233] https://help.elitehrv.com/article/67-what-are-r-r-intervals
[234] https://journals.plos.org/plosone/article?id=10.1371/journal.pone.0006642
[235] https://www.frontiersin.org/articles/10.3389/fpubh.2017.00258/full
[236] https://www.whoop.com/thelocker/heart-rate-variability-hrv/
[237] https://www.england.nhs.uk/coronavirus/wp-content/uploads/sites/52/2020/06/C0445-remote-monitoring-in-primary-care-jan-2021-v1.1.pdf
[238] https://info.patientmpower.com/faq-covid/
[239] Racial Bias in Pulse Oximetry Measurement , N Engl J Med 2020; 383:2477-2478 DOI: 10.1056/NEJMc2029240
[240] Gottlieb ER, Ziegler J, Morley K, Rush B, Celi LA. Assessment of Racial and Ethnic Differences in Oxygen Supplementation Among Patients in the Intensive Care Unit. JAMA Intern Med. 2022;182(8):849–858. doi:10.1001/jamainternmed.2022.2587
[241] https://mindfield-esense.com/esense-respiration-en/

[242] https://www.temptraq.com/News/University-Hospitals-expands-use-of-TempTraq%C2%AE-syst

[243] Li, Xiao et al. "Digital Health: Tracking Physiomes and Activity Using Wearable Biosensors Reveals Useful Health-Related Information." PLoS biology vol. 15,1 e2001402. 12 Jan. 2017, doi:10.1371/journal.pbio.2001402

[244] https://techcrunch.com/2020/03/23/kinsas-fever-map-could-show-just-how-crucial-it-is-to-stay-home-to-stop-covid-19-spread/

[245] Richardson, S. et al. Presenting characteristics, comorbidities and outcomes among 5,700 patients hospitalized with COVID-19 in the New York City area.JAMA 323, 2052–2059 (2020).

[246] https://www.webmd.com/cold-and-flu/news/20200117/could-your-fitbit-help-detect-the-flu

[247] M. J. Tobin, F. Laghi, A. Jubran, Why COVID-19 silent hypoxemia is baffling to physicians. Am. J. Respir. Crit. Care Med. 10.1164/rccm.202006-2157CP , (2020)

[248] https://journals.plos.org/plosbiology/article?id=10.1371/journal.pbio.2001402

[249] https://jamanetwork.com/journals/jamanetworkopen/fullarticle/2784555

[250] https://www.thelancet.com/journals/landig/article/PIIS2589-7500(19)30222-5/fulltext

[251] https://www.nature.com/articles/s41591-020-1123-x

[252] https://www.nature.com/articles/s41598-020-78355-6

[253] https://osher.ucsf.edu/news/51m-awarded-tempredict

[254] https://www.mdpi.com/2076-393X/10/2/264/htm

[255] https://www.mountsinai.org/about/newsroom/2021/mount-sinai-study-finds-wearable-devices-can-detect-covid19-symptoms-and-predict-diagnosis-pr

[256] https://www.jmir.org/2021/2/e26107

[257] https://www.medrxiv.org/content/10.1101/2021.06.13.21258795v1.full-text

[258] https://journals.plos.org/plosone/article?id=10.1371/journal.pone.0243693

[259] https://www.covid-red.eu/en/

[260] https://www.avawomen.com/

[261] https://corona-datenspende.de/

[262] https://www.nature.com/articles/s41746-020-00363-7

[263] https://www.whoop.com/thelocker/covid-health-monitoring-tips-resources/ as at Feb 2022

[264] https://www.statnews.com/2019/07/24/fitbit-accuracy-dark-skin/

[265] Again for full disclosure purposes, these are my personal devices and I have no affiliation with Fitbit, Whoop or Oura.

[266] https://www.nature.com/articles/s41467-021-22663-6

[267] https://ysph.yale.edu/news-article/wearable-air-sampler-detects-personal-exposure-to-sars-cov-2/

[268] https://twitter.com/yalesph/status/1483501739768696838

[269] Zimmer, A.J., Ugarte-Gil, C., Pathri, R. et al. Making cough count in tuberculosis care. Commun Med 2, 83 (2022). https://doi.org/10.1038/s43856-022-00149-w

[270] Laguarta, J., Hueto, F. & Subirana, B. COVID-19 artificial intelligence diagnosis using only cough recordings. IEEE Open J. Eng. Med. Biol. 1, 275–281 (2020)

[271] Forsad Al Hossain, Andrew A. Lover, George A. Corey, Nicholas G. Reich, and Tauhidur Rahman. 2020. FluSense: A Contactless Syndromic Surveillance Platform for Influenza-Like Illness in Hospital Waiting Areas. <i>Proc. ACM Interact. Mob. Wearable Ubiquitous Technol.</i> 4, 1, Article 1 (March 2020), 28 pages.

DOI:https://doi.org/10.1145/3381014
[272] https://www.embs.org/ojemb/articles/covid-19-artificial-intelligence-diagnosis-using-only-cough-recordings/
[273] Chan, J., Rea, T., Gollakota, S. et al. Contactless cardiac arrest detection using smart devices. npj Digit. Med. 2, 52 (2019). https://doi.org/10.1038/s41746-019-0128-7
[274] https://www.science.org/doi/10.1126/sciadv.abd4794
[275] Yang, Y., Yuan, Y., Zhang, G. et al. Artificial intelligence-enabled detection and assessment of Parkinson's disease using nocturnal breathing signals. Nat Med (2022). https://doi.org/10.1038/s41591-022-01932-x
[276] https://www.frontiersin.org/articles/10.3389/fdgth.2020.00008/full
[277] J. Am. Chem. Soc. 2022, 144, 25, 11226–11237. Publication Date:June 8, 2022. https://doi.org/10.1021/jacs.2c02537
[278] https://novabiomedical.com/statstrip-glu/index.php
[279] https://pubs.acs.org/doi/10.1021/acs.jproteome.0c01042
[280] https://pubmed.ncbi.nlm.nih.gov/34006662/
[281] Lippé, Roger. "Flow Virometry: a Powerful Tool To Functionally Characterize Viruses." Journal of virology vol. 92,3 e01765-17. 17 Jan. 2018, doi:10.1128/JVI.01765-17
[282] https://www.ncbi.nlm.nih.gov/pmc/articles/PMC3754246/
[283] https://www.ncbi.nlm.nih.gov/pmc/articles/PMC5411592/
[284] https://www.ncbi.nlm.nih.gov/pmc/articles/PMC4744565/
[285] Zhang F.; Abudayyeh O. O.; Gootenberg J. S. A protocol for detection of COVID-19 using CRISPR diagnostics (v.20200321). Broad Institute of MIT and Harvard. www.broadinstitute.org/files/publications/special/COVID-19%20detection%20(updated).pdf
[286] Broughton J. P.; et al. CRISPR–Cas12-based detection of SARS-CoV-2. Nat. Biotechnol. 2020, 10.1038/s41587-020-0513-4
[287] https://sherlock.bio/platforms/inspectr/
[288] https://wyss.harvard.edu/technology/inspectr-a-direct-to-consumer-molecular-diagnostic/
[289] Metsky, H.C., Welch, N.L., Pillai, P.P. et al. Designing sensitive viral diagnostics with machine learning. Nat Biotechnol (2022). https://doi.org/10.1038/s41587-022-01213-5
[290] https://www.ncbi.nlm.nih.gov/pmc/articles/PMC7860141/
[291] https://www.ncbi.nlm.nih.gov/pmc/articles/PMC7302192/
[292] Ackerman, Cheri M et al. "Massively multiplexed nucleic acid detection with Cas13." Nature vol. 582,7811 (2020): 277-282. doi:10.1038/s41586-020-2279-8
[293] https://www.science.org/doi/10.1126/sciadv.abh2944
[294] https://www.cell.com/cell/fulltext/S0092-8674(20)31623-8
[295] Electric field-driven microfluidics for rapid CRISPR-based diagnostics and its application to detection of SARS-CoV-2, Ramachandran, Ashwin et al. doi: 10.1073/pnas.2010254117, Proceedings of the National Academy of Sciences, https://doi.org/10.1073/pnas.2010254117. 2022/08/22
[296] https://www.ncbi.nlm.nih.gov/pmc/articles/PMC7498250/
[297] Najafabadi, Zeinab Yousefi et al. "The Trend of CRISPR-Based Technologies in COVID-19 Disease: Beyond Genome Editing." Molecular biotechnology, 1–16. 29 Jan. 2022, doi:10.1007/s12033-021-00431-7

[298] https://www.ncbi.nlm.nih.gov/pmc/articles/PMC7189862/
[299] Shihong Gao, David et al. "Development and application of sensitive, specific, and rapid CRISPR-Cas13-based diagnosis." Journal of medical virology vol. 93,7 (2021): 4198-4204. doi:10.1002/jmv.26889
[300] Shademan, Behrouz et al. "CRISPR Technology in Gene-Editing-Based Detection and Treatment of SARS-CoV-2." Frontiers in molecular biosciences vol. 8 772788. 11 Jan. 2022, doi:10.3389/fmolb.2021.772788
[301] T. Rajesh, M. Jaya, 7 - Next-Generation Sequencing Methods, Editor(s): Paramasamy Gunasekaran, Santosh Noronha, Ashok Pandey, Current Developments in Biotechnology and Bioengineering, Elsevier,
2017, Pages 143-158, ISBN 9780444636676, https://doi.org/10.1016/B978-0-444-63667-6.00007-9.
[302] Slatko, Barton E et al. "Overview of Next-Generation Sequencing Technologies." Current protocols in molecular biology vol. 122,1 (2018): e59. doi:10.1002/cpmb.59
[303] https://en.wikipedia.org/wiki/Viral_phylodynamics
[304] https://www.illumina.com/systems/sequencing-platforms.html
[305] https://nanoporetech.com/how-it-works
[306] https://www.whatisbiotechnology.org/index.php/science/summary/nanopore/nanopore-sequencing-makes-it-possible-to-decode-the
[307] https://nanoporetech.com/products/minion-comparison
[308] https://www.journalofinfection.com/article/S0163-4453(21)00308-X/fulltext
[309] https://www.sciencedirect.com/science/article/pii/B9780123751560000102
[310] Gorzynski, John E. et al., Ultrarapid Nanopore Genome Sequencing in a Critical Care Setting,
New England Journal of Medicine,
https://www.nejm.org/doi/full/10.1056/NEJMc2112090, February 17, 2022 386(7):700
[311]
https://www.nejm.org/doi/suppl/10.1056/NEJMc2112090/suppl_file/nejmc2112090_appendix.pdf
[312] Kaelin EA, Rodriguez C, Hall-Moore C, et al. Longitudinal gut virome analysis identifies specific viral signatures that precede necrotizing enterocolitis onset in preterm infants. Nat Microbiol. Published online April 21, 2022:1-10. doi:10.1038/s41564-022-01096-x
[313]
https://docs.google.com/document/d/1kP2w_uTMSep2UxTCOnUhh1TMCjWvHEY0sUUpkJHPYV4/edit
[314] Yelagandula, Ramesh et al. "Multiplexed detection of SARS-CoV-2 and other respiratory infections in high throughput by SARSeq." Nature communications vol. 12,1 3132. 25 May. 2021, doi:10.1038/s41467-021-22664-5
[315] https://www.biorxiv.org/content/10.1101/2020.04.06.025635v2
[316] https://www.notion.so/Octant-SwabSeq-Testing-9eb80e793d7e46348038aa80a5a901fd
[317] https://www.fda.gov/medical-devices/medical-device-regulatory-science-research-programs-conducted-osel/microfluidics-program-research-microfluidics-based-medical-devices
[318] Ganguli, A., Ornob, A., Yu, H. et al. Hands-free smartphone-based diagnostics for simultaneous detection of Zika, Chikungunya, and Dengue at point-of-care. Biomed Microdevices 19, 73 (2017). https://doi.org/10.1007/s10544-017-0209-9

[319] Ye X, Li L, Li J, Wu X, Fang X, Kong J. Microfluidic-CFPA Chip for the Point-of-Care Detection of African Swine Fever Virus with a Median Time to Threshold in about 10 min. ACS Sens. 2019 Nov 22;4(11):3066-3071. doi: 10.1021/acssensors.9b01731. Epub 2019 Oct 24. PMID: 31602971.

[320] Magro L., Jacquelin B., Escadafal C., Garneret P., Kwasiborski A., Manuguerra J.C., Monti F., Sakuntabhai A., Vanhomwegen J., Lafaye P., Tabeling P. Paper-based RNA detection and multiplexed analysis for Ebola virus diagnostics. Sci. Rep. 2017;7(1):1347

[321] Qin P., Park M., Alfson K.J., Tamhankar M., Carrion R., Patterson J.L., Griffiths A., He Q., Yildiz A., Mathies R., Du K. Rapid and fully microfluidic Ebola virus detection with CRISPR-cas13a. ACS Sens. 2019;4(4):1048–1054.

[322] Glynn M.T., Kinahan D.J., Ducrée J. Rapid, low-cost and instrument-free CD4+ cell counting for HIV diagnostics in resource-poor settings. Lab Chip. 2014;14(15):2844–2851.

[323] Zhuang, Jianjian et al. "Advanced "lab-on-a-chip" to detect viruses - Current challenges and future perspectives." Biosensors & bioelectronics vol. 163 (2020): 112291. doi:10.1016/j.bios.2020.112291

[324] Wu, J., Dong, M., Rigatto, C. et al. Lab-on-chip technology for chronic disease diagnosis. npj Digital Med 1, 7 (2018). https://doi.org/10.1038/s41746-017-0014-0

[325] Jiang K, Jokhun DS, Lim CT. Microfluidic detection of human diseases: From liquid biopsy to COVID-19 diagnosis. J Biomech. 2021;117:110235. doi:10.1016/j.jbiomech.2021.110235

[326] Hemmig E, Temiz Y, Gökçe O, Lovchik RD, Delamarche E. Transposing Lateral Flow Immunoassays to Capillary-Driven Microfluidics Using Self-Coalescence Modules and Capillary-Assembled Receptor Carriers. Anal Chem. 2020 Jan 7;92(1):940-946. doi: 10.1021/acs.analchem.9b03792. Epub 2019 Dec 20. PMID: 31860276.

[327] Lin, Qiuyuan et al. "Microfluidic Immunoassays for Sensitive and Simultaneous Detection of IgG/IgM/Antigen of SARS-CoV-2 within 15 min." Analytical chemistry vol. 92,14 (2020): 9454-9458. doi:10.1021/acs.analchem.0c01635

[328] Li, Ziyue et al. "Instrument-free, CRISPR-based diagnostics of SARS-CoV-2 using self-contained microfluidic system." Biosensors & bioelectronics vol. 199 (2022): 113865. doi:10.1016/j.bios.2021.113865

[329] http://europepmc.org/article/MED/33461849

[330] Chen, L., Ying, B., Song, P., Liu, X., A Nanocellulose-Paper-Based SERS Multiwell Plate with High Sensitivity and High Signal Homogeneity. Adv. Mater. Interfaces 2019, 6, 1901346. https://doi.org/10.1002/admi.201901346

[331] https://www.cell.com/matter/fulltext/S2590-2385(20)30553-1

[332] Abdulhadee Yakoh, Umaporn Pimpitak, Sirirat Rengpipat, Nattiya Hirankarn, Orawon Chailapakul, Sudkate Chaiyo, Paper-based electrochemical biosensor for diagnosing COVID-19: Detection of SARS-CoV-2 antibodies and antigen, Biosensors and Bioelectronics, Volume 176, 2021, 112912, ISSN 0956-5663, https://doi.org/10.1016/j.bios.2020.112912.

[333] Li X, Qin Z, Fu H, et al. Enhancing the performance of paper-based electrochemical impedance spectroscopy nanobiosensors: An experimental approach. Biosensors & Bioelectronics. 2021 Apr;177:112672. DOI:

10.1016/j.bios.2020.112672. PMID: 33461849; PMCID: PMC7550100
[334] Taylor R F et al 1991 Antibody- and receptor-based biosensors for detection and process control Anal. Chim. Acta 249 67-70
[335] Magar, Hend S et al. "Electrochemical Impedance Spectroscopy (EIS): Principles, Construction, and Biosensing Applications." Sensors (Basel, Switzerland) vol. 21,19 6578. 1 Oct. 2021, doi:10.3390/s21196578
[336] https://doi.org/10.1016/j.ma tt.2021.05.003
[337] https://biologicalproceduresonline.biomedcentral.com/articles/10.1186/s12575-020-00134-4/tables/1
[338] Maeda, Tomoya et al. 2022/02/10, Bio-Interface on Freestanding Nanosheet of Microelectromechanical System Optical Interferometric Immunosensor for Label-Free Attomolar Prostate Cancer Marker Detection. 10.3390/s22041356 - Sensors
[339] https://www.achiko.com/products/aptamex
[340] Zou, Xinran et al. "Application of Aptamers in Virus Detection and Antiviral Therapy." Frontiers in microbiology vol. 10 1462. 3 Jul. 2019, doi:10.3389/fmicb.2019.01462
[341] surface plasmon resonance (SPR) aptasensors, colorimetric aptasensors, chemiluminescence (CL) aptasensors, fluorescence aptasensors, surface-enhanced Raman scattering (SERS) aptasensors, and interferometry aptasensors
[342] Nidzworski, D., Siuzdak, K., Niedziałkowski, P. et al. A rapid-response ultrasensitive biosensor for influenza virus detection using antibody modified boron-doped diamond. Sci Rep 7, 15707 (2017). https://doi.org/10.1038/s41598-017-15806-7
[343] Turbé, V., Gray, E.R., Lawson, V.E. et al. Towards an ultra-rapid smartphone-connected test for infectious diseases. Sci Rep 7, 11971 (2017). https://doi.org/10.1038/s41598-017-11887-6
[344] Zhao J, Yang Y, Huang H. Relationship between the ABO blood group and the COVID-19 susceptibility. Clin Infect Dis. 2021;73:328–331
[345] Kim, Young et al. "Relationship between blood type and outcomes following COVID-19 infection." Seminars in vascular surgery vol. 34,3 (2021): 125-131. doi:10.1053/j.semvascsurg.2021.05.005
[346] https://www.ncbi.nlm.nih.gov/pmc/articles/PMC7751038
[347] https://aacrjournals.org/mcr/article/14/10/898/135577/Cell-free-DNA-cfDNA-Clinical-Significance-and
[348] https://www.ncbi.nlm.nih.gov/pmc/articles/PMC5711344/
[349] https://doi.org/10.1016/j.medj.2021.01.001
[350] https://apnews.com/article/science-business-health-hodgkin-lymphoma-oregon-ca899bb9c4c7f1859d4e9ce16a1cf78d
[351] Danwang C, Endomba FT, Nkeck JR, Wouna DLA, Robert A, Noubiap JJ. A meta-analysis of potential biomarkers associated with severity of coronavirus disease 2019 (COVID-19). Biomark Res. 2020;8:37. Published 2020 Aug 31. doi:10.1186/s40364-020-00217-0
[352] Henry BM, de Oliveira MHS, Benoit S, Plebani M, Lippi G. Hematologic, biochemical and immune biomarker abnormalities associated with severe illness and mortality in coronavirus disease 2019 (COVID-19): a meta-analysis. Clin Chem Lab Med. 2020;58(7):1021-1028. doi:10.1515/cclm-2020-0369
[353] Demichev V, Tober-Lau P, Nazarenko T, Lemke O, Kaur Aulakh S, Whitwell HJ,

et al. (2022) A proteomic survival predictor for COVID-19 patients in intensive care. PLOS Digit Health 1(1): e0000007. https://doi.org/10.1371/journal.pdig.0000007

[354] https://somalogic.com/massive-scale-proteomics-for-covid-19/

[355] Biomarkers for progression from latent to active tuberculosis identified in multiplexed proteomic assay (SOMAscan™) of human plasma (MPF6P.657) Urs Ochsner, Thomas Hraha, David Sterling, Mary De Groote, Kirsten Wall, Nebojsa Janjic, Daniel Zak, Ethan Thompson, Adam Penn-Nicholson, Thomas Scriba, The Journal of Immunology May 1, 2015, 194 (1 Supplement) 202.15

[356] Berlin, D. A., Gulick, R. M. & Martinez, F. J. N. Engl. J. Med. 383, 2451–2460 (2020).

[357] Roberts, G.H.L., Partha, R., Rhead, B. et al. Expanded COVID-19 phenotype definitions reveal distinct patterns of genetic association and protective effects. Nat Genet 54, 374–381 (2022). https://doi.org/10.1038/s41588-022-01042-x

[358] Karlsen, T.H. Understanding COVID-19 through genome-wide association studies. Nat Genet 54, 368–369 (2022). https://doi.org/10.1038/s41588-021-00985-x

[359] https://www.sec.gov/Archives/edgar/data/1569568/000149315220017609/ex99-1.htm

[360] Yoo YJ, Ko JH, Lee GJ, et al. Gires–Tournois immunoassay platform for label-free bright-field imaging and facile quantification of bioparticles. Adv Mater. 2022:2110003. doi: 10.1002/adma.202110003

[361] Molecularly Imprinted Polymer Nanoparticles Enable Rapid, Reliable, and Robust Point-of-Care Thermal Detection of SARS-CoV-2. Jake McClements, Laure Bar, Pankaj Singla, Francesco Canfarotta, Alan Thomson, Joanna Czulak, Rhiannon E. Johnson, Robert D. Crapnell, Craig E. Banks, Brendan Payne, Shayan Seyedin, Patricia Losada-Pérez, and Marloes Peeters. ACS Sensors 2022 7 (4), 1122-1131. DOI: 10.1021/acssensors.2c00100

[362] Anal. Chem. 2019, 91, 22, 14552–14560. Publication Date:October 8, 2019 https://doi.org/10.1021/acs.analchem.9b03612

[363] Jackson CB, Zhang L, Farzan M, Choe H. Functional importance of the D614G mutation in the SARS-CoV-2 spike protein. Biochem Biophys Res Commun. 2021;538:108-115. doi:10.1016/j.bbrc.2020.11.026

[364] https://www.sciencedirect.com/science/article/pii/S1074761321005082

[365] https://jamanetwork.com/journals/jama/fullarticle/2775006

[366] https://www.biorxiv.org/content/10.1101/2022.04.12.487379v1

[367] https://assets.publishing.service.gov.uk/government/uploads/system/uploads/attachment_data/file/1007566/S1335_Long_term_evolution_of_SARS-CoV-2.pdf

[368] https://www.the-scientist.com/news-opinion/plenty-of-evidence-for-recombination-in-sars-cov-2-69156

[369] https://twitter.com/PeacockFlu/status/1504158873938272269

[370] https://scitechdaily.com/what-are-virus-variants-explaining-viral-mutations-covid-and-vaccines/

[371] https://scitechdaily.com/covid-omicron-variant-how-did-it-emerge-and-is-it-more-contagious-than-delta-a-virus-evolution-expert-explains

[372] https://www.nature.com/articles/d41586-020-02544-6

[373] https://bit.ly/3jDIOzP

[374] R. S. Creager et al., "RADx Variant Task Force Program for Assessing the Impact of Variants on SARS-CoV-2 Molecular and Antigen Tests," in IEEE Open Journal of

Engineering in Medicine and Biology, vol. 2, pp. 286-290, 2021, doi: 10.1109/OJEMB.2021.3116490
[375] https://www.medtechdive.com/news/fda-update-covid-tests-fail-detect-omicron-variant/611617/
[376]
https://assets.publishing.service.gov.uk/government/uploads/system/uploads/attachment_data/file/1039644/Omicron_SGTF_case_update_FINAL.pdf
[377] https://www.bmj.com/content/375/bmj.n3133/rr
[378] https://www.fda.gov/medical-devices/coronavirus-covid-19-and-medical-devices/sars-cov-2-viral-mutations-impact-covid-19-tests#omicronvariantimpact
[379]
https://assets.publishing.service.gov.uk/government/uploads/system/uploads/attachment_data/file/1042688/RA_Technical_Briefing_32_DRAFT_17_December_2021_2021_12_17.pdf
[380] Discordant SARS-CoV-2 PCR and Rapid Antigen Test Results When Infectious: A December 2021 Occupational Case Series: Blythe Adamson, Robby Sikka, Anne L. Wyllie, Prem Premsrirut
medRxiv 2022.01.04.22268770; doi: https://doi.org/10.1101/2022.01.04.22268770

[381] https://time.com/6138928/swab-throat-nose-covid-19-rapid-tests/
[382] https://www.help.senate.gov/hearings/addressing-new-variants-a-federal-perspective-on-the-covid-19-response
[383] https://hub.jhu.edu/2021/07/19/andrew-pekosz-delta-variants/
[384] https://www.who.int/en/activities/tracking-SARS-CoV-2-variants/
[385] https://www.cdc.gov/coronavirus/2019-ncov/variants/variant-classifications.html
[386] Zhang, T., Deng, R., Wang, Y. et al. A paper-based assay for the colorimetric detection of SARS-CoV-2 variants at single-nucleotide resolution. Nat. Biomed. Eng 6, 957–967 (2022). https://doi.org/10.1038/s41551-022-00907-0
[387] Yang K, Schuder DN, Ngor AK, Chaput JC. Revealr-based genotyping of sars-cov-2 variants of concern in clinical samples. J Am Chem Soc. 2022;144(26):11685-11692. doi: 10.1021/jacs.2c03420
[388] Smyth, D.S., Trujillo, M., Gregory, D.A. et al. Tracking cryptic SARS-CoV-2 lineages detected in NYC wastewater. Nat Commun 13, 635 (2022). https://doi.org/10.1038/s41467-022-28246-3
[389] https://covid.cdc.gov/covid-data-tracker/#wastewater-surveillance (as at March 13 2022).
[390] Michael A. Jahne et al, Droplet digital PCR quantification of norovirus and adenovirus in decentralized wastewater and graywater collections: Implications for onsite reuse. Water Research, Volume 169, 2020, 115213, ISSN 0043-1354, https://doi.org/10.1016/j.watres.2019.115213.
(https://www.sciencedirect.com/science/article/pii/S004313541930987X)
[391] Sangeet Adhikari, Rolf U. Halden, Opportunities and limits of wastewater-based epidemiology for tracking global health and attainment of UN sustainable development goals, Environment International, Volume 163, 2022, 107217, ISSN 0160-4120, https://doi.org/10.1016/j.envint.2022.107217.
[392] https://www.cdc.gov/nndss/index.html
[393] https://www.cimit.org/
[394] https://www.biorxiv.org/content/10.1101/2021.12.24.474095v1

[395] Ford Colby T., Jacob Machado Denis, Janies Daniel A., Predictions of the SARS-CoV-2 Omicron Variant (B.1.1.529) Spike Protein Receptor-Binding Domain Structure and Neutralizing Antibody Interactions, Frontiers in Virology, Vol 2, 2022, URL=https://www.frontiersin.org/article/10.3389/fviro.2022.830202, DOI=10.3389/fviro.2022.830202 , ISSN=2673-818X

[396] https://news.microsoft.com/innovation-stories/microsoft-premonition/

[397] https://www.cdc.gov/forecast-outbreak-analysis/

[398] https://www.nytimes.com/2022/04/27/science/pandemic-viruses-machine-learning.html

[399] Han et al, Rodent reservoirs of future zoonotic diseases, 2015, Proceedings of the National Academy of Sciences, Page 7039-7044, Vol 112, doi:10.1073/pnas.1501598112, https://www.pnas.org/doi/abs/10.1073/pnas.1501598112

[400] https://www.who.int/news/item/03-02-2022-2022-celebrating-70-years-of-gisrs-(the-global-influenza-surveillance-and-response-system)

[401] https://www.ncbi.nlm.nih.gov/pmc/articles/PMC5935243/

[402] https://www.ted.com/talks/bill_gates_we_can_make_covid_19_the_last_pandemic

[403] https://www.aarp.org/health/conditions-treatments/info-2021/at-home-covid-tests.html

[404] Baron S, Fons M, Albrecht T. Viral Pathogenesis. In: Baron S, editor. Medical Microbiology. 4th edition. Galveston (TX): University of Texas Medical Branch at Galveston; 1996. Chapter 45. Available from: https://www.ncbi.nlm.nih.gov/books/NBK8149/

[405] Wu, Zhonglan et al. "The unique features of SARS-CoV-2 transmission: Comparison with SARS-CoV, MERS-CoV and 2009 H1N1 pandemic influenza virus." Reviews in medical virology vol. 31,2 (2021): e2171. doi:10.1002/rmv.2171

[406] Ke, R., Martinez, P.P., Smith, R.L. et al. Daily longitudinal sampling of SARS-CoV-2 infection reveals substantial heterogeneity in infectiousness. Nat Microbiol (2022). https://doi.org/10.1038/s41564-022-01105-z

[407] Lloyd-Smith, J. O., Schreiber, S. J., Kopp, P. E. & Getz, W. M. Superspreading and the effect of individual variation on disease emergence. Nature 438, 355–359 (2005)

[408] https://uniogen.com/news-page/abacus-diagnostica-launches-new-genomera-assay-kit-for-rapid-detection-of-viruses-causing-viral-meningitis/

[409] Qavi AJ, Meserve K, Aman MJ, et al. Rapid detection of an Ebola biomarker with optical microring resonators. Cell Rep Methods. 2022:100234. doi: 10.1016/j.crmeth.2022.100234

[410] https://www.cdc.gov/globalhealth/stories/2019/world-deadliest-animal.html

[411] Jankelow AM, Lee H, Wang W, et al. Smartphone clip-on instrument and microfluidic processor for rapid sample-to-answer detection of Zika virus in whole blood using spatial RT-LAMP. Analyst. 2022:10.1039.D2AN00438K. doi: 10.1039/D2AN00438K

[412] Zhang, X.-A. et al. N. Engl. J. Med. 387, 470–472 (2022).

[413] https://www.nature.com/articles/nm0110-11a

[414] https://www.rand.org/content/dam/rand/pubs/research_briefs/2007/RAND_RB9293.pdf

[415] https://www.cdc.gov/malaria/about/faqs.html

[416] https://www.who.int/teams/global-malaria-programme/case-management/diagnosis/rapid-diagnostic-tests

[417] histidine-rich protein-2 (HRP2), plasmodium lactate dehydrogenase (pLDH)
[418] Cunningham, J., Jones, S., Gatton, M.L. et al. A review of the WHO malaria rapid diagnostic test product testing programme (2008–2018): performance, procurement and policy. Malar J 18, 387 (2019). https://doi.org/10.1186/s12936-019-3028-z
[419] von Fricken, Michael E et al. "Performance of the CareStart glucose-6-phosphate dehydrogenase (G6PD) rapid diagnostic test in Gressier, Haiti." The American journal of tropical medicine and hygiene vol. 91,1 (2014): 77-80. doi:10.4269/ajtmh.14-0150
[420] Ocker, Ronja et al. "MALARIA DIAGNOSIS BY LOOP-MEDIATED ISOTHERMAL AMPLIFICATION (LAMP) IN THAILAND." Revista do Instituto de Medicina Tropical de Sao Paulo vol. 58 (2016): 27. doi:10.1590/S1678-9946201658027
[421] https://www.cdc.gov/globalhealth/newsroom/topics/tb/index.html
[422] https://academic.oup.com/jid/article/205/suppl_2/S191/806449
[423] Kivihya-Ndugga, Lydia et al. "Comparison of PCR with the routine procedure for diagnosis of tuberculosis in a population with high prevalences of tuberculosis and human immunodeficiency virus." Journal of clinical microbiology vol. 42,3 (2004): 1012-5. doi:10.1128/JCM.42.3.1012-1015.2004
[424] Steingart KR, Schiller I, Horne DJ, Pai M, Boehme CC, Dendukuri N. Xpert® MTB/RIF assay for pulmonary tuberculosis and rifampicin resistance in adults. Cochrane Database Syst Rev. 2014;2014(1):CD009593. Published 2014 Jan 21. doi:10.1002/14651858.CD009593.pub3
[425] The Use of Loop-Mediated Isothermal Amplification (TB-LAMP) for the Diagnosis of Pulmonary Tuberculosis: Policy Guidance. Geneva: World Health Organization; 2016. Available from: https://www.ncbi.nlm.nih.gov/books/NBK384520/
[426] https://unitaid.org/assets/2017-Unitaid-TB-Diagnostics-Technology-Landscape.pdf
[427] Wood BR, Ballenger C, Stekler JD. Arguments for and against HIV self-testing. HIV AIDS (Auckl). 2014;6:117-126.
[428] To Catch a Virus, p.181
[429] Updated recommendations on HIV prevention, infant diagnosis, antiretroviral initiation and monitoring [Internet]. Geneva: World Health Organization; 2021 Mar. 3, CLINICAL GUIDELINES: DIAGNOSTICS AND TREATMENT MONITORING. Available from: https://www.ncbi.nlm.nih.gov/books/NBK569324/
[430] ibid
[431] Malik Yashpal Singh etal, Advances in Diagnostic Approaches for Viral Etiologies of Diarrhea: From the Lab to the Field. Frontiers in Microbiology, Vol. 10, 2019. https://www.frontiersin.org/article/10.3389/fmicb.2019.01957
[432] https://www.nytimes.com/2022/08/21/opinion/even-a-single-case-of-polio-is-a-threat.html
[433] Alex Shaw, Catherine Troman, Joyce Akello, Erika Bujaki, Manasi Majumdar, Javier Martin, Nick Grassly 2022. Poliovirus direct detection and nanopore sequencing (DDNS) FAQs. protocols.io https://dx.doi.org/10.17504/protocols.io.b5ggq3tw
[434] https://www.who.int/news/item/16-06-2022-new-agreement-under-c-tap-aims-to-

improve-global-access-to-covid-19-testing-technologies
[435] https://www.ncbi.nlm.nih.gov/pmc/articles/PMC4016042/
[436] https://www.who.int/teams/control-of-neglected-tropical-diseases
[437] https://www.ncbi.nlm.nih.gov/pmc/articles/PMC4438894/
[438] https://www.cepheid.com/en/tests/Critical-Infectious-Diseases/Xpert-MTB-RIF
[439] Arumugam, A.; Faron, M.L.; Yu, P.; Markham, C.; Wu, M.; Wong, S. A Rapid SARS-CoV-2 RT-PCR Assay for Low Resource Settings. Diagnostics 2020, 10, 739. https://doi.org/10.3390/diagnostics10100739
[440] Lin EE, Razzaque UA, Burrows SA, Smoukov SK (2022) End-to-end system for rapid and sensitive early-detection of SARS-CoV-2 for resource-poor and field-test environments using a $51 lab-in-a-backpack. PLoS ONE 17(1): e0259886. https://doi.org/10.1371/journal.pone.0259886
[441] https://jamanetwork.com/journals/jamanetworkopen/fullarticle/2788464?resultClick=3
[442] https://www.ncbi.nlm.nih.gov/pmc/articles/PMC4756427/
[443] https://www.who.int/publications/m/item/covid-19-target-product-profiles-for-priority-diagnostics-to-support-response-to-the-covid-19-pandemic-v.0.1
[444] Silva, Severino Jefferson Ribeiro da et al. "Loop-Mediated Isothermal Amplification (LAMP) for the Diagnosis of Zika Virus: A Review." Viruses vol. 12,1 19. 23 Dec. 2019, doi:10.3390/v12010019
[445] https://www.who.int/news/item/15-11-2021-new-reduced-costs-of-dual-hiv-syphilis-rapid-tests-to-accelerate-progress-toward-emtct-of-hiv-and-syphilis
[446] https://unitaid.org/covid-19-old/act-accelerator/#en
[447] Median values of 7-day rolling averages in each income group. Data correct as at 7 January 2021, www.finddx.org/covid-19/test-tracker
[448] Breman JG, Henderson DA. Poxvirus dilemmas--monkeypox, smallpox, and biologic terrorism. N Engl J Med. 1998 Aug 20;339(8):556-9. doi: 10.1056/NEJM199808203390811. PMID: 9709051.
[449] Weaver JR, Isaacs SN. Monkeypox virus and insights into its immunomodulatory proteins. Immunol Rev. 2008 Oct;225:96-113. doi: 10.1111/j.1600-065X.2008.00691.x. PMID: 18837778; PMCID: PMC2567051.
[450] Riccò M, Ferraro P, Camisa V, Satta E, Zaniboni A, Ranzieri S, Baldassarre A, Zaffina S, Marchesi F. When a Neglected Tropical Disease Goes Global: Knowledge, Attitudes and Practices of Italian Physicians towards Monkeypox, Preliminary Results. Trop Med Infect Dis. 2022 Jul 14;7(7):135. doi: 10.3390/tropicalmed7070135. PMID: 35878146; PMCID: PMC9316880.
[451] https://www.npr.org/2022/07/12/1110897541/monkeypox-outbreak-testing-vaccine-cases
[452] https://twitter.com/CDCDirector/status/1555283178625159169/photo/2
[453] https://www.finddx.org/mpx-test-directory/
[454] https://cordx.com/press-releases/ce-mark-applied-to-cordxs-latest-monkeypox-diagnostic-test/
[455] https://doi.org/10.1016/S0140-6736(21)02724-0
[456] https://ukhsa.blog.gov.uk/2021/12/24/reflecting-on-a-year-responding-to-covid-19/
[457] Lim, YW., Steinhoff, M., Girosi, F. et al. Reducing the global burden of acute lower respiratory infections in children: the contribution of new diagnostics. Nature 444, 9–18 (2006). https://doi.org/10.1038/nature05442
[458] Enrique Valera et al, ACS Nano 2021, 15, 5, 7899–7906. Publication Date:May 13,

2021. https://doi.org/10.1021/acsnano.1c02981
[459] https://www.thelancet.com/commissions/diagnostics
[460] https://www.thelancet.com/journals/lancet/article/PIIS0140-6736(21)00673-5/fulltext
[461] https://www.cdc.gov/coronavirus/2019-ncov/hcp/testing-overview.html
[462] Joung SY, Ebinger JE, Sun N, et al. Awareness of SARS-CoV-2 Omicron Variant Infection Among Adults With Recent COVID-19 Seropositivity. JAMA Netw Open. 2022;5(8):e2227241. doi:10.1001/jamanetworkopen.2022.27241
[463] https://www.cdc.gov/vhf/nipah/about/index.html
[464] Longitudinal analysis reveals high prevalence of Epstein-Barr virus associated with multiple sclerosis, Alberto Ascherio et al. 2022/01/21, doi: 10.1126/science.abj8222. American Association for the Advancement of Science
[465] Cairns DM, Itzhaki RF, Kaplan DL. Potential Involvement of Varicella Zoster Virus in Alzheimer's Disease via Reactivation of Quiescent Herpes Simplex Virus Type 1. J Alzheimers Dis. 2022;88(3):1189-1200. doi: 10.3233/JAD-220287. PMID: 35754275.
[466] https://www.alzdiscovery.org/news-room/announcements/dxa2
[467] https://twitter.com/michaelmina_lab/status/1329659618621054976
[468] Viking, 2022. ISBN: 0241510538
[469] St Martin's Press, 2021. ISBN: 1250770165
[470] Penguin, 2022. ISBN: 0241579600
[471] https://www.nytimes.com/2022/08/17/us/politics/cdc-rochelle-walensky-covid.html
[472] Grammatopoulos DK, Young L, Anderson NR. Transforming the UK's diagnostics agenda after COVID-19. Lancet. 2022 Apr 23;399(10335):1606. doi: 10.1016/S0140-6736(22)00169-6. PMID: 35461555; PMCID: PMC9022999.
[473] https://www.abhi.org.uk/media/2768/diagnostics-a-future-roadmap.pdf
[474] https://dianews.roche.com/rs/106-RRW-330/images/The%20Future%20of%20Diagnostics%20Delivery%20in%20the%20UK%20report.pdf
[475] Nelson, Philipp P et al. "Current and Future Point-of-Care Tests for Emerging and New Respiratory Viruses and Future Perspectives." Frontiers in cellular and infection microbiology vol. 10 181. 29 Apr. 2020, doi:10.3389/fcimb.2020.00181
[476] https://talk.ictvonline.org/ictv-reports/ictv_online_report/introduction/w/introduction-to-the-ictv-online-report/425/hosts-vertebrates
[477] https://www.ncbi.nlm.nih.gov/pmc/articles/PMC8306705/
[478] https://jamanetwork.com/journals/jamaotolaryngology/fullarticle/2770786
[479] https://pubmed.ncbi.nlm.nih.gov/29174837/
[480] Swetha Pinninti, Connie Trieu, Sunil K Pati, Misty Latting, Joshua Cooper, Maria C Seleme, Sushma Boppana, Nitin Arora, William J Britt, Suresh B Boppana, Comparing Nasopharyngeal and Midturbinate Nasal Swab Testing for the Identification of Severe Acute Respiratory Syndrome Coronavirus 2, Clinical Infectious Diseases, Volume 72, Issue 7, 1 April 2021, Pages 1253–1255, https://doi.org/10.1093/cid/ciaa882
[481] https://www.ncbi.nlm.nih.gov/pmc/articles/PMC8291630/
[482] https://www.medrxiv.org/content/10.1101/2020.10.21.20206078v1.full
[483] https://assets.publishing.service.gov.uk/government/uploads/system/uploads/attachment_data/file/951021/technical-validation-report_Abbot_ID_Now.pdf

[484] Freire-Paspuel Byron, et al, Cotton-Tipped Plastic Swabs for SARS-CoV-2 RT-qPCR Diagnosis to Prevent Supply Shortages, Frontiers in Cellular and Infection Microbiology, V. 10, 2020.
URL=https://www.frontiersin.org/article/10.3389/fcimb.2020.00356, DOI=10.3389/fcimb.2020.00356
[485] Song, J., Korunes-Miller, J., Banerji, R., Wu, Y., Fazeli, S., Zheng, H., Orr, B., Morgan, E., Andry, C., Henderson, J., Miller, N. S., White, A., Grinstaff, M. W., On-Site, On-Demand 3D-Printed Nasopharyngeal Swabs to Improve the Access of Coronavirus Disease-19 Testing. Global Challenges 2021, 5, 2100039. https://doi.org/10.1002/gch2.202100039
[486] https://jamanetwork.com/journals/jamaotolaryngology/fullarticle/2779393
[487] Glenn Patriquin, Ian Davis, Charles Heinstein, Jimmy MacDonald, Todd F. Hatchette, Jason J. LeBlanc,
Exploring alternative swabs for use in SARS-CoV-2 detection from the oropharynx and anterior nares,
Journal of Virological Methods, Volume 285, 2020, 113948, ISSN 0166-0934, https://doi.org/10.1016/j.jviromet.2020.113948.
(https://www.sciencedirect.com/science/article/pii/S0166093420302007)
[488] Evaluation of Saline, Phosphate-Buffered Saline, and Minimum Essential Medium as Potential Alternatives to Viral Transport Media for SARS-CoV-2 Testing, Rodino Kyle G. et al, doi: 10.1128/JCM.00590-20, Journal of Clinical Microbiology, 2022/03/06
[489] https://www.ncbi.nlm.nih.gov/pmc/articles/PMC8402664/
[490] https://www.sciencedirect.com/science/article/pii/S0166354216304016?via%3Dihub

List of Figures

Figure 1: Number of Virus Species discovered
Figure 2: Comparative Viral sizes. Source: PBS
Figure 3: Common virus morphologies. Source: Artasensi et al, 2021
Figure 4: The 6 Virus Realms sorted by number of species. Source: ICTV
Figure 5: The expanded Taxonomy view showing the classification of species: SARS-CoV
Figure 6: Electron Microscope view of a Coronavirus (229E) - Source: CDC Public Domain Image
Figure 7: Alpha and Beta Coronaviruses that affect humans and their discovery date
Figure 8: Structure of SARS-CoV-2 Source: Bioengineering 2021
Figure 9: SARS-CoV-2 compared to Influenza. Images from USA Today
Figure 10: A simplified overview of the main viral infections and the most notable involved species. Source: Häggström, Mikael (2014)
Figure 11: the RADx approach to speeding diagnostic developments. Source:

NIH
Figure 12: US Monthly testing capacity as at Q1, 2022.
Figure 13: Daily Covid Testing in January 2022. Source: Our World In Data
Figure 14: UK daily testing, as reported by BBC
Figure 15: Disparities in testing by income
Figure 16: Testing Tradeoffs by Location of Testing
Figure 17: The FDA guidance flowchart for test manufacturers
Figure 18: Nasal/Oral sample collection sites
Figure 19: An Oropharyngeal swab. Source: CDC Image
Figure 20: Breakdown of Sample Types submitted to RADx program
Figure 21: Public Understanding of Test Indications
Figure 22: An automated swabbing machine to protect HCP from exposure during sample collection
Figure 23: TTR study in the US in 2020
Figure 24: The variety of swabs supplied with consumer test kits (Apple Watch for Scale)
Figure 25: FoodMarble Aire Digestive tester and Lumen Metabolic Analyser, (Apple Watch for Scale)
Figure 26: SpiroNose device
Figure 27: Google Searches for PCR before and during the COVID-19 pandemic
Figure 28: The Ingredients for an RT-PCR Test for an RNA Virus. Source: Mayo Clinic
Figure 29: What a PCR Test result looks like. Source:
Figure 30: A Feb. 2022 headline reporting on concerns about PCR cycle thresholds
Figure 31: A study of EUA-approved SARS-CoV-2 assays
Figure 32: Growing interest in LAMP
Figure 33: Google Searches for Lateral Flow
Figure 34: Image showing top and side view of a typical LFT
Figure 35: Variety of LFTs (including SARS-CoV-2, Ag, Ig; Vitamin D and Troponin examples) with Apple Watch for Scale
Figure 36: POC BD Veritor Plus Device and 2 LFT cartridges. Source: BD
Figure 37: Antibodies, Paratopes & Epitopes. Source
Figure 38: (L) EUA antibody tests by target antibody and (R) by detection antigen used
Figure 39: SARS-CoV-2 S and N antigens are most used to identify antibodies for them
Figure 40: Antigenic Targets of Antibodies by Vaccination Status. Source: CDC
Figure 41: Typical timing of different antibody responses POS
Figure 42: Testing Technologies used in Antibody Tests for SARS-CoV-2.

Source.

Figure 43: ROC curve for comparative diagnostic performance of urine- and serum-based ELISA for COVID-19

Figure 44: SARS-CoV-2 antibody detection in blood donations received between February 2020 and September 2020. Error bars represent 95% confidence intervals.

Figure 45: Combined Immune System Response. Source: https://www.tspotcovid.com

Figure 46: 2018: In Vitro Diagnostics: Technologies and Global Markets

Figure 47: Abbott & Cephid POC NAAT Devices

Figure 48: A Visby handheld NAAT for SARS-CoV-2

Figure 49: Cue Reader device and 3 test cartridges

Figure 50: Cue Future Testing Menu

Figure 51: Cue Development Timeline

Figure 52: Detect Reader Device

Figure 53: Circle's HealthPod device

Figure 54: The Lucira COVID-19 Kit

Figure 55: Domestic NAAT reader devices: From L to R: Detect, Circle, Cue Reusable Readers and the single use Lucira device. With an Apple Watch for Scale

Figure 56: Some Wearable Sensors

Figure 57: An Aktiia PPG Continuous Blood Pressure strap (top) and a fingertip Pulse Oximeter (bottom)

Figure 58: RR Intervals. Source:

Figure 59: the Mindfield eSense Respiration sensor offers dedicated respiratory rate tracking

Figure 60: An example WHOOP report showing an increase in respiration per minute that might indicate illness. Source: WHOOP

Figure 61 - Kinsa data showing unexpected increase in tracked incidences of fever as COVID-19 emerged in 2020

Figure 62: Trackers can notice changes before onset of symptoms

Figure 63: Indicators (HR, RR, HRV and Temperature) before and after vaccination

Figure 64: changes in HRV values observed in the study

Figure 65: Example of an Alert triggered 2 days before onset of symptoms based on RHR

Figure 66: HRV Changes before symptom onset

Figure 67: The Yale Fresh Air Clip. Source: Yale.

Figure 68: An example of the VitalConnect platform

Figure 69: Comparing Glucometer Antibody testing results vs lab test

Figure 70: An illustration of Flow Virometry workflow

Figure 71: Image from Mammoth Biosciences' white paper comparing the diagnostic workflow times with DETECTR, SHERLOCK, and typical CDC/WHO gold standard RT-qPCR method

Figure 72: Low cost CRISPR - $15 battery-powered device

Figure 73: Categories of research using CRISPR for SARS-CoV-2

Figure 74: Rapid progress in genetic sequencing techniques

Figure 75: A screenshot of GISAID analysis of sequences uploaded from researchers

Figure 76: (L) An Illumina iSeq 100 benchtop device and (R) an Oxford Nanopore MinIon device

Figure 77: RAPID 1.0 with handheld device

Figure 78: Growing interest in the role and use of Aptamers in the last 20 years

Figure 79: The Sight OLO® is a point-of-care blood analyser that performs a 5 part Complete Blood Count (CBC)

Figure 80: Proteomics on PubMed

Figure 81: SARS-CoV-2 mutations. Source: ibid

Figure 82: SARS-CoV-2 Phylogeny tree from GISAID data, generated April 9th by the Author (see web for hi-res colour version)

Figure 83: An example of the NWSS reporting available via the CDC.

Figure 84: A Microsoft "Premonition" device to capture mosquitoes for automated analysis

Figure 85: CDC's Center for Forecasting and Outbreak Analytics (CFA)

Figure 86: Earlier Diagnosis than typical is desirable (target shaded area)

Figure 87: Viral Load vs When Types of Test are Positive (+)

Figure 88: Diagnostics for Enteric Viruses

Figure 89: (L) Mesa Biotech Accula and (R) Talis One

Figure 90: LAMP for Diagnosis of Zika Virus: A Review

Figure 91: US National Monkeypox weekly laboratory testing capacity in mid-2022 grew from 8k to 80k. Source: CDC

Figure 92: August 2022 Available Monkeypox tests

Figure 93: Virus Taxa from ICTV

Figure 94 - NP Swabbing - Insert Horizontally, not Upwards

Figure 95: Immunology Learnings from SARS-CoV and MERS-CoV

www.ingramcontent.com/pod-product-compliance
Lightning Source LLC
Chambersburg PA
CBHW071350210526
45465CB00001B/53